Down's Anomaly

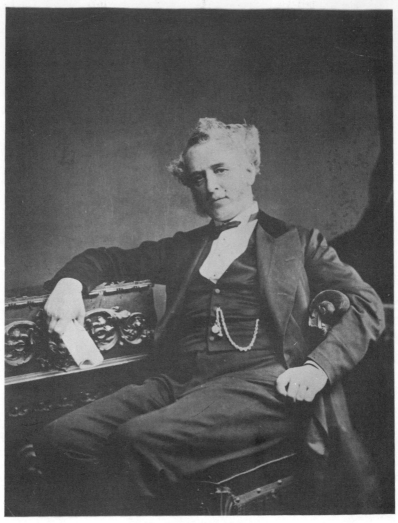

Dr. J. Langdon Down.

Down's Anomaly

G. F. SMITH, M.D.
Director of Genetics, Otago Medical
School, Dunedin, New Zealand

J. M. BERG, M.B., B. Ch., M. Sc., M.R.C. Psych.
Professor of Psychiatry and Associate Professor
of Medical Genetics, University of
Toronto; Director of Genetic Services,
Surrey Place Centre, Toronto

SECOND EDITION

CHURCHILL LIVINGSTONE
Edinburgh London and New York 1976

CHURCHILL LIVINGSTONE

Medical Division of Longman Group Limited

Distributed in the United States of America by Longman
Inc., 19 West 44th Street, New York, N.Y. 10036
and by associated companies, branches and
representatives throughout the world.

© Longman Group Limited, 1976

First Edition 1966
Second Edition 1976

ISBN 0 433 01398 5

˥ιο 030587 -4

Library of Congress Cataloging in Publication Data
Smith, George F   1924-
Down's anomaly.

First ed. by L. S. Penrose and G. F. Smith.

Bibliography: p.
Includes index.

1. Mongolism. I. Berg, J.M., joint author.
II. Penrose, Lionel Sharples. Down's anomaly
III. Title.

RC571.P4   1976   616.8'58842   75-33992

Printed and bound in the United States of America

Preface to the First Edition

A hundred years have passed since Langdon Down first described mongolism. During this time an enormous amount of relevant literature has accumulated all over the world. The object of this book is to provide information about Down's anomaly for students, physicians and research workers. The material which has been selected covers a wide field and the book is intended to be useful as a reference manual. It has been the aim of the authors to present the data as objectively as possible, but their own interests have no doubt unavoidably introduced bias. Nevertheless, though the reader's indulgence is requested if there is unevenness in treatment of various parts of the subject, it is hoped that the great advances, which have taken place during a century, have been demonstrated in a way which will stimulate future researches.

The name 'mongolism' has been used extensively in the world literature and there has been no general agreement on an alternative, consequently it has been retained here. If physicians should find the name offensive, the present writers would ask them to remember that its use carries no racial implication. Since the book is written for professional personnel rather than for laymen, the term should not cause any distress to parents or relatives of patients. The eponymous title, Down's Anomaly, can be used in personal contacts.

Though the book has been jointly prepared by the two writers, Smith has been mainly responsible for presenting the clinical and pathological aspects and Penrose (who deplores the too frequent reference to his own papers) for the mathematical elaborations. The writers wish to thank all those people who have been helpful during the preparation of the book. Sections of it have been read, and very useful comments provided by Dr. J. M. Berg, Dr. J. R. Ellis, Dr. Sarah B. Holt, Dr. C. Kupfer, Dr. Ursula Mittwoch, Dr. J. H. Ottaway, Dr. A. Shapiro, Professor C. A. B. Smith and Dr. J. Stern. We would also like to thank Miss Judith Dowdeswell and Mrs. Prudence M. Smith for secretarial assistance and Mr. A. J. Lee for excellent drawings and charts. To Miss Helen Lang-Brown we owe a special debt of gratitude for her assistance in all phases of preparation of the text and the organization of the bibliography. Our gratitude is extended to Dr. A. G. Bearn, Lord Brain, Dr. J. L. German, Mr. J. L. Hamerton, Dr. D. J. McDonald and Professor A. H. Sturtevant for supplying material used in illustrations. In addition we acknowledge the kindness and help provided by Dr. H. O. Åkesson, Mr. R. Brinsden, Professor H. Forssman, Dr. B. Hall, Dr. E. Hinden, Dr. R. Langdon-Down, Dr. E. Matsunaga, Dr. S. Milham, Dr. J. Øster and Dr. A. Stoller.

One of the writers (G, F. S.) had special fellowship awards, during the early period of the preparation of the text, from, first, the National Institute of Neurological Diseases and Blindness and then from the National Institute of Child Health and Human Development of the United States Public Health Service.

Kennedy-Galton Centre,   L. S. PENROSE
Harperbury Hospital,   G. F. SMITH
nr. St. Albans.

January 1966

Preface to the Second Edition

In the ten years since the first edition of this book was written, a remarkably extensive array of additional literature and new observations with refined techniques have been published on Down's syndrome. Indeed, the amount of material on the subject which has appeared in print during the past decade approximates to, and may even exceed, that which was available in the previous century. Though the crucial aetiology of the syndrome still remains elusive, important contributions have been made towards the greater understanding of nearly all facets of the condition. These developments have led to more effective preventive, therapeutic and rehabilitative procedures, as well as to a more general awareness of the disorder and its implications.

A new edition intended to reflect these advances and changing circumstances therefore seemed timely. In the interval between this and the first edition, Lionel Penrose unhappily has died and the surviving original co-author has been joined by another. The basic format and much of the content, albeit modified, of the initial edition has been retained. However, a great deal of new material has been added throughout, including two extra chapters (on immunological and rehabilitative aspects) and a substantially larger bibliography.

Though the intent of the present authors has been to provide as comprehensive an account as possible and to objectively reflect current trends, their own outlooks and experiences inevitably will have influenced the emphasis and scope of the presentation. Whatever the shortcomings, it is hoped that the text, like its predecessor, may serve as a useful source of reference for students, physicians, research workers and other professionals and that it may provide indications of gaps in knowledge which call for further research.

Both authors had the privilege and good fortune of a long and close association with the late Professor Penrose and acknowledge here with pleasure the beneficial impact of his ideas and views in the formulation of this volume. Particular thanks are expressed also to Mrs. Patricia Smith for her admirable and tireless editorial efforts, and to Miss Marika Korossy for her efficient and good-natured assistance in the preparation of the typescript. In addition, thanks are due to Miss Maryanne Doherty for librarial services and to Mrs. Ann Sanders for illustrations.

1976   G. F. SMITH
                                                  J. M. BERG

Contents

		Page
	Preface to the First Edition	v
	Preface to the Second Edition	vii
1	Historical	1
2	Physical Signs	14
3	Bones and Muscles	42
4	Mental Development	61
5	Dermatoglyphs	76
6	Haematology	100
7	Biochemistry	119
8	Immunology	141
9	Clinical Diagnosis	149
10	Cytology	169
11	Vital Statistics	234
12	Aetiology	251
13	Prevention and Treatment	265
14	Social and Educational Considerations	275
	References	279
	Index	335

1. Historical

THE FIRST DESCRIPTIONS

It is a remarkable fact that a condition as clinically distinct and, at least in modern times, as relatively frequent as Down's syndrome was recognized as a definite entity only little more than a century ago. The condition was described, and named mongolian idiocy, by Langdon Down (1866) in a paper published in the London Hospital Reports. Early authorities (Ireland 1877, Shuttleworth 1883, Kovalesky 1906, Comby 1917) all agreed in crediting him with the discovery of a clinical entity. Before Down's paper, however, there had been isolated descriptions in the medical literature of patients who, in retrospect, can be seen to have belonged to the same category. Seguin (1866), in his account of cretinism, described a furfuraceous type "with its milk-white, rosy, and peeling skin; with its shortcomings of all the integuments, which give an unfinished aspect to the truncated fingers and nose; with its cracked lips and tongue; with its red ectopic conjunctiva, coming out to supply the curtailed skin at the margin of the lids". There are, moreover, descriptions of patients which are suggestive of Down's syndrome in earlier works of Seguin (1846) and even one doubtful example from Esquirol (1838). There are also indications of isolated observations in early notes by other observers. In the case books of Earlswood Hospital, where Langdon Down was Medical Superintendent from 1858 until 1868, the same class of patients had been referred to as "strumous cretins" (Shuttleworth 1909). At the Eastern Counties' Asylum for Idiots and Imbeciles, Duncan (1866) had noted a female child with a small round head, Chinese-looking eyes, projecting lower lip and large tongue, who knew only a few words but could sing.

Preceding written descriptions, appearances of children in several works of art have been considered as suggestive of Down's syndrome. A fifteenth century painting by Andrea Mantegna (Ruhräh 1935), referred to on page 5, and others by Jacob Jordaens in the seventeenth century (Zellweger 1968a) are cases in point. The first pictorial illustration of a person with Down's syndrome in a medical text (see Fig. 1) was published by Fraser & Mitchell (1876).

CLINICAL SURVEYS

After 1866, there seem to have been no publications on Down's

1

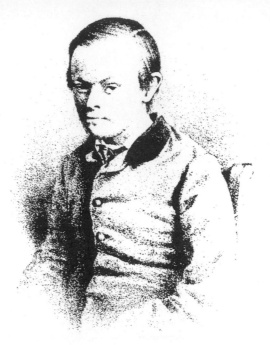

Fig. 1. Photograph of the first pictorial illustration of a person with Down's syndrome (after Fraser & Mitchell 1876).

syndrome until the combined papers of Fraser & Mitchell (1876). Although these writers referred to their patients as Kalmuck idiots, they gave no indication that they knew of Langdon Down's paper. In fact, Fraser stated that he had reviewed the literature and found no prior publication on this type of patient. He reported a case and gave an excellent description of autopsy of the brain. Mitchell drew attention to brachycephaly and increased maternal age.

Many clinical reports followed, notably those of Ireland (1877), Beach (1878), Shuttleworth (1883, 1886) and Shuttleworth & Beach (1899). Shuttleworth, who was considered to be the leading authority on the subject at that time, referred to Down's syndrome individuals as "unfinished children". By this phrase he did not intend to imply that they were born prematurely, but meant that some influence had depressed the maternal powers so that development was incomplete.

Jones (1890) described the brain, Oliver (1891) studied the eyes, Smith (1896) observed the curved little finger as characteristic of Down's syndrome and this was discussed also by West (1901). Garrod (1894) described the association with congenital heart disease and this also studied by Thomson (1898) and by Fennell (1904).

Soon papers on Down's syndrome appeared frequently in medical journals all over the world. Bourneville (1902, 1903), Bourneville & Royer (1906), Comby (1903, 1906, 1907) and Babonneix (1909), in France, made observations on large numbers of cases. In Germany and Austria, Neumann (1899), Kassowitz (1902) and Siegert (1906, 1910) made substantial contributions to the literature. Other investigators at that time were Alberti (1904) in Italy, Barr (1904) and Herrman (1905) in the United States, Hjorth (1907) in Denmark, Kovalesky (1906) and Medovikoff (1910) in Russia, Taillens (1908) in Switzerland, Cafferata (1909) in Argentina, Wood (1909) in Australia, Cordero (1911) in Equador, Hultgren (1915) in Sweden and van der Scheer (1919a) in Holland.

The next decade was marked by a series of surveys each of which emphasized a different aspect of the condition. Brushfield (1924) was primarily concerned with clinical details and their presence or absence in different cases. In a discussion of survival in Down's syndrome, Rosenberg (1924) mentioned, without details, a woman whom he considered to have the syndrome who had given birth to two normal children. Orel (1927) recorded familial data which included notes on ABO blood groups and microsymptoms in relatives. A comprehensive work by van der Scheer (1927) surveyed the families of 259 cases and recorded many statistical and genetical data. Greig (1927) made a remarkable study of three Down's syndrome skulls. In Brousseau & Brainerd's (1928) general account of the subject, which contained detailed information about cases, an extensive list of previous literature was provided.

Surveys, which paid attention to mother's age, familial recurrence of Down's syndrome and incidence of other peculiarities in patients and their relatives, were carried out by Turpin & Caratzali (1934), Lahdensuu (1937) and by Doxiades & Portius (1938). A convenient summary of the literature from 1928 to 1942 was provided by Jervis (1942), and a selective review was undertaken by Beidleman (1945). A comprehensive and critical account of Down's syndrome, which also presented much new data, was given by Øster (1953). An even more extensive account, concerned with 800 cases, was that provided by Hanhart (1960a). A clinical and sociological study was made by Mengoli *et al.* (1957), and a psychological one by Beley *et al.* (1958). Recently, Koch (1973) has published a comprehensive bibliography on Down's syndrome containing over 3,000 references.

EARLY IDEAS ON CAUSATION

Down perceived correctly that, in the syndrome, there was an unusual biological phenomenon which required a special explanation. His scheme for an ethnic classification of idiots was in harmony with contemporary scientific thought which had been influenced by Darwin's work on evolution. Down suggested that if disease could break down racial barriers this helped to demonstrate the unity of the human species. The ethnic theory never became popular but the terms "mongolian" and "mongol" came into general use, although it was admitted by most authorities that the patients so named showed no true resemblance to Mongolian peoples (Tredgold 1908). Down's concept of reversion to an earlier phylogenetic type, however, was supported energetically by Crookshank (1924), an imaginative writer who thought that Down's syndrome was a regression, not merely to a primitive Oriental human type but also to the orang-utan. Crookshank's ideas received some attention at the time (e.g. Hermann 1925). However, they were not well founded and are now seldom referred to except in relation to such peculiarities as the so-called "simian" flexion crease on the palm.

An intensive aetiological study of 350 cases was made by Shuttleworth (1909). The advanced age of the mother at the time of gestation was emphasized and also the fact that Down's syndrome individuals tended to be the last born in a large family. Shuttleworth was unable to decide which of the two related factors was the more important, advanced maternal age or exhaustion produced by a long series of pregnancies. He rejected syphilis as a cause. This had been suggested by Sutherland (1899), but Hjorth (1907) had failed to find any evidence of syphilitic infection in the cases which he studied. However, advocates of the theory of syphilis as a cause of Down's syndrome persisted (Stevens 1915, 1916, Babonneix & Villette 1916). Familial tuberculosis had been observed by Down and by Shuttleworth (1906) and this disease seemed to them the probable cause. As patients with Down's syndrome themselves so frequently died of tuberculosis, often of the miliary type, this assumption appeared not unreasonable (Tredgold 1908, Potts 1909).

Parental alcoholism, incriminated as a cause of other forms of mental retardation, was invoked by Cafferata (1909) to explain Down's syndrome. Other influences suggested as causes were indicated by the occurrences, in close relatives, of epilepsy, insanity, nervous instability and mental retardation (Tredgold 1908, Caldecott 1909). Maternal emotional distress or worry during pregnancy periodically also was considered of possible aetiological significance.

Implicitly, Down had recognized that mongolism was a disease which developed very early in life. Garrod (1894, 1898, 1899) and Thomson (1898) had noted an association of cardiac defects with the syndrome. This association strengthened the argument localizing the time of onset in the early months of gestation. The same kind of reasoning was employed much later when it had been found that those with Down's syndrome had characteristic dermatoglyphic patterns (Cummins 1936). Dermal ridge patterns are fixed by the tenth week of gestation, so the abnormal process must have started before that time.

Since Down's syndrome had formerly been confused with cretinism, it is not surprising to find that thyroid deficiency was sometimes considered to be the cause (Stoeltzner 1919). In these connections, reference may be made here to a remarkable painting of a Madonna and Child by Andrea Mantegna (1431-1506) which was illustrated and described by Ruhräh (1935). He drew attention to some features of Down's syndrome, as well as of cretinism, displayed by the child and noted the presence of a small goitre in the mother. Many physicians had tried thyroid gland preparations for treatment, but had afterwards commented that they found them of little or no value. Clark's (1929) notion that fetal hyperthyroidism was the main aetiological factor obtained little credence, though Myers (1938) found some evidence of maternal dysthyroidism. Other writers drew attention to endocrine disturbances in Down's syndrome and attributed primary causal significance to them. Hypoplasia of the adrenal glands was noted by Vas (1925), dysfunction of the pituitary gland by Benda & Bixby (1939) and abnormality of the thymus by Barnes (1923). Brown (1954) argued that damage to fetal adrenals by maternal infections, anoxia or ionized air could result in the development of Down's syndrome.

Another suggestion was Jansen's (1921) theory that the amniotic sac was too small to allow the fetus to grow properly during the sixth and seventh weeks of gestation. A factor sometimes blamed was the use of chemical contraceptives. Curettage was suspected by Mayerhofer (1939) and by Engler (1949) and faulty implantation by Bennholdt-Thomsen (1932).

Among the more favoured hypotheses were those based upon theoretical degeneration of the ovum (Jenkins 1933, Rosanoff & Handy 1934, Bleyer 1934). Such inferences could be drawn from the observed relationship of the incidence to maternal age. However, there were no biological data, experimental or of natural occurrence, to support views of this kind. Searches for ovarian dysfunction in mothers of Down's syndrome children gave equivocal results (Geyer 1939, Schröder 1940). The dangers of maternal-fetal incompatibility increase with each successive pregnancy, but a serological survey of patients with Down's syndrome and their parents gave no suggestion that this could be a causal factor here (Lang-Brown *et al.* 1953).

TRENDS OF RECENT RESEARCHES

During the last 40 years investigations into the aetiology of Down's syndrome have been increasingly concerned with the genetical aspects of the subject. The first necessity was to establish the frequency of the condition at birth. Estimates were provided by Jenkins (1933) and by Malpas (1937) and subsequent observations have confirmed their figures. The sex ratio sometimes indicates predominance of males (Hug 1951). The recognition of cases in non-European populations was an important step forward.

Barbour (1902), Bleyer (1925), Brahdy (1927) and Dunlap (1933) recorded Negro patients and Bleyer (1932, 1934) noted that Down's syndrome occurred in American and Mexican Indians. An affected Chinese boy was described by Tumpeer (1922). Other instances in Chinese children and many among Japanese were reported by Sweet (1934). Chand (1932) mentioned cases in India and Illing (1939) in Malaya. Down's syndrome among the Bantu races of South Africa was reported only relatively recently (Lötter 1955, Kaplan 1955), and instances among Ugandan Africans were noted at about the same time (Luder & Musoke 1955).

The familial incidence was the next important problem and numerous scattered examples had been recorded in surveys of patients. It was agreed that the concentration of cases in families was slight and some investigators found no evidence at all for its existence (Goddard 1914). With such a relatively common disease (that is, one with an incidence of 1 in about 700 at birth), the significance of a family group containing two affected members was difficult to evaluate. However, three facts indicated that hereditary influence could be genuine in some circumstances.

The first was that dizygotic twins had been found to be unequally and monozygotic twins equally affected (Halbertsma 1923, Reuben & Klein 1926). Many similar reports were published subsequently which lent further support to the view that hereditary influence was critical and they included a few examples in which the members of a clearly dizygotic twin pair were both affected with Down's syndrome (Keay 1958). The second fact was that the syndrome could be directly transmitted from mother to child (Lelong et al. 1949, Rehn & Thomas 1957). The third was that, when more than one member of a family was affected, the dependence upon mother's age was weakened (Penrose 1951, 1953). This was especially noticeable when inheritance came apparently through the mother. The existence of cases with hereditary origin and with incidence independent of the mother's age could be postulated.

The precise nature of the association between the incidence of Down's syndrome and the ages of the parents was independently investigated by Jenkins (1933) and by Penrose (1933a). It was shown that, in pooled samples of cases, the age of the father, by itself, was of no significance. The less tractable problem of separating the effects of birth order from those of the mother's age was investigated by Penrose (1934b) and the influence of birth order, by itself, also was shown to be insignificant.

A great deal of interest has been focussed upon the question of incomplete, partial, abortive or vestigial Down's syndrome (Tredgold 1908). Some writers have denied the existence of such conditions (Fanconi 1939) and others have diagnosed them frequently (Malz 1937). If it were accepted that incomplete forms existed and that individual signs, characteristic of Down's syndrome, could be found in normal members of the population, two genetical questions were raised. First, are the characteristic traits heritable variations? Secondly, are these characters of significantly more frequent occurrence in close relatives of patients than in the general population? Examples of qualitative investigations were the study of furrowed tongue by Turpin & Caratzali (1933) and the analysis of data on the transverse palmar crease by Erne (1953). The genetics of the position of the palmar triradius t was studied quantitatively by Penrose (1954a). The results of these and other comparable investigations have indicated that the "mongol" traits under consideration were, indeed, by themselves, familial; they also showed increased incidence among relatives of patients as compared with controls.

On the more strictly clinical side advances have been made in a variety of fields often facilitated by new technical developments. For example, Kreezer (1939) examined the electroencephalogram in Down's syndrome and Himwich & Fazekas (1940) showed that the rate of oxygen utilization in the brain was lowered as compared with normal controls. Extensive biochemical tests in Down's syndrome were carried out on the blood (Bixby 1941) and the urine (Bixby & Benda 1942) and the results showed no constant abnormalities. However, Stern & Lewis (1958, 1962) found low blood calcium and pseudocholinesterase levels. Exact tests for thyroid gland function were made by Kearns & Hutson (1951) and by Kurland *et al.* (1957), but no specific peculiarities were identified.

A deficiency of lobulation in polymorphonuclear leucocytes was observed by Benda (1946) and by Turpin & Bernyer (1947). Leukaemia in Down's syndrome was studied by Krivit & Good (1956, 1957) and the association of the two conditions was demonstrated statistically by Stewart *et al.* (1958). More recently the amount of alkaline phosphatase in leucocytes was found to be somewhat increased in the syndrome (Trubowitz *et al.* 1962). The results of ABO blood group typing by many observers have been studied critically by Kaplan *et al.* (1964) and it is clear that the distributions do not differ from those in control populations.

The value of a particular trait for purposes of diagnosis depends upon its frequency in Down's syndrome as compared with that in the general population. Provided that such traits are not too closely correlated they can be used in combination. In an early attempt, Penrose (1933b) used ten such traits and found that the presence of any four of them in one person made the diagnosis probable. An extension of this method was used by Ford Walker (1957) with dermatoglyphic data, and a number of discriminative dermatoglyphic indices have been devised subsequently (see page 95). Many other characters have now been studied which could be used in combination for diagnostic purposes, such as angles measured, in X-ray photographs, of pelvic bones (Caffey & Ross 1956). Some of the most effectively discriminative traits can be observed at birth (Carter & MacCarthy 1951, Hall 1964). The eye if carefully studied shows numerous features which are highly characteristic (Lowe 1949). So far, however, no attempt has been made to combine all the tests from different clinical aspects into a single diagnostic criterion though this is theoretically possible.

In Down's syndrome a universal characteristic is diminution of the intellectual powers, but this is not the only mental change. Early investigators noticed that the personality was somewhat different from that in other patients. Shuttleworth (1895) described the powers of mimicry, love of music and rhythm in persons with Down's syndrome. Writing, drawing and simple industrial tasks were within their scope, but not the higher intellectual operations. The temperament is also usually considered to be distinctive, but some observers have denied that there is any well-defined type (Blacketer-Simmonds 1953). However, differential abilities between Down's syndrome and other retarded patients have been recognized by carefully planned testing (O'Connor & Hermelin 1963).

THE CHROMOSOMES

It was suspected for a long time that some chromosomal aberration might be implicated in the pathology of Down's syndrome. Waardenburg (1932) suggested non-disjunction as an explanation, but at that time there was difficulty in accepting this for two reasons. First, there was no evidence from experimental genetics to suggest that non-disjunction could be strongly influenced by maternal age, the most critical causal factor in the syndrome. Secondly, familial cases often indicated transmission through normal carriers. This pattern of inheritance suggested the transmission of an abnormal chromosome sometimes producing offspring with unbalanced chromatin content (Penrose 1939). Meanwhile trisomy had been discussed by Bleyer (1934).

In his studies of normal testicular tissue, Painter (1921) reported chromosome numbers ranging from 45 to 48. At the time he noted that, even though the counts ranged from 45 to 48, the clearest equatorial plate he studied showed 46 chromosomes. Two years later Painter (1923) finally decided that the correct chromosome number was 48. Mittwoch (1952) studied spermatogenesis in an individual with Down's syndrome and concluded that, at diakinesis, there were 24 chromosomal masses, but because the correct diploid number was considered to be 48 at the time, this finding was not thought to be unusual.

In 1956, Tjio & Levan, working with cultures of lung fibroblasts derived from human embryos and using a greatly improved technique, found that the normal diploid chromosomal number was 46. This finding was shortly afterwards confirmed in observations on human spermatocytes by Ford & Hamerton (1956), who found that the haploid number was 23.

Studies of the karyotype in various pathological conditions started independently in several laboratories, but advances were held up by the difficulty of finding suitable tissues for routine testing. There was a delay of over two years and then Lejeune et al. (1959a) showed that persons with Down's syndrome had an extra acrocentric chromosome and a total diploid chromosomal number of 47 in cultures from fibrous tissue. Moreover, Jacobs & Strong (1959) had found an extra chromosome, in bone marrow cells of a case of Klinefelter's syndrome, which was interpreted as an additional X.

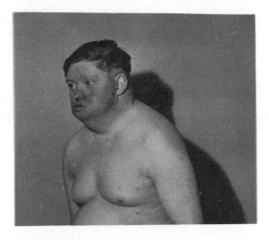

Fig. 2. Appearance of first recorded Down's syndrome individual with double aneuploidy: Down-Klinefelter syndromes (48,XXY,21+) (Ford *et al.* 1959a, Harnden *et al.* 1960).

Ford *et al.* (1959a) examined the bone marrow of a patient with both Down's and Klinefelter's syndromes (see Fig. 2) and showed that he had 48 chromosomes, which included 44 autosomes, an extra acrocentric, and an XXY pattern. Jacobs *et al.* (1959), again using bone marrow cells, reported on three male and three female cases of Down's syndrome, all of whom had 47 chromosomes. Böök *et al.* (1959) obtained similar results, using both bone marrow cells and skin.

It now became a matter of urgent interest to investigate familial cases and also young mothers of Down's syndrome children who were not exposed to the effect of increasing age. Polani *et al.* (1960) examined the chromosomes of a Down's syndrome child, selected because of the youthful age of the mother (21 years) at the time of the child's birth. Only 46 chromosomes were present, four in the 21—22 group, five in the 13—15 group and an extra one in the 6—12 group. The extra chromosome was found to be a translocation, a centric fusion of two chromosomes. Familial transmission of this type of translocation was demonstrated in a family with two Down's syndrome sibs by Penrose *et al.* (1960). The translocated chromosomes (15:21) were shown to be present in three generations of the family.

Another type of translocation had been found by Fraccaro *et al.* (1960). They reported a case of Down's syndrome with 46 chromosomes, but with only three in group 21—22 and an additional one in group 19—20. They concluded that the extra chromosome was either an isochromosome of 21 or a translocation between chromosomes 21 and 22.

Mosaicism had by now been established in sex chromosomal abnormalities (Ford 1960a) and it was timely that, in 1961, Clarke *et al.* reported definite mosaicism, in both blood and skin cultures, of a two-year-old female of almost normal intelligence but with some physical characteristics of Down's syndrome. At about the same time Hanhart *et al.* (1961) reported chromosomal studies on a trisomic Down's syndrome female and her similarly trisomic child. This was the first demonstration of secondary or inevitable non-disjunction in man. A report by Levan & Hsu (1960) had shown also that a trisomic Down's syndrome female could give birth to a child with a normal karyotype. It could now be surmised that certain mothers of Down's syndrome individuals were themselves mosaic for normal and trisomic cells. This situation was actually found by Blank *et al.* (1962) and they reported trisomic mosaicism in a mother of a standard trisomic case of Down's syndrome.

A number of rare atypical chromosomal findings have been reported in Down's syndrome. Day *et al.* (1963), for example, found a triple-X Down's syndrome female with 48 chromosomes. Workers in many laboratories had suspected that persons with both Down's and Turner's syndrome should be found and this combination was eventually reported by van Wijck *et al.* (1964), whose patient was a Down's syndrome female with features of Turner's syndrome. She had X/XX mosaicism in addition to trisomy of a small acrocentric.

Gagnon *et al.* (1961) described a patient with Down's syndrome who was also trisomic for chromosome 18. Another Down's syndrome patient was found to be also trisomic for a chromosome in the 13–15 group (Becker *et al.* 1963), and yet another was observed to have an XYY sex chromosome complement (Verresen & van den Berghe 1965). Numbers of examples of such combined chromosomal errors have subsequently been reported. Most unexpected of all was the finding of de Wolff *et al.* (1962). They reported monozygotic twins one of whom was physically normal with 46 chromosomes and a normal karyotype. The second twin was a typical case of Down's syndrome with 47 chromosomes.

Makino *et al.* (1960) examined 10 Japanese cases of Down's syndrome and found them all to be standard trisomics, and similar results were soon reported from other countries.

COMPARATIVE STUDIES

It is remarkable that a condition of such significance in man as trisomy of a small acrocentric should have so few parallels in lower animals. The set of 12 trisomic conditions described by Blakeslee (1923), one for each chromosome pair in *Datura stramonium,* is a demonstration that, in plants, aberrations of this kind need not be harmful. In *Drosophila melanogaster* trisomy of the very small chromosome IV produces a fly which is slightly smaller than the normal (Fig. 3 and see Chapter 10), but which is neither obviously abnormal nor infertile (Morgan *et al.* 1925). Only relatively recently have trisomic mammals other than man been discovered.

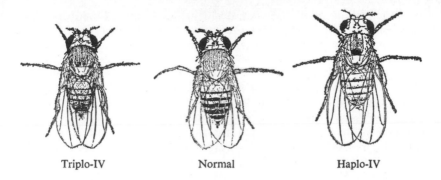

| Triplo-IV | Normal | Haplo-IV |

Fig. 3. *Drosophila melanogaster* females. Triplo-IV has dark colour and narrow wings, whereas Haplo-IV has pale colour and wide wings (Morgan *et al.* 1925).

Cattanach (1964) described a mouse of normal appearance but sterile with trisomy of one of the smaller autosomes. A female chimpanzee (*Pan troglodytes*) with trisomy of a small acrocentric chromosome, arbitrarily designated as No. 22, was reported by McClure *et al.* (1969). The chimpanzee showed clinical features which included the following: a slow growth rate, retarded postural development, hypotonia, congenital heart defects and prominent epicanthus. She was born to a comparatively young mother and both her parents had apparently normal chromosome complements.

The origin of trisomy in experimental animals or plants has not been shown to have any connection with the age of the maternal germ cells and thus no clue was provided by comparative study which might have suggested trisomy as an explanation of Down's syndrome. Some information about genetical causation of trisomics was provided by the work of Sturtevant (1929) and of Lewis & Gencarella (1952), who found that certain recessive genes in the mother could produce non-disjunction in *Drosophila*. Also Beadle (1932) showed that a gene called "sticky" in maize could induce aberrations, including trisomy at meiosis and also in mitotic cell divisions. The trisomic mouse, referred to earlier, occurred after its father had been exposed to a chemical mutagen.

NOMENCLATURE

Many alternative designations have been suggested for the condition. Since Down introduced a name for the Mongolian type of idiocy, variations have arisen which have included mongol, mongolism, mongoloid, mongolian imbecile and mongoloid idiot. Mongoloid deformity was recommended by van der Scheer (1927). Kalmuck idiocy was used by Fraser & Mitchell (1876) and shortly after this the word Tartar began to appear in the literature.

"Unfinished child" was suggested by Shuttleworth (1886) and "ill-finished" by Thomson (1907). Acromicria was introduced by Neumann (1899) and, later, this name was approved by Benda (1946, 1960). Generalized fetal dysplasia was suggested by Penrose (1949a) and peristatic amentia by Engler (1949). Down's disease, which had been for a long time and is still used in Russia (Davidenkova et al (1964), has recently been more widely adopted in other countries. Variations now recognized are Down's or Langdon-Down's syndrome, Down's anomaly, Down's deformity, and the Down-Seguin or Seguin-Down syndrome. Trisomy 21 anomaly has been proposed (Lejeune 1964) on the assumption, at the time, that the larger of the two small acrocentric pairs is always implicated. Mosaic mongol, incomplete or partial mongol and para-mongoloid are terms that have been used for special classifications of the syndrome. The writers here have used chiefly the term Down's syndrome.

TEXTS OF GENERAL INTEREST

Texts on Down's syndrome of particular interest to parents and the general public have been published from time to time, especially in recent years. Dale Evans Rogers (1963) has written a personal account, first published in 1953, about her Down's syndrome daughter who lived for only two years. Mary Rita Lynch (1960) has recounted her own experiences in similar circumstances. Nancy and Bruce Roberts (1968), a husband and wife writer-photographer team, have collaborated in an excellently illustrated text about their son with Down's syndrome. A remarkable autobiographical essay, written by Nigel Hunt (1967), a young man with Down's syndrome, provides an unusually interesting view of events as seen by an affected person. Recently, Smith & Wilson (1973) have described the characteristics of Down's syndrome, for parents and others, and provided useful guidance to them. The book contains a series of appealing photographs of individuals with the syndrome from infancy to adulthood. Another helpful booklet for parents, also well illustrated, has been written by Pitt (1974). A practical parental guide, with contributions by a mother, a physician, a language therapist and teachers, is now available as well (Horrobin & Rynders 1974). Down's syndrome also has attracted the attention of fiction writers as witnessed by Slavitt's (1973) novel in which the hero is a youth with the syndrome who developed extraordinary talents.

L. S. PENROSE

We think it appropriate to refer here to the special place occupied by the late Lionel S. Penrose in the history of Down's syndrome. No one has contributed more to the elucidation of its many mysteries than he, and few have maintained as extensive an interest in the subject during a whole professional lifetime (Smith & Berg 1974, Berg 1975).

He realized early in his career that comprehensive scientific study of the condition was important not only for the purposes of understanding its nature, but as a means of throwing light on biological obscurities about man in general. Not least of all, he had genuine regard for affected persons themselves so that, in all his endeavours, concern for their well-being was constantly present.

Many of Penrose's ideas and references to his work are contained in this book, not simply because he was co-author of the first edition but because they are of abiding value.

2. Physical Signs

In this chapter the physical signs which are characteristic of Down's syndrome are described mainly in so far as they concern the surface of the body and soft tissues. Anomalies of the face are very noticeable and, as in many other syndromes, a high proportion of cases can be immediately recognized by them. Though observations are often based on subjective impressions, an increasing number of metrical techniques are being applied (Joseph & Dawburn 1970).

LIPS

Morphologically, the lips are not considered unusual. At birth and in early infancy, they are similar to those of normal infants. Changes that occur are usually thought to be secondary, and probably are related to the mouth being held open and to the habitual protrusion of the tongue which allows the lips to be excessively bathed with saliva and afterwards to become cracked and dry. Butterworth *et al.* (1960) noted a whitening and thickening of the membrane of the lips which was followed by vertical fissuring (see Fig. 4) and gradual but persistent enlargement. Scaling and crusting were not infrequent. Other writers have suggested that the abnormal lips seen in Down's syndrome are due to actinic factors damaging anatomically imperfect skin. Avitaminosis has also been suggested as a possible cause of the pathology of the lips but, in general, vitamin therapy has not been successful. Butterworth *et al.*, however, did note some improvement after prescribing a combination of vitamins and hormones. Rhagades may be seen at the corners of the mouth. Permanent changes are most frequently found in males during the third decade of life.

ORAL CAVITY

The mouth has usually been described as small, the palate high and narrow and the maxilla underdeveloped. However, Redman *et al.* (1965) produced measurements which indicated that the palatal vault in Down's syndrome is not abnormal when the diminished size of the bones of the skull is taken into account. In a subsequent study, Shapiro *et al.* (1967) made direct measurements of palatal height, width and length in 153 Down's syndrome patients, ranging in age from 7 to 66 years, and

14

compared these with data from normal subjects. They concluded that the palatal vault in Down's syndrome is probably not increased in height, but that the Down's syndrome palate is narrower, and distinctly shorter, than normal. Kisling (1966) reported reduction in palatal height, as well as in width and length, in adult males with Down's syndrome compared to controls; palatal shape was much the same in the two groups. Austin *et al.* (1969) measured the length of the hard palate, from lateral skull roentgenograms, in 10 newly born infants with Down's syndrome and in controls. They found shorter hard palates in the Down's syndrome babies and felt that, in a full-term infant, a hard palate length of 26 mm. or less was a sign of Down's syndrome whereas a length of 29 mm. or more was against the diagnosis. In Jensen *et al.*'s (1973) survey, the palatal height in Down's syndrome was found to be consistently smaller than normal at all ages and in both sexes.

The majority of patients habitually hold their mouths open. Øster (1953) reported this finding in 67 per cent of his cases, most of whom were in the 5 to 14 year age group. Barnes (1923) explained that the mouth is held open because of the relatively narrow nasopharynx and unusually enlarged tonsils and adenoids. A similar explanation for the open mouth and tongue protrusion, related to the need to provide an airway, was suggested by Ardran *et al.* (1972). Others regard the open mouth as secondary to the protrusion of the enlarged tongue. Cleft palate and hare lip each occur in about 0.5 per cent of persons with Down's syndrome (McMillan & Kashgarian 1961), a frequency substantially higher than in the general population. Schendel & Gorlin (1974) examined 389 Down's syndrome patients and found a submucous cleft palate in 3 (0.8 per cent) and some degree of bifid uvula in 18 (4.6 per cent), incidences also greater than in the general population. They considered these anomalies to be micromanifestations of the more severe isolated cleft palate.

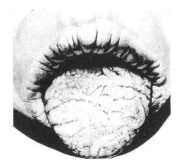

Fig. 4. The tongue and upper lip of a Down's syndrome male aged 24 years.

TONGUE

As early as 1876 Mitchell considered fissuring of the tongue (see Fig. 4) as an important clinical finding in Down's syndrome. The tongue is normal at birth but later develops hypertrophy of the vallate papillae (Thomson 1907). The papillary hypertrophy usually does not begin before the second year and fissuring supposedly begins at about 4 years (Engler); however, Thomson found papillary hypertrophy in the first year of life. Occasionally, fissuring may begin as early as 6 months of age. A large number of the patients, reported by Øster, had papillary hypertrophy, but he found that it was difficult to differentiate between this and furrowed tongue. In his series of patients those with furrowed tongue, as a rule, also had papillary hypertrophy. The tongue was furrowed in 59 per cent of his cases. This abnormality was present in all age groups but showed an increasing frequency with age. It has been reported (Engler) that all cases of Down's syndrome over 5 years of age have furrowed tongues but this observation has not been confirmed (Benda 1960).

The cause of the papillary hypertrophy and furrowing is unknown. One of the reasons frequently given for these conditions is the excessive sucking of the tongue. There is evidence that it is a genetical trait in some families (Seiler 1938). Turpin & Caratzali (1933) noted an increased incidence of fissuring of the tongue in the relatives of individuals with Down's syndrome.

Øster (1953) reported that the tongue seemed too large in 57 per cent of his cases. Many authors, however, consider that the tongue is normal in size and that it is enlarged only in rare instances. In a radiographic examination of 8 patients with Down's syndrome, aged from 5 to 15 years, Ardran et al. found that none had generalized enlargement of the tongue, though 5 showed localized enlargement in the region of the lingual tonsil.

TEETH

There are an increasing number of reports in the literature referring to teeth and gum anomalies in Down's syndrome. One of the earliest reports was by Jones (1890) who commented on the irregular development of teeth. A comprehensive review was provided recently by Shapiro (1970).

Eruption. The deciduous teeth are frequently late in erupting and the pattern can be different from that occurring in normals (Brousseau & Brainerd 1928). The first incisors may not appear until 9 months whereas, in normal infants, they usually appear at about 6 months. Eruption of the first tooth can be delayed till 20 months or later. Completion of the deciduous dentition may not occur until 4–5 years of age. The pattern of eruption may be disturbed so that the molars appear before all the incisors have erupted. In some cases the pattern of eruption is peculiar because certain deciduous and permanent teeth are absent. Øster (1953) observed the age of first tooth eruption for 267 persons with Down's syndrome. He found that only 19 had their first tooth before or during the sixth month of life, while 161 did not have their first tooth till the twelfth month or later. In a more recent study of the eruption of deciduous teeth, Roche & Barkla (1964) found that the age interval over which the first teeth erupted was shorter than that previously reported. The youngest child with Down's syndrome in whom a tooth had erupted was aged 8.5 months and the oldest in whom a tooth had not erupted was aged 13.9 months. Among normal children, the corresponding ages were 4.4 and 15.5 months. Abnormal sequence of eruption was also noted.

The permanent teeth tend to appear more regularly than the temporary teeth. However, delayed or irregular eruption of the permanent teeth has been noted by numbers of observers (Brousseau & Brainerd, Silimbani 1962, Kaczmarczyk 1964, Barkla 1966a, Orner 1973). Barkla found that in fewer than 5 per cent of cases of Down's syndrome examined did any particular tooth erupt within the normal age range. In Orner's study, the Down's syndrome children showed also a consistent tendency towards later mean age of eruption for each tooth type, whereas their sibs resembled other normal children in these regards.

Missing teeth. Congenital absence or fusion of deciduous teeth is not unusual in Down's syndrome children (Barkla 1963). In Barkla's series these findings always involved the lateral incisors. Early shedding of the deciduous teeth, especially of the lateral and central incisors, is quite common. Furthermore, congenital absence of certain permanent teeth has been reported (Greig 1927, Ingalls & Butler 1953, Barkla 1966b, Orner 1971). The maxillary permanent lateral incisor is often affected. This tooth was noted by Ingalls & Butler to be congenitally absent in 25 per cent, or stunted in 10 per cent. They pointed out that a third of Down's syndrome children have congenitally missing or defective upper lateral permanent incisors. This was interpreted as evidence of injury to the primordium.

Abnormality of shape. The teeth in Down's syndrome are considered to be microdontic and to show abnormalities of shape, such as being "pegged" or having malformation of the crown. Measurements of mesiodistal width of permanent teeth have shown, in general, reduction in size compared to controls (Kisling 1966, Gekiauskas & Cohen 1970). Examination of extracted teeth indicated that the roots were much shorter than would be expected (McMillan & Kashgarian 1961). On the basis of X-ray examination of the teeth, Spitzer & Robinson (1955) reported aplasia of the enamel. Later, Spitzer *et al.* (1961) noted that 86 per cent of a small group of Down's syndrome patients had changes of dental structure.

Periodontal disease. In general terms, periodontal disease destroys the surrounding and supporting tissues of the teeth. These are the periodontal membrane which is located between the root of the tooth and the bony wall of the socket, the alveolar process which is a projection of bone forming a socket for the root of the tooth, and the gingiva or gum tissue (Dow 1951).

Benda (1946) quotes Nash who found 90 per cent of Down's syndrome cases with some evidence of periodontal disease. In Cohen et al.'s (1960) study, all 100 individuals with Down's syndrome examined, ranging in age from 3 to 18 years, had periodontal involvement. In addition to periodontis, superimposed necrotizing gingivitis was noted in many cases. Similarly high frequencies of periodontal disease in Down's syndrome were observed by Julku et al. (1962), Johnson & Young (1963), Kisling & Krebs (1963), Sznajder et al. (1968) and by Jensen et al. (1973). It is noteworthy that Swallow (1964) and Cutress (1971a) each found a relatively low prevalence of periodontal disease in persons with Down's syndrome living at home as opposed to institutions.

Periodontal disease, which may begin as early as 3 years of age, can cause loss of deciduous incisors before the age of 5 years (Brown & Cunningham 1961). The severity of the condition seems to increase steadily with age, and the mandibular incisors are usually the first to be affected. Later the process spreads to the other teeth. In young patients the first indication of the onset usually is severe gingivitis with ulcerations and sloughing of the interdental papillae and gingival margins. In older subjects severe bone loss and gingival recession are the most marked features (Brown & Cunningham). Sometimes alveolar bone loss and consequent loosening of the teeth precedes the onset of gingivitis (MacFarland 1964).

The cause of the periodontal disease is not clear. Dow thought that local factors cannot explain the condition and considered that anoxia resulting from poor circulation is a possible cause. Others have suggested that susceptibility to infection, nutritional factors or poor oral hygiene may be causes, but it is doubtful if any of these is of primary importance. Evidence of a relationship between periodontal disease and blood citric acid levels, which has been noted in normal persons (Tsunemitsu 1963, Simon et al. 1968) has not been established in Down's syndrome (Cutress et al. 1971).

Caries. Numbers of investigators, including Rapaport (1957), Johnson et al. (1960), McMillan & Kashgarian (1961), Winer & Cohen (1961, 1962) and Jensen et al. have reported that dental caries is relatively uncommon in Down's syndrome. Delayed eruption of teeth may partially or largely account for such findings (Johnson et al., Swallow, Cutress 1971b). Rapaport noted that, in an area of low fluorine content in the water (0.1 mg. per litre), dental caries was found in 45.1 per cent of cases of Down's syndrome and 82.9 per cent of controls; while in an area where the fluorine in the water was higher (1 mg. per litre) dental caries occurred in 21.6 per cent of Down's syndrome cases and 43.4 per cent of controls. He speculated on the action of enzymatic inhibitors to account for this difference.

Malocclusion. Brown & Cunningham reported that 64 per cent of Down's syndrome patients over the age of 11 years had class III malocclusion, and that almost all of them also had a cross-bite in the posterior region, with the lower incisors anterior to the upper incisors. Similar findings were reported by Jensen *et al.* who also noted that interdental spacing tended to increase with advancing age in Down's syndrome compared to a decrease in controls. In an analysis of the occlusion of the teeth in 68 adult males with Down's syndrome, Kisling found mandibular overjet, anterior open bite and posterior cross-bite as typical malocclusions. At least one of these anomalies was present in all the cases. Prognathism has been attributed to the tongue's pushing against the lower teeth (Gosman 1951). In Down's syndrome, however, this would seem to be the inevitable result of the projecting mandible which is relatively better developed than the maxilla.

VOICE

Though there have been a few suggestions to the contrary, based on studies of relatively small numbers of children (Michel & Carney 1964, Hollien & Copeland 1965, Weinberg & Zlatin 1970), the voice in Down's syndrome has, in most cases, usually been considered to be guttural and low-pitched; in addition to this, articulation is generally faulty. Spectrographic analyses of the vocal responses to pain stimuli of 30 infants with Down's syndrome, undertaken by Lind *et al.* (1970), showed several abnormal acoustic characteristics, including low pitch, flat melody form and nasality. In a comparison of 20 Down's syndrome children with normal controls, Montague & Hollien (1973) found that the Down's syndrome children exhibited considerably more breathiness, roughness of the voice and nasality than did the controls. There is no adequate explanation of these various voice changes. In studying the larynx of several patients, Benda (1960) found the mucosa thickened and fibrotic. The larynx seemed higher in the neck than usual. Brousseau & Brainerd thought that the harshness and faulty articulation might be due, in part, to organic defects, such as high palate, nasal obstruction and shortness of the buccal cavity. More particularly, they considered that it reflected a lack of control of the movements of the mouth, tongue and lips. Novàk (1972) attributed voice characteristics in Down's syndrome to a combination of hypotonia, inadequate control of the glottis, poor respiratory function and, especially, alteration in the shape of the resonating cavities.

NOSE

The shape of the nose is variable in Down's syndrome; however, certain features are consistently observed. One characteristic is the flatness of the nose bridge associated with underdevelopment or even absence of the nasal bones. This is most noticeable in the age group 0–4 years. Kisling (1966) found nasal bone aplasia in 9 out of 68 adult males with Down's syndrome. The nose is considered to be small in about half the cases. The cartilaginous part may be wide and triangular, producing a "pug nosed" appearance. In many cases the anterior nares point forward instead of downwards. The nasal mucosa tends to be thickened and a mucous discharge is frequently present.

EYES

Palpebral fissures. One of the outstanding features in Down's syndrome is that the palpebral fissures are often oblique and narrow laterally. The normal outer canthus is slightly higher than the inner and this difference may give the appearance of a slant. Solomons *et al.* (1965) found such a slant in 91 per cent of 93 Down's syndrome patients below the age of 10 years and in 58 per cent of 123 older patients, compared to a 14 per cent incidence in 150 normal controls. The slant is usually, but not always, bilateral and, occasionally, in the opposite direction. Gifford (1928) pointed out that in the Mongolian peoples the axis of the palpebral fissure is no different from that in Europeans. In Orientals, the palpebral fissures are said to be almond-shaped because the widest part is near the inner angle, and the fissure narrows and tapers laterally. In addition, an epicanthic fold exists normally in Orientals (Komoto 1892), which, by itself, gives an impression of obliquity.

The cause of the obliquity of the palpebral fissures in Down's syndrome is uncertain. Van der Scheer (1919a) considered the cause to be malformation of the nasal bones. Benda (1960) suggested that under-development of the facial bones causes the orbits to be egg-shaped, and to slant laterally, and determines the shape of the palpebral apertures. Lowe (1949), however, found on examination of four skulls of Down's syndrome adults that the orbital axis was inclined downwards and outwards, as in normal Europeans. He explained that the upward slope of the orbital axis in Down's syndrome, observed by Benda, could be a retardation of development which was corrected as the patient grew older. He also pointed out that the slope of the palpebral fissures and that of the orbital axes changed at different times during development so that they must be independent processes. He attributed the obliquity of the palpebral fissures to changes in the skin and gave examples of other skin conditions (ectodermal defects, dermatomyositis and scleroderma) which could produce changes in alignment which resembled those in Down's syndrome.

Epicanthic folds. Epicanthic folds in Down's syndrome have been variously reported to occur in from 20 to over 80 per cent of cases (Solomons *et al.*). In their own study, Solomons *et al.* noted a substantial difference in incidence in both Down's syndrome and normal individuals when age was taken into account (see Table 1). The folds are usually bilateral but are found unilaterally in some instances. Epicanthic folds are

Table 1. Bilateral or Unilateral Epicanthic Folds in Down's Syndrome and Normal Controls (After Solomons *et al.* 1965)

| | Age below 10 years | | Age 10 years and over | |
	No.	With folds	No.	With folds
Down's syndrome	93	56(60%)	123	11(9%)
Normal controls	60	12(20%)	90	3(3%)

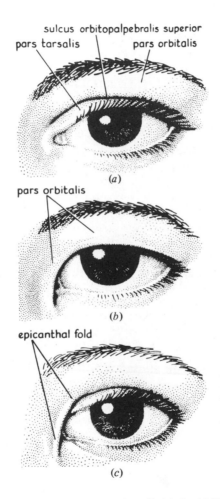

Fig. 5. Epicanthic variations (Solnitzky 1962).

(a) Absence of epicanthic fold;
(b) Epicanthic fold in Oriental populations;
(c) Epicanthic fold in Down's syndrome.

of great interest in Down's syndrome since their presence helped Down to conclude that these patients were in some way a reversion to a Mongolian race. Usher (1935) gives credit for naming these folds to von Ammon in 1831 even though the folds were described as early as 1828 by Schön, as noted by Sichel (1851). In 1860 von Ammon described some special types.

For the purpose of recognizing the folds which are characteristic of Down's syndrome a different classification is perhaps more useful. Figs. 5, a, b and c show anatomical variations of the epicanthic area. In Fig. 5a, no epicanthic fold is present. This type of epicanthic area is usual in European races, but it also occurs in many Oriental people (Gifford) and in some Down's syndrome adults. In Fig. 5b, the epicanthic fold is continuous with the pars orbitalis and hides a large part of the pars tarsalis. This type of fold occurs frequently in normal Oriental persons and in some Orientals with Down's syndrome. In Fig. 5c, the epicanthic fold is smaller than that seen in Fig. 5b. The fold arises from the inner region of the pars orbitalis. This type of epicanthic fold is very often found in Down's syndrome, especially at a young age. It also occurs in normal Europeans and especially in children, and can occur in normal Orientals and in Orientals with Down's syndrome.

The epicanthic folds in normal Oriental people tend to differ widely from individual to individual (Gifford, Wagner 1962). The folds in Oriental children with Down's syndrome may be almost the same as those found in normal Oriental children (Wagner, Tsuang 1964) though somewhat intensified.

The reasons for the variations in epicanthic folds are not well understood. In Orientals they are attributed to extra tissue in epicanthic areas (von Ammon 1841) or to underdevelopment of the nasal bones (Sichel 1851, Jansen 1921). With stronger development of the nasal and facial bones in Down's syndrome, epicanthic folds become less obvious or completely disappear (Lowe). Noticeable epicanthus occurs in about 30 per cent of normal newly born infants and may persist until about the age of 4 years or longer. In a small number of normal Europeans, the folds may be present throughout life and in these cases they may have specific genetical determination (Usher). According to Waardenburg (1932) epicanthic folds are fetal characteristics which can be carried on into postnatal life.

Iris. Speckled iris, commonly referred to as "Brushfield's spots", was described in Down's syndrome by Thomas Brushfield (1924). It should be noted that, as early as 1908, Tredgold observed that speckled irides were very common in the syndrome, and Tredgold gave credit to R. Langdon Down for calling this observation to his attention. The spots are characterized by white, or lightly coloured, slightly elevated areas on the surface of the iris. They appear to be aggregates of stromal fibres which have become densely packed. The area between the spots appears to have less than the normal number of stromal fibres. The spots are usually

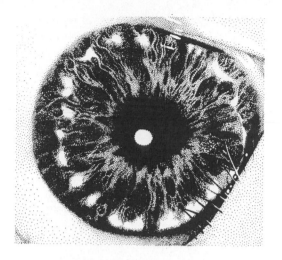

Fig. 6. Brushfield's spots: speckling and moderate hypoplasia of the iris periphery (after Donaldson 1961).

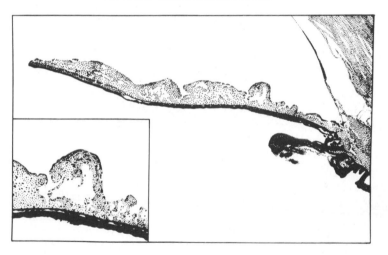

Fig. 7. Drawing of photomicrograph of a Down's syndrome iris sectioned through a Brushfield's spot (X 25). Note thinning of the peripheral iris stroma. Inset illustrates the spot at higher magnification (X 60). Note dense anterior border layer with local elevation of the iris (after Donaldson 1961).

arranged in a ring concentric with the pupil and are frequently located near the junction of the middle and outer third on the iris surface (see Fig. 6). On histological examination (see Fig. 7) the spots consist of well demarcated connective tissue condensations of the anterior stromal layer and are composed of normal iris elements (Purtscher 1958).

Speckled irides are very frequently present at birth in Down's syndrome (Wallis 1951, Purtscher) and are a useful diagnostic sign. They have to be carefully differentiated from similar spots which are seen in normal newborns. Some have considered that speckled irides are substantially less frequent in brown eyes (Solomons *et al.*). However, Donaldson (1961) found that the spots occurred with similar frequency in brown irides (77 per cent) as in blue ones (93 per cent). Because of the increased pigmentation in brown irides, the spots may be less obvious and may require magnification to be recognized. Donaldson pointed out that the spots in Down's syndrome are different from those found in normal individuals in that they are located closer to the pupillary margin and that they are more numerous and more distinct. He found speckling in 85 per cent of 180 cases of Down's syndrome compared to a 24 per cent incidence in the irides of normal controls (see Table 2). Rather lower, though not dissimilar, percentages were reported by Solomons *et al.*

Table 2. Comparison of Iris Speckling in Down's Syndrome and Controls. (After Donaldson 1961).

Description		Down's syndrome No.		Controls No.	
(a) Location of spots	Mid zone	49 ⎫		2 ⎫	
	Mixed	73 ⎬ (85%)		6 ⎬ (24%)	
	Peripheral	31 ⎭		30 ⎭	
	Absent	27	(15%)	119	(76%)
	Total	180		157	
(b) Distinctness of spots	Grade 5*	8	(4%)	0	
	Grade 4	41	(23%)	0	
	Grade 3	41	(23%)	8	(5%)
	Grade 2	46	(26%)	16	(10%)
	Grade 1	17	(9%)	14	(9%)
	Absent	27	(15%)	119	(76%)
	Total	180		157	
(c) Incidence of hypoplasia of iris		146	(81%)	14	(9%)

*Grade 5 = most distinct; Grade 1 = least distinct.

Lowe observed hypoplasia or thinning of the peripheral third of the iris, in addition to speckling, in Down's syndrome. He considered hypoplasia a more prominent feature than speckled iris. In his series hypoplasia was present at an early age and occurred in 95 per cent of patients. Speckling, which occurred in 90 per cent, was frequently associated with, but not dependent upon, iris hypoplasia. Hypoplasia of the peripheral portion of the iris to the same degree as in Down's syndrome is unusual in normal individuals (Lowe, Donaldson).

Table 3. Iris Colour in Down's Syndrome and Mentally Defective Controls.
(After Berg 1958)

Iris Shade	Brown	Blue	Total
Martin colour scale	1–8	9–16	
Down's syndrome	34	60	94
Controls	42	52	94
Total	76	112	188

Eye colour. Berg (1958) found that there was no statistical difference in the number of brown and blue eyed persons with Down's syndrome as compared with a control population (see Table 3). Solomons *et al.* observed also that eye colour distribution in the syndrome was essentially the same as in normal controls.

Lens. Pearce *et al.* (1910) and Ormond (1912) were among the first to describe in detail the lens opacities in Down's syndrome. Ormond reported on 42 cases of the syndrome and found that 59.5 per cent showed some lens opacity. Van der Scheer (1919b) noted lens opacities in 36 out of 60 Down's syndrome patients. In addition he found no lens opacities in patients below 8 years of age and thus he confirmed Ormond's observation of the absence of such opacities in young children with Down's syndrome. An indication of the distribution, by age, of lens opacities in the syndrome is provided in Table 4.

Table 4. Lenticular Changes in Down's Syndrome
(After Igersheimer 1951)

Age in years	No. of patients	Lenticular changes Present	Absent
1-5	7	0	7
6-10	35	8	27
11-15	34	21	13
16-20	21	20	1
21-30	19	19	0
31-40	9	9	0
Totals	125	77	48

Lowe noted that lens opacities in Down's syndrome could be placed in four main categories. In general, they can be classified as arcuate opacities, sutural opacities, flake opacities and congenital cataracts. Arcuate opacities are the earliest to develop, as they show plainly within the fetal nucleus. The simplest form is seen as a small white arc deep within the lens (see Fig 8b). Sutural opacities are seen with the Y sutures of the fetal nucleus (see Fig. 8a & c). Flake opacities are sharply localized in the

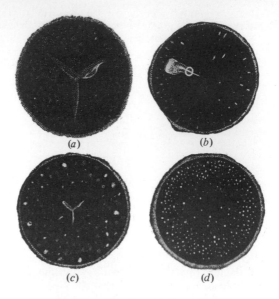

Fig. 8 Lens opacities found in Down's syndrome.

(a) Y-suture and small flakes;
(b) arcuate and flakes;
(c) Y-suture and large flakes;
(d) numerous flake opacities, near the periphery especially.

infantile and adult nuclei and they are rarely found near the lens surface (see Fig. 8d). Congenital cataracts may be directly associated with Down's syndrome or they may have independent causes. Lowe also noted the occasional presence in the syndrome of thick bilateral lamellar cataracts and typical posterior polar cataracts.

Arcuate opacities are specially characteristic of Down's syndrome. They are extremely rare in individuals who are normal or who have other diseases. The sutural and flake cataracts are much more common in Down's syndrome patients than arcuate opacities, but they are also commonly found in normal people and in those with other diseases. Congenital cataracts of the types seen in persons without Down's syndrome have been described in Down's syndrome infants (Jeremy 1921), but they are considered to be rare. Skeller & Øster (1951), however, found 6 cases of Down's syndrome with congenital cataracts among 32 with opacities of the lens. Engler found only 4 congenital cataracts in 300 Down's syndrome individuals, and cataracts were recorded at birth in only 6 of 2,421 children with Down's syndrome surveyed by Fabia & Drolette (1970b).

The frequency of lens opacities in the syndrome is considered high by all authors who have investigated the problem thoroughly (see Table 5). The different proportions with lens opacities reported can probably be partially explained by the different age groups of the patients investigated, and the methods used.

Table 5. Incidence of Lens Opacity in Down's Syndrome

Source	Number of patients	Number with lens opacity
Ormond (1912)	42	25
van der Scheer (1919b)	60	36
Lowe (1949)*	52	45
Igersheimer (1951)	125	77
Øster (1953)	69	32
Spitzer et al. (1961)	33	31

*Only evaluated for flake opacities.

Lowe investigated 52 Down's syndrome patients, 31 of whom were between 20 and 51 years of age, and Spitzer et al. (1961) investigated 33 patients, who were between the ages of 8 and 44 years, with a mean age of 26 years. The types of lens opacities found in these two studies can be seen in Table 6.

Table 6. Types of Lens Opacities found in Down's Syndrome

	No. of patients	Number with each type*		
		Arcuate	Sutural	Flake
Lowe (1949)	52	8	14	45
Spitzer et al. (1961)	33	10	20	28

*In some patients more than one type was found

Arcuate opacities, which are the earliest to develop and are in the region of the fetal nucleus, were found in 15 per cent of Down's syndrome patients by Lowe and in 31 per cent by Spitzer et al. Sutural opacities, which occur in the Y sutures of the fetal nucleus, were found in 27 per cent by Lowe. In all his cases, this type of opacity occurred in both eyes. Spitzer et al. had a much higher percentage (60 per cent) with this finding, and in all their cases the opacities were bilateral. In six eyes the sutural opacities occurred to an equal extent in the anterior and posterior Y sutures; in six eyes they were more marked in the anterior Y sutures and in eight eyes in the posterior Y sutures. Flake opacities, of which there are two types, blue smoky-grey minute flakes and white or light brown radial spokes, usually occur in the outer nuclear layers, and were found in 86 per cent of cases by Lowe. If he included only those over 14 years of age these opacities occurred in 92 per cent. Spitzer et al. had an equally high percentage (85 per cent) of patients with this type of opacity. Arcuate, sutural and flake opacities may all be found in the same lens.

Lowe thought that arcuate opacities are caused by an abnormal capsulopupillary vessel, during early fetal life, and are different from the other distinct cataracts found in Down's syndrome since they are probably opaque lens fibres and are not opacities between the fibres. The peculiar shapes of the sutural and flake cataracts are probably due to fluid and debris between the lens fibres. Occasionally, they are associated with metabolic and/or endocrine disturbances; however, a satisfactory explanation will have to wait until more is known about the biochemistry and physiology of the lens.

Interpupillary distance. The interpupillary distance is a useful diagnostic feature because it can be recorded as an exact measurement rather than a clinical impression. It is of significance mainly in hypertelorism and in Down's syndrome. Barr (1904) noted the proximity of the eyes in the syndrome and Brushfield (1924), on the basis of actual measurements, made the same observation. Lowe assumed the eyes of persons with Down's syndrome to be about 5 mm. closer together than those of normal adults, though this had to be considered in relation to the sizes of their heads and reduction of their measurements generally. Other observers have reported that the eyes are too far apart or were unable to find any difference from the normal.

Kerwood *et al.* (1954) resolved the problem of the interpupillary distance by correlating it with head width. On this basis it was shown that the interpupillary distance was reduced and that the ratio of interpupillary distance to head width was a useful clinical index (see Fig. 9). This ratio,

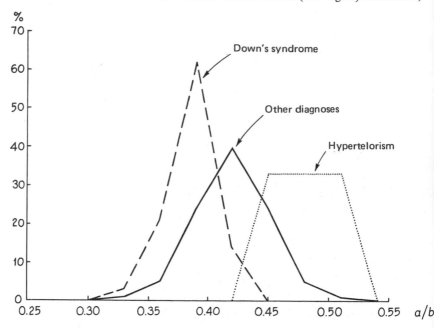

Fig. 9. Distributions of the ratio of interpupillary distance, *a*, to head breadth, *b*.

which was a normal value of 0.42 with a standard deviation of 0.02, is much increased in hypertelorism (0.48) and diminished in Down's syndrome (0.38). It has been suggested (Øster 1953) that exophthalmos is a frequent sign in Down's syndrome, but subsequent studies (Mosier & Dingman 1963) have not confirmed this observation.

Strabismus. Strabismus is common in Down's syndrome (Sutherland 1899, Ormond, Brushfield, Lowe, Cowie 1970, Hiles *et al.* 1974); it is usually convergent, though divergent strabismus has been reported. Opinions vary on its frequency. Part of the difficulty arises from superficial clinical observations because marked obliquity of the palpebral apertures and the epicanthal folds in Down's syndrome can mislead in evaluating strabismus. However, Lowe reported that, of 67 patients with the syndrome examined, 22 had constant strabismus. This is at least 20 times the incidence in the general population. If he included the inconstant squints and spontaneous or irregular convergences, then some form of noticeable ocular muscular anomaly was found in more than half of the patients. Cowie noted constant or variable strabismus more often in older than in younger Down's syndrome infants. It was present in 23 per cent of Down's syndrome babies under 14 weeks and in 36 per cent of the children above that age (see Table 7). The deviation was always found to

Table 7. Strabismus in Down's Syndrome Infants (After Cowie 1970)

Age in weeks	Strabismus + or ±		Total Observations
<14	21	70	91
16-45	34	63	97
Total	55	133	188

+ = Constant	± = Variable	− = Absent

be convergent. Lowe thought that, unlike many of the features of Down's syndrome, strabismus could be readily explained. In his opinion the inconstant and variable aberrations of convergence were due to insufficient harmonization of accommodation and convergence reflexes and to the patient's attempts to obtain clear images according to the demands of the frontal cortex. The most important causes of constant strabismus were uncorrected high myopia and lens opacities and these occurred in approximately one-third of cases of Down's syndrome. Strabismus from other causes is probably as frequent as in the general population. In approximately two-thirds of the cases strabismus corrects itself in later life (Benda 1960).

Nystagmus. Nystagmus has often been recorded in Down's syndrome (Sutherland 1899, Muir 1903, Ormond 1912, Lowe 1949). So-called pseudo-nystagmus in the syndrome has been attributed to strabismus, obliquity of the palpebral apertures, and lack of keen interest in the surroundings (Lowe). Pronounced nystagmus is probably most frequently related to ocular defect (lens opacity or myopia) but in rare cases the causes are within the central nervous system. In a large ophthalmological study on Down's syndrome, Eissler & Longenecker (1962) found nystagmus in 15 per cent.

Refraction. Visual acuity studies are difficult in Down's syndrome persons on account of their mental retardation. Uncorrected refractive errors have to be taken into consideration first. Lowe found that one-third of a small group of patients with Down's syndrome whom he studied had myopia and Gardiner (1967) noted myopia in half of his series, but Øster (1953) reported that myopia was comparatively rare. Hypermetropia is not infrequent. Regardless of which error is the commoner a reduction in visual acuity in Down's syndrome individuals is to be expected and, therefore, any such individual who is to receive special schooling should also have a full ophthalmological examination and be provided with spectacles where appropriate. Substantial impairment of dark adaptation in a small group of Down's syndrome patients was reported by Griffiths & Behrman (1967) and was thought to be possibly due to disordered Vitamin A metabolism. Colour vision in Down's syndrome is considered to be normal.

Obvious blindness in one or both eyes was found in 10 of 143 cases of Down's syndrome, aged 14 to 54 years, examined by Cullen (1963). It was usually secondary to complications associated with cataract formation and occurred mainly in patients over 30 years old. Keratoconus, which occurred in about 6 per cent of the patients (Cullen & Butler 1963), was also a cause of blindness. Woillez & Dansaut (1960) also noted a relatively high incidence of keratoconus in Down's syndrome. According to Falls (1970), acute keratoconus and/or acute hydrops of the cornea is more frequent in Down's syndrome than in any other known disorder. He suggested that keratoconus may reflect a connective tissue disturbance and superimposed constant rubbing trauma by the patient.

Retinal vessels. Williams *et al.* (1973) found significantly more retinal vessels crossing the margin of the optic nerve head in Down's syndrome patients than in controls. They considered this, combined with an unusual spoke-like appearance of the retinal vasculature, as a helpful sign in the clinical diagnosis of the syndrome.

Eyelids. The eyelids, as such, are not particularly unusual in Down's syndrome. However, Falls noted that the highest point in the arch of the upper eyelid margin occurs in the centre of the lid, whereas in the normal eyelid it is at the junction of the inner and middle third. Total eversion of the upper eyelids, which is a rare event in the newborn child, seems to occur with increased frequency in Down's syndrome (Gilbert *et al.* 1973, Stern *et al.* 1973). The mechanism of the congenital eversion is uncertain, but pressure from overdeveloped epicanthic folds, absence of effective lateral canthal ligaments, eyelid laxity consequent on hypotonia and oedema of the conjunctival tissues are among explanations which have been suggested.

EARS

Ear anomalies have been frequently described (Bourneville 1903a, Brousseau & Brainerd, Levinson *et al.* 1955, Benda 1960, Beckman *et al.* 1962); however, there has been a marked difference of opinion regarding the types of anomalies which are most characteristic and the frequencies with which they occur. It is of interest that anomalies of the ear are noted in many other conditions associated with abnormal physical development.

Part of the difficulty which arises when discussing anomalies of the ear comes from complexity of its structure (see Fig. 10). Nearly all the deformities that have been described show great variation in expression;

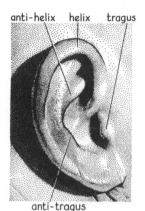

anti-helix   helix   tragus

anti-tragus

Fig. 10. Normal ear.

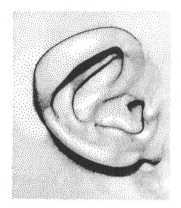

Fig. 11. Angular overlapping helix and small ear lobe in Down's syndrome.

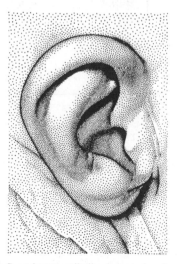

Fig. 12. Prominent antihelix and overlapping helix.

they grade into one another and the natural margin between what is normal and what is abnormal is uncertain. Another difficulty is the relative lack of quantitative measurements. For example, many authors describe the ear in Down's syndrome as being "small," while some mention that occasionally it is "large." However, some direct measurements have been made. Betlejewski *et al.* (1966), Thelander & Pryor (1966) and Aase *et al.* (1973) found substantial reduction in ear length (i.e. longitudinal dimension of the pinna) in Down's syndrome persons of various ages compared to controls. Reduction in ear breadth has also been noted in Down's syndrome (Betlejewski *et al.*, Thelander & Pryor) though considerable variation occurs in individual instances. In Betlejewski *et al.*'s series of 100 Down's syndrome children and 200 normal children, the length of the ear lobule also was measured and no significant difference between the two groups was found. Wallis (1955) drew attention to smallness of the external auditory meatus in Down's syndrome infants.

In spite of shortcomings, some useful information about ear deformities in Down's syndrome is available. Possibly one of the most characteristic findings is the angular overlapping helix (see Fig. 11). The usefulness of this finding has been pointed out by several investigators. Beckman *et al.* found that folded ears of this sort occur very often in Down's syndrome as compared with patients with mental defect of unknown aetiology or normal individuals (see Table 8). A prominent antihelix seems to be a

Table 8. Incidence of Folded Helix
(After Beckman *et al.* 1962)

Sample	Present Bilaterally	Present Unilaterally Right	Present Unilaterally Left	Absent	Total
Down's syndrome males	13	1	5	40	59
Down's syndrome females	22	3	3	27	55
Male adults ⎫	0	1	1	98	100
Female adults ⎬ controls	3	3	0	94	100
Children ⎭	1	0	1	98	100

common finding (see Fig. 12). Another deformity which has been observed often in Down's syndrome is a small or absent ear lobe (Brousseau & Brainerd). This does seem to occur with unusual frequency in the syndrome (Beckman *et al.*). It should be noted that normal females have a higher frequency of attached lobes than normal males; however, this sex difference seems to be accentuated in Down's syndrome.

Prominent or projecting ears are said to be frequent in the syndrome, but, here again, the finding is to a large extent based on arbitrary definition. It has been suggested that the location of the ears varies (Brousseau & Brainerd, Benda 1960), but Øster (1953) refuted this. Other deformities of the ear have been described such as "lop ears" and "funnel-shaped ears", but these seem to be rare. Significant bilateral differences between the ears are extremely rare also.

Hearing loss in Down's syndrome has been reported from time to time (Rigrodsky *et al.* 1961, Glovsky 1966, Fulton & Lloyd 1968, Brooks *et al.* 1972) with considerable variation in findings on the type and frequency of loss. Brooks *et al.* found a higher incidence of conductive, mixed and sensorineural hearing losses in Down's syndrome patients compared to controls with other varieties of mental retardation. The frequency for each of these types of hearing loss was about double that observed by Fulton & Lloyd. Conductive hearing loss was the commonest type and this was thought by Brooks *et al.* to be due primarily to exudative otitis media.

NECK

The neck tends to be short and broad. According to Forssman (1965) the posterior aspect of the neck and sloping shoulders is exceedingly characteristic. The impression, that of a "Raglan" style tunic, is unmistakable. The appearance is exaggerated by the flat occiput. In young infants there may be looseness of the skin over the neck and shoulders. The hair line reaches further down the back of the neck than is usual in normals. Webbing of the neck occurs in Down's syndrome, but it is rare.

HEART

Garrod (1894, 1898, 1899) was the first observer to recognize clearly a definite association between cardiac anomalies and Down's syndrome. By the turn of the century this association was sufficiently well established for Sutherland (1900) to be able to list the frequency of congenital cardiac defects in Down's syndrome as one of the features differentiating the syndrome from cretinism. Since then there has been a marked difference of opinion concerning the incidence of congenital heart disease in the syndrome. Incidence figures have varied from 7.1 to 70.8 per cent (most reports give between 12 and 44 per cent with an average of 19 per cent) (Berg *et al.* 1960). Some of the reasons for the wide range, listed by the various authors, are given by Rowe & Uchida (1961). First, early evaluations were limited to clinical examination before present-day diagnostic techniques were available. Secondly, in many series, only older children and adults with Down's syndrome were examined, and a high percentage of Down's syndrome patients with congenital cardiac anomalies die during the first year of life. Thirdly, autopsy studies may give a spuriously high frequency since, in general, Down's syndrome individuals with congenital heart anomalies are more likely to be in hospitals than those without them. Fourthly, clinical studies on institutional or hospital cases also involve samples not necessarily representative of those in the general population. The incidence of congenital cardiac anomalies might vary in samples from different countries, as some reports suggest.

There is fair agreement on the incidence of cardiac anomalies in Down's syndrome in recent studies. From clinical and autopsy observations Benda (1960) estimated that cardiac anomalies occurred in 60 per cent of all cases. On autopsy studies alone Berg *et al.* found 79 with cardiac anomalies out of 141 individuals with Down's syndrome (56 per cent). Another pathological survey of 55 cases of Down's syndrome with congenital heart disease (Tandon & Edwards 1973) showed a similar variety of malformations to that in Berg *et al.*'s study, although there were some differences in the relative frequency of particular defects, perhaps because of differences in the age distribution of the two series. Rowe & Uchida studied the problem in an out-patient clinic using advanced diagnostic techniques, including angiocardiography. They followed 184 Down's syndrome patients and found 104 with no evidence of cardiac anomalies, 70 (40 per cent) with cardiac anomalies (Table 9) and 10 in

Table 9. Cardiac Malformation Types found in 70 Down's Syndrome Patients
(Rowe & Uchida 1961)

Defects		No.	%
Atrioventricular canal defects:			
Atrioventricularis communis	22 ⎫	25	36
Ostium primum	3 ⎭		
Ventricular septal defect		23	33
Patent ductus arteriosus		7	10
Secundum atrial septal defect		6	9
Isolated aberrant subclavian artery		5	7
Tetralogy of Fallot		1	1
Simple pulmonary stenosis		1	1
Equivocal type		2	3
	Totals	70	100

whom the diagnosis was uncertain. A rather similar investigation, by Matsuo *et al.* (1972), of 106 Japanese children with Down's syndrome, ranging in age from 2 days to 5 years, revealed that 55 per cent had major congenital cardiac defects. So far, all these studies have contained some element of bias and, therefore, the true incidence figure is unknown but probably somewhere between 40 and 60 per cent.

There is, however, general agreement that there is a high mortality in Down's syndrome infants with cardiac anomalies. Esen (1957) reported that 9 out of 12 affected infants with such anomalies died within the first two years of life, but only 3 out of 19 without cardiac anomalies died during the same period. Evans (1950) found that a preponderance of cardiac cases died between the second and fifth months. The high mortality of Down's syndrome individuals with cardiac anomalies during the first year of life was demonstrated in the case material of Berg *et al.* They found that, from 2 to 11 months, 44 per cent (35 of 79) of cases with such anomalies died. In the same age group only 25.8 per cent (16 of 62) without cardiac anomalies died (see Table 10). These findings agree

Table 10. Age at Death of 141 Cases of Down's Syndrome with and without Congenital Heart Defects. (After Berg *et al.* 1960)

Period during which death occurred	With C.H.D.*		Without C.H.D.†	
Stillborn	2	(2.5)	2	(3.2)
1st 24 hours	6	(7.6)	3	(4.8)
2nd–7th day	7	(8.9)	2	(3.2)
8th–31st day	6	(7.6)	4	(6.5)
2nd–11th month	35	(44.3)	16	(25.8)
2nd year	8	(10.1)	6	(9.7)
3rd year	8	(10.1)	5	(8.1)
4th–10th year	5	(6.3)	22	(35.5)
11th–27th year	2	(2.5)	2	(3.2)
Totals	79	(99.9)	62	(100.0)

*Percentage of total with C.H.D. (79) in brackets.
†Percentage of total without C.H.D. (62) in brackets.

with those of Rowe & Uchida who studied the age at death of 53 patients with Down's syndrome of whom 32 had cardiac anomalies, 1 had some other form of heart disease and 20 had normal hearts. More recently, life tables of Down's syndrome children for the first 10 years of life, constructed by Fabia & Drolette (1970a), showed a much higher mortality among those with congenital heart defects than among those without such defects (see p. 242).

Just as there had been a marked difference of opinion concerning the incidence of congenital heart anomalies in Down's syndrome, so too, there had been no agreement about the frequencies of the particular types of cardiac lesions found. Abbott (1924, 1936) drew attention to the persistent ostium primum and persistent ostium atrioventricularis communis as cardiac anomalies characteristic of Down's syndrome. Ventricular septal defect is a frequent cardiac malformation in the syndrome (Keith *et al.* 1958, Liu & Corlett 1959, Berg *et al.,* Rowe & Uchida, Cullum & Liebman 1969) but it is not as characteristic as atrioventricularis communis (Rowe & Uchida). Rosenquist *et al.* (1974) examined 14 heart specimens from patients with Down's syndrome in whom neither ventricular septal defect nor atrioventricular valve abnormalities were present. They found significant enlargement of the membranous ventricular septum as compared to that in hearts of normal individuals. They considered that this might predispose Down's syndrome patients to congenital heart disease.

In a pathological survey of 79 persons with Down's syndrome and 300 controls, all of whom had congenital heart disease, Berg *et al.* demonstrated that ventricular septal defect, alone or in combination with other cardiac defect, was the most common abnormality in both the Down's syndrome and control patients. Moreover, atrioventricularis communis, persistent ostium secundum and anomalies of the mitral and triscuspid valves were more frequent in the Down's syndrome than in the control sample. Among other types, Fallot's tetralogy, Eisenmenger's complex, transposition of the great vessels, coarctation of the aorta and anomalies of the aortic and pulmonary valves were more frequent in the control population. Patent ductus arteriosus was almost as common in Down's syndrome as in controls.

Strauss (1953) noted an increased incidence of isolated aberrant subclavian artery in Down's syndrome, and this finding has been confirmed by others (Rowe & Uchida, Liu & Corlett). It is estimated that the malformation occurs in 1.3 per cent of normal (Anson 1959) and 5.6 per cent of Down's syndrome individuals (Rowe & Uchida). Benda (1960) has stressed the general infantilism of the vascular system; the aorta is thin and narrow and all the main vessels are undersized.

The serious implications of cardiac anomalies in Down's syndrome are emphasized by the high death rate in infancy. Modern cardiac surgery undoubtedly could save some of these infants; however, because of their poor general physical condition, one would not expect the results to be as successful as in normal infants. Using modern investigative techniques,

Table 11. Other Congenital Malformations in 79 Down's Syndrome Cases with, and 62 without, Congenital Heart Defects (C.H.D.) (Berg *et al.* 1960).

Non-cardiac malformations	79 cases with C.H.D.	62 cases without C.H.D.
Cleft palate and/or harelip	1	4
Duodenal stenosis or atresia	5	5
Stenosis of common bile duct	–	1
Partial agenesis of pancreas	1	–
Kidney agenesis or hypoplasia	2	2
Hypoplastic adrenal; dislocated hip	1	–
Meningocoele; horseshoe kidney	–	1
Hydrocephalus; hydrocoele vaginalis	–	1
Absent corpus callosum; absent radius and thumb	1	–
Syndactyly; polydactyly	1	2
Webbed neck	–	1
Diaphragmatic hernia	1	–
Excessive pulmonary lobation	1	–
Malformed costal cartilages	1	–
Talipes equino-varus	2	–
Total	17	17

including cardiac catheterization and angiocardiography, Shaher *et al.* (1972) reviewed the clinical course and haemodynamic features of 39 Down's syndrome children with congenital heart disease. Infants with the syndrome, free from significant cardiac anomalies, and those with cardiac anomalies, both have the highest death rate in the first month of life. The high death rate continues for those infants with cardiac anomalies but, after the first year and a half, Down's syndrome individuals with cardiac anomalies and those with normal hearts again have about the same death rate (Rowe & Uchida). Associated congenital malformations seem to be no more frequent in Down's syndrome persons with cardiac anomalies than in those with normal hearts (see Table 11), although this has not been the case in all reported studies (Fabia & Drolette 1970b). A slight increase in the mean maternal age of mothers of Down's syndrome children with cardiac anomalies as compared with others was noted in the series of Rowe & Uchida; however, Liu & Corlett and Fabia & Drolette did not find this age difference in their respective series of cases. Down's syndrome individuals with cardiac anomalies have been reported to weigh more at birth than those with normal hearts (Liu & Corlett); a tendency in the opposite direction was observed by Fabia & Drolette.

It is of interest that two other trisomic conditions (17–18, 13–15) also have a high incidence of cardiac anomalies. In both these conditions, ventricular septal defects and patent ductus arteriosus appear to be particularly common (Warkany *et al.* 1966).

LUNGS

The observation has often been made that persons with Down's syndrome are prone to develop respiratory tract, including pulmonary, infections. Such infections are a frequent cause of death (see Table 105). However, malformations of the lung appear to be uncommon. Abnormal pulmonary lobation, hypoplasia of the lungs and other such defects are occasionally reported and diaphragmatic hernia sometimes contributes to respiratory difficulties. There is no evidence of a particular connection of any of these anomalies with Down's syndrome. On rare occasions (Milunsky 1968, Vertrella *et al.* 1969), respiratory problems in a Down's syndrome child have been found to be connected with the presence of cystic fibrosis.

ABDOMEN

The abdomen in Down's syndrome tends to be prominent, especially in children. This is probably related to the hypotonia of the abdominal muscles which allows distension. Umbilical hernia was reported in approximately 12 per cent of cases of the syndrome (Øster 1953) and is much more frequent in children than in adults. Diastasis recti was observed in approximately 11 per cent of patients (Øster); this is most likely to be found in the age group 0–4 years. Levinson *et al.* (1955), however, reported a very much higher incidence (76 per cent) of diastasis recti.

Abnormalities of the intestine occur in Down's syndrome which can affect the shape of the abdomen. Microcolon, megacolon, duodenal bands, ileal and jejunal atresia, malrotation of the bowel, oesophageal and pyloric stenosis, and malformations of the rectum and anus have all been reported. An association of Hirschsprung's disease with Down's syndrome has been noted on a number of occasions (Vacher *et al.* 1956, Wolf & Zweymüller 1962, Bodian & Carter 1963, Emanuel *et al.* 1965, Graivier & Sieber 1966, Kilcoyne & Taybi 1970), and several authors have suggested that this association is not fortuitous.

The relative frequency of congenital duodenal obstruction in Down's syndrome was recognized some years ago by Lanman (1949), Grove & Rasmussen (1950) and Bodian *et al.* (1952). Bodian *et al.* described 10 cases. In rare instances, manifestations are first noted in early adulthood, as in the 18 and 19 year old patients described by Gross (1959) and by Chandler & Gay (1967) respectively. Louw (1952) observed that the association with Down's syndrome was particularly frequent when the obstruction in the duodenum was situated at or above the biliary papilla. In an Australian series of 70 children with duodenal obstruction admitted to hospital, 14(20 per cent) had Down's syndrome (Nelson 1963). A more extensive United States survey of 503 patients with congenital duodenal obstruction revealed that 150 of them (30 per cent) had Down's syndrome (Fonkalsrud *et al.* 1969). The occurrence of duodenal obstruction was ascertained in 63 out of 2,421 Down's syndrome children (2.6 per cent) surveyed by Fabia & Drolette (1970b). They estimated that the risk of duodenal obstruction in Down's syndrome was more than 300 times that in other persons. Annular pancreas may be relatively frequently associated with duodenal obstruction in Down's syndrome (Salzer *et al.* 1961, Hyatt 1962, Milunsky & Fisher 1968). Of the 63 Down's syndrome patients with duodenal obstruction in Fabia & Drolette's series, 15 had annular pancreas.

SKIN AND HAIR

A large number of skin abnormalities have been reported but these all occur in the general population also; a few of them seem to occur especially frequently in Down's syndrome.

The integument appears to be too large for the skeleton. This may be most noticeable at the wrists and ankles in adults and at the back of the neck and shoulders in newly born babies. The skin is usually soft in infants; however, it may be thick, dry and rough, particularly when there are other signs of hypothyroidism. The cheeks often show circumscribed areas of redness. Marmoration, localized to the distal parts of the extremities, occurs in approximately 43 per cent of cases of Down's syndrome (Øster 1953). Acrocyanosis is also a frequent finding (Zeligman & Scalia 1954). Vitiligo is sometimes noted.

Kersting & Rapaport (1958) described localized chronic hyperkeratotic lichenification in 75 per cent of their cases. The most frequent site was the dorsum of the upper arm, including the elbow; other areas were the anterior surfaces of the thighs, the ankles, the wrists, the back of the neck and the knuckles. The lesions consisted of well defined plaques of thickened, corrugated, lichenified, slightly reddened skin covered with a firm grey scale. Xerosis (xeroderma or asteatosis) was another skin disorder which occurred in 90 per cent of the Down's syndrome patients they examined. These patients had dry skin, with abnormality varying in degree from slight asteatosis to severe dryness with a fine brittle scale. Elastosis perforans serpiginosa, a dermatological condition in which localized or disseminated hyperkeratotic papules develop, has been reported in a number of Down's syndrome patients (Mehregan 1968, Rasmussen 1972), though it is not clear whether the incidence of the condition is increased in such patients. Localized eczema and lichen simplex chronicus was found to be associated with Ehlers-Danlos syndrome in Down's syndrome patients (Schachter 1947). Allergic conditions involving the skin and other tissues occur in Down's syndrome (Casa 1961, Coghlan & Evans 1964, Romanski & Walczynski 1966, Weiss & Grolnick 1967) but there is no good evidence that the incidence or manifestations are unusual.

Reference may be made here to so-called "mongolian spots". These are gradually disappearing, irregular areas of bluish pigmentation often noted in infants, usually dark-skinned ones, in the lumbo-sacral region and elsewhere (Frier 1962, Wallis 1954, 1962, Wood 1962, Brouwer 1962). Despite the rather unfortunate nomenclature, they have no particular connection with Down's syndrome.

The hair is generally considered to be fine and soft; however, curly or wavy hair is also seen. All shades and colours have been reported (Øster 1953). Europeans with Down's syndrome supposedly lack pigmentation of the hair (Benda 1960). However, dark hair is common, particularly as age increases (Smith *et al.* 1963). Spencer (1973) noted a distinctive white lock of hair over the occiput in 3 out of 45 women with Down's syndrome whose head hair was otherwise black or brown. Kiil (1948) reported differences in frontal hair direction in Down's syndrome individuals compared to controls. In particular, he observed an absence of upwardly directed hair streams (type III) in the Down's syndrome cases which he thought might be due to growth retardation in the region of the head. Partial or total alopecia of the head hair is occasionally noted in Down's syndrome (Wunderlich & Braun-Falco 1965).

SECONDARY SEX CHARACTERISTICS

Males. In Down's syndrome male infants, the penis and scrotum appear poorly developed. In pubertal and adult males these organs are also considered small. A few cases have been reported where the penis was enlarged and this has been noticed in patients after prolonged treatment with testicular hormone. Benda (1960) reported that, in about 50 per cent of cases, the testes are not descended at birth and that, in these cases, they do not descend. This is a higher figure than reported by Øster (1953) who found cryptorchidism in 27 per cent of patients in the age groups 0 to 9 years and 14 per cent of those over 15 years of age. Rundle & Sylvester (1962) measured testicular size in 35 adults with Down's syndrome and found it to be significantly reduced in comparison with control groups of other types of mentally retarded males. Adult males tend to have increased subcutaneous fatty tissue in the breast areas and round the abdomen. The pubic hair is invariably straight (Forssman 1965) and silky, and axillary hair is scanty. The beard tends to be slight and thinly distributed. Libido is much diminished. Reduced sperm counts in semen have been reported in adult patients (Stearns *et al.* 1960) and there is no proven case of a fully affected individual with Down's syndrome fathering a child. On a few occasions, precocious sexual development has been noted in both males and females with Down's syndrome and this may be associated with hypothyroidism (Pabst *et al.* 1967).

Females. Bleyer (1937) pointed out that the labia majora are frequently over-sized and rounded in Down's syndrome females. In adult females, the labia minora are frequently enlarged and protruding. The clitoris also tends to be enlarged, but Engler found hypoplasia to be more common. On the basis of autopsy reports, the ovaries and uterus are considered to be small in adults. The secondary sexual characteristics are usually late in appearing and also poorly manifested. Smith *et al.* (1963) noted a retarded rate of development of axillary hair and a tendency to lose this hair at a relatively early age. In post-pubertal females with Down's syndrome, as well as in females with other forms of mental retardation, absence of axillary hair was found by Shelley & Butterworth (1955) to be associated with underdevelopment or absence of axillary apocrine glands. As in males, the pubic hair is invariably straight (Forssman). Engler reported that the onset of menstruation was at the normal age; Øster (1953) found the mean age of onset to be 13 years 9 months in Danish girls with Down's syndrome. In this group the youngest was 11 years old and the oldest was aged 20 years. The control mean for the menarche in Denmark was given as 14 years 9 months. However, van Gelderen & Dooren (1963) found, in their study of mentally retarded females, that menstruation was often absent in girls who showed physical signs of maturation. In their experience it was not unusual to find that mentally retarded girls, who had been menstruating normally at home, showed amenorrhoea after having been admitted to an institution. In an investigation of 13 women with Down's syndrome residing in an institution (Tricomi *et al.* 1964), repeated vaginal smear examinations showed evidence of ovulation to be definite in 5, probable or possible in another 4 and absent in the remaining 4 patients.

During puberty the breasts remain small, but in adults they may be enlarged and contain excessive subcutaneous fat and reduced glandular tissue. The areola is indistinct and the nipple small.

ENDOCRINE GLANDS

Although clinicians often tend to diagnose thyroid or pituitary dysfunction in Down's syndrome, there is little evidence of morphological abnormality in the endocrine glands apart from that reported by Benda (1946). Biochemical studies on thyroid activity are described in Chapter 7. Degenerative changes were observed by Bourneville (1903b) and some degree of colloid goitre was found by Benda to be associated with hypoplasia. Assessment of such findings is often difficult because of lack of control material. Only 4 definite instances of primary hypothyroidism, and only 15 of hyperthyroidism, in patients with Down's syndrome, were found in the literature by Hayles *et al.* (1965) who reported another example of each. Unlike the experience of Øster, who found no instances of thyroid gland enlargement in 526 cases of Down's syndrome, Ruvalcala *et al.* (1969) noted 5 cases of goitre among 307 Down's syndrome patients compared with none in a control group of 327 patients from the same institution.

The pituitary gland is also considered to be underdeveloped in Down's syndrome by Benda and to lack sufficient secretory cells. The adrenals are also abnormal according to Hirning & Farber (1934). This view is supported by Benda who found hypoplasia of the cortex and medulla with hypertrophy of the boundary zone. The thymus gland in Down's syndrome infants, though its lymphoid tissue appears normal, contains, according to Benda & Strassmann (1965), abnormally large Hassal corpuscles.

3. Bones and Muscles

As shown in Chapter 2, a distinctive feature of Down's syndrome is the widespread involvement of many tissues and organs resulting in significant alterations in morphology and in function. The bones and muscles are no exception and an account of them is provided in this chapter.

OSSEOUS DEVELOPMENT

Although it is agreed that a generalized disturbance of growth is characteristic of Down's syndrome, there is a divergence of opinion as to whether or not osseous development is delayed. Kassowitz (1902) could not demonstrate any delay. However, some authors reported normal development usually but noted delay in some patients (Siegert 1910, Hefke 1940, Dutton 1959a, Engler 1949, Øster 1953). Predominance of developmental delay has been noted by Bullard (1911), Clift (1922), Brousseau & Brainerd (1928), Menghi (1954), Benda (1960), Pozsonyi *et al.* (1964), Rarick *et al.* (1964) and by Roche (1964). Certain cases with advanced development have also been mentioned (Bullard, Siegert, Hefke, Benda, Pozsonyi *et al.*). Considerable differences among Down's syndrome individuals in skeletal maturation rates (Roche) probably account for some of the apparent discrepancies which have been reported. It seems likely also, as Rundle *et al.* (1972) suggested, that another reason for such discrepancies is the various age groups studied in view of a variable rate of skeletal development at different ages in the syndrome.

Hefke examined the hands and wrists roentgenologically and reported that the osseous development in 57 (49 per cent) of 72 Down's syndrome children up to 15 years of age was normal. There was a slight advance in 10 cases (14 per cent) and a slight delay in 5 (7 per cent). Among 87 affected persons studied radiographically for the development of ossification centres, Øster found 66 normal, 19 delayed and 2 advanced. Dutton, using what he called a "skeletal quotient", found that, although stature was markedly reduced, skeletal development was essentially normal. Benda, however, reported that the appearance of the ossification centres was irregular and frequently retarded. In some cases he observed that the capitate and hamate bones were present at 2 or 3 months after birth and that, after the first three centres had appeared, new centres were usually delayed until the age of 4 or 5 years. He reported that, at 4 to 5 years of age, many children with Down's syndrome had a bone age of 6 to 12 months. Currarino & Swanson (1964) noted two ossification centres, instead of one, in the manubrium sterni more frequently in Down's syndrome children under 5 years (27 out of 30) than in a control group (20 out of 100), and suggested this as a useful diagnostic sign in doubtful cases of the syndrome. Similar findings were reported by Horns & O'Loughlin (1965).

Pozsonyi et al. studied the skeletal maturation of 100 Down's syndrome patients between the ages of 2 weeks and 15 years. They found that delayed skeletal maturation was present until about 8 years of age; after this it assumed, on the average, a position in advance of normal. The acceleration of osseous development continued until termination of bone growth at the early age of 15 years. Correlation studies failed to show any relationship between the skeletal maturation rate and birth weight, neonatal illnesses, nutritional status, sex or intelligence level. The work of these authors suggests that, in Down's syndrome, there is an endogenous early ageing process. Evaluation of this idea is difficult since Rarick et al. had somewhat different findings. They reported that, in the age group 12 to 14 years, the bone maturation was a little over one year behind that of normal controls. They studied 64 persons with Down's syndrome for a period of 4 years and X-rays of the hands and wrists of each subject were obtained annually. It was found that the mean skeletal age between 7 and 9 years was approximately 3 years retarded and that this skeletal retardation had decreased by the time the age 12 to 14 years had been attained. One patient in six reached the mean skeletal age of normal children and such patients, then, were fairly close to puberty. The authors concluded that the onset of puberty and skeletal maturation tend to occur simultaneously in Down's syndrome as in normal children. In a subsequent report, Rarick et al. (1966) provided details of tibial length measured from radiographs taken annually, over an 8 year period, in 68 Down's syndrome children of both sexes. These children ranged in age, at the beginning of the study, from 6 to 12 years. Although, at 7 years, both the boys and girls were about 4 years behind normal children in tibial length, their annual incremental gains were within normal limits. Epiphyseal closure tended to occur late, though the period between onset and completion of fusion was substantially less than in normal children. The data indicated that the time of onset of epiphyseal fusion was closely related to the time when evidence of puberty became apparent in both Down's syndrome and normal children, thus strengthening the conclusion of the authors in their earlier study.

Osseous abnormalities may occasionally be found because of the presence of coincidental pathology as, for example, in the rare event of the same child having both Down's syndrome and achondroplasia (Sommer & Eaton 1970).

CRANIUM

The outstanding clinical feature of the head in Down's syndrome is brachycephaly (Mitchell 1876). There is shortening of the anteroposterior diameter and also flattening of the occiput, especially noticeable in a profile view, and the occipital proturberance is reduced or absent (see Fig. 13). The biparietal diameter (width) is only slightly reduced as compared

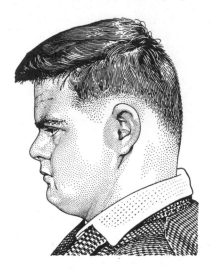

Fig. 13. Flat occiput in Down's syndrome.

Table 12. Mean Head Measurements (in millimetres) in Groups of Adult Males. (Penrose 1963b).

	Cephalic Breadth (i)	Length (ii)	Height (iii)	Cephalic index (i)/(ii)
11 Down's syndrome patients	142.5	174.6	125.7	0.82
5 Acrocephalics	153.4	180.8	136.6	0.85
10 Microcephalics	131.6	180.8	115.5	0.73
All types of defectives of comparable grades	146.9	188.3	131.2	0.78
General hospital population (Goring 1913)	149.3	190.4	132.9	0.78
Australian control population (Berry & Porteus 1920)	152.5	193.7	134.6	0.78

with the normal (see Table 12). The cephalic index (width/length) is correspondingly increased; normally the cephalic index lies between 0.75 and 0.80, but in Down's syndrome it is usually 0.80 or over and, in rare instances, it exceeds 1.00 (Engler 1949, Roche *et al.* 1961b). Cranial capacity of the head also is reduced as compared with the normal and Down's syndrome individuals are occasionally referred to as being microcephalic; however, this designation is not universally accepted. Brousseau & Brainerd (1928) pointed out that, in the syndrome, the forehead is prominent and normally shaped and the cranial vault globular; whereas in true microcephaly the head is long and the vault is flattened. Other abnormalities in the shape of the head have been occasionally reported, including brachyoxycephaly (Engler), hydrocephaly (Desgeorges 1905), dolichocephaly (Garrod & Langmead 1906) and trigonocephaly (De Myer & Palmer 1965).

Many explanations have been put forward to account for the shape of the head in Down's syndrome but none is adequate. It was even held, at one time, that the anteroposterior shortening at the base of the skull was the primary error. Sutherland (1899), however, found no evidence for premature ossification and, therefore, concluded that imperfect development of the basal parts of the encephalon led to deficient expansion of the base of the skull. Howells (1957) has pointed out some of the complex factors that affect the size and shape of the cranial vault. Martin & Saller (1958) showed that, in normal adults, the maximal head length is positively correlated with body length and proposed that the short stature of persons with Down's syndrome might partly explain their low maximal head length. Brothwell (1960), in his report of finding an eighth or ninth century Saxon skull, which he considered to be that of an individual with Down's syndrome, drew attention to the difficulties of making a diagnosis of the syndrome when only the skull is measured.

The general thinness of the skull bones, seen in X-ray photographs, has been confirmed by pathological examinations (Greig 1927, Lowe 1949, Roche & Sunderland 1960). This has been attributed by some to an absence of diploë formation of the flat bones, though Roche & Sunderland found that the proportion of diploë present appeared to be normal.

In infants with Down's syndrome the fontanelles may be large and the sutures broad. The frontal suture may extend far down towards the glabella (Øster 1953). A wide separation may be present at the vertex. Delayed closing of the fontanelles (Kassowitz 1902, Hellmann 1909, Øster, Roche & Sunderland) may be found in children. Øster reported that the anterior fontanelle was still open in 25 out of 77 Down's syndrome children in the age groups 2 years to 4 years 11 months. At ages over 3 years the frequency of a closed fontanelle began to increase but, even in the age group 5 years and over, the fontanelle was open in 5 instances. In infants a third fontanelle, a depression caused by absence of bone, may be found along the sagittal suture (Hoyle & Franklin 1954).

In the newly born infant, the head measurements are within normal range except for rare cases (Benda 1960, Roche et al. 1961a), and flattening of the occiput may not be obvious. Hall (1964), however, found that the head circumference and length were significantly smaller in Down's syndrome infants than normal newly born controls (see Table 13). Persistence of a relatively small head circumference was noted in a follow-up study (Hall 1966). The head width remains nearly normal, until

Table 13. Mean Head Measurements (in millimetres) of Newly Born Down's Syndrome Infants and Controls. (After Hall 1964)

Measurement	Down's syndrome	Controls
Circumference	330	338
Length	108	115
Width	91	92

about 1 year of age, after which it increases slowly as compared with controls; the length, however, grows even more slowly until, at 5 years of age, it is on the average 3–4 S.D. below normal (Roche *et al.* 1961a) (see Fig. 14 and Table 14).

Table 14. Head Measurements in Down's Syndrome Males and Females. (After Roche *et al.* 1961a)

Chronological Age (yr.)	Males Number	Head Width (cm.)	Head Length (cm.)	Chronological Age (yr.)	Females Number	Head Width (cm.)	Head Length (cm.)
0.1	2	9.9	12.2	0.1	2	9.8	11.9
0.5	3	11.2	12.8	0.3	2	10.8	12.1
0.7	6	11.8	13.0	0.5	3	10.9	12.2
1.3	4	12.5	14.2	0.7	4	11.7	13.2
2.6	9	12.8	14.8	1.1	3	11.9	14.1
3.0	3	12.7	14.8	1.5	8	12.2	13.9
3.4	3	13.2	14.3	2.0	3	12.0	14.2
3.8	2	12.4	15.8	2.4	2	12.2	14.5
4.7	1	13.2	14.6	3.5	2	12.4	14.0
5.3	6	13.6	15.7	5.3	5	13.3	15.7
6.7	5	13.4	15.9	7.0	2	13.3	15.6
8.7	2	14.0	16.2	8.4	2	13.3	15.9
9.5	1	14.4	16.2	9.3	2	13.0	16.8
11.4	1	14.6	16.5	10.1	1	15.8	15.6
13.5	2	14.3	16.6	11.5	5	13.4	16.1
14.6	3	14.6	16.6	12.6	5	13.6	16.2
15.8	2	14.0	16.3	13.6	4	13.3	16.1
16.6	1	14.6	16.4	14.2	6	13.8	16.5
17.4	2	14.4	17.4	15.3	1	14.6	16.5
				16.1	1	13.9	16.9
				17.5	3	13.9	16.4

The earliest anatomical description of a skull from a person with Down's syndrome was given by Fraser (1876) but Greig (1927) made one of the most comprehensive studies. He gave average measurements of three Down's syndrome skulls and compared them with the average measurements of three microcephalic skulls (see Table 15). From a comparison of these measurements the differences are quite obvious, and substantiate the clinical observations of Brousseau & Brainerd on differences between the heads of Down's syndrome and microcephalic individuals. From his

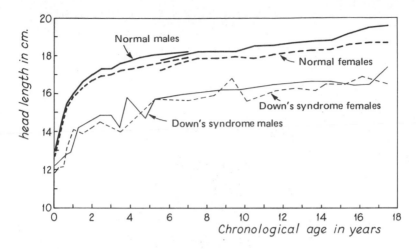

Fig. 14. Head lengths in Down's syndrome and normal controls (Roche *et al* 1961b).

Table 15. Comparison of average Measurements of Down's Syndrome Skulls
with those of Microcephalic Skulls (Greig 1927)
(Linear measurements in millimetres).

Measurement	Down's syndrome*	Microcephaly†
Circumference	444	375
Length	150	135
Breadth	129	104
Cephalic index	85.7	77.3
Height	112	101
Altitudinal index	87.6	74.8
Basinasal length	78	87
Basialveolar length	74	86
Gnathic index	94.6	98.6
Nasal height	33	38
Nasal width	19	20
Orbital height	33	31
Orbital width	32	33
Orbital index	95.1	93.1
Ophryo-mental length	96	117
Bizygomatic width	102	99
Total facial index	94.2	118.9
Ophryo-alveolar length	68	85
Superior facial index	69.9	86.4
Cranial capacity (c.c.)	982	543
Weight (grams)	316.6	311.8

*Average measurements taken from three Down's syndrome females, ages
5, 14 and 16 years.

†Average measurements taken from two females, ages 16, 19, and one
male, 9 years.

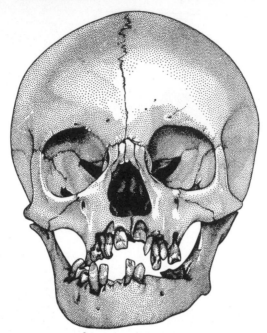

Fig. 15 Skull of a 14-year-old female with Down's syndrome showing persistent metopic suture, decreased length and breadth of the maxillae, small nasal bones and irregular dentition.

Table 16. Summary of Skull Abnormalities emphasized by Greig and Lowe
Greig (1927) (3 Down's syndrome skulls)*

Poorly developed diploë.
Brachycephaly with increased zygomatic breadth.
Early basilar synostosis.

Limited growth of maxillae and facial bones, retaining infantile character.
Flat palate.

Relatively well developed mandible.

Lowe (1949) (4 Down's syndrome skulls)†

General thinness of skull bones.
Shortness of sagittal diameter.
Open metopic sutures.

Small maxillae.
Flattened orbital ridges.
Orbits reduced in depth with anteroposterior axes inclined at 75° instead of 45° and lateral axes sloping downwards and outwards.
Small or absent nasal bones and limited development of sinuses.

   *Females aged 16, 14 and 5 years.
   † Ages 31, 35, 42 and 52 years.

observations of the skulls, Greig came to the conclusion that Down's syndrome seems to be a defect in growth (fetal) rather than a defect in development (embryonic) (see Fig. 15). Lowe (1949) examined four adult Down's syndrome skulls and made some observations that were similar and others that were different from those made by Greig (see Table 16). Lowe concluded that the skull in Down's syndrome contains so many peculiarities that it is difficult to separate the secondary effects from those of a more fundamental nature.

SKULL: X-RAY

Examinations by X-rays of skulls in Down's syndrome expose a variety of abnormalities. Some of them have not been properly assessed or lack substantiation, and are therefore difficult to evaluate. None of them seems to be entirely characteristic of the syndrome nor is found in all cases. Øster (1953) studied skull X-rays of 30 affected persons and found abnormalities in only 9, and in these, the changes were indefinite. In general, an X-ray photograph shows the head to be slightly reduced in size and gives evidence of brachycephaly (Bullard 1911) with flattening of the occiput, though these features may not be seen in infants (Benda 1960, Hall 1964). In a radiological study of the lateral view of the skulls of Down's syndrome and normal individuals, Seward et al. (1961) found no departure from the normal contour of the posterior portion of the skull in Down's syndrome. These skulls, however, had significantly low values for both height and length. This suggested that the flattened occiput which is seen clinically may be the effect of the soft tissue covering the posterior part of the skull and the neck.

The metopic suture, which usually closes shortly after birth, may remain open for many years (Greig 1927). Spitzer & Quilliam (1958) noted persistence of the metopic suture in 15 out of 20 Down's syndrome patients ranging from 4 to 14 years in age. In a study of patients over 10 years of age, Roche et al. (1961b) found a patent metopic suture in 67 per cent of the males and 42 per cent of the females; in the general population a similar finding occurred in 8.8 per cent of males and 12.3 per cent of females. The sinuses may be absent or poorly developed. All 20 of Spitzer & Quilliam's patients referred to above had absent frontal sinuses and subsequently Spitzer et al. (1961) found that the frontal sinuses were absent in 24 out of 29 cases that they examined. Similar findings were noted by Roche et al. (1961b) in 30 out of 31 males with Down's syndrome and 48 out of 56 females, and by Betlejewski et al. (1964) in 61 out of 77 patients with the syndrome ranging in age from 1 to 24 years. Le Double (1903) noted that the absence of frontal sinuses was more common in skulls with a persistent metopic suture than in skulls in which the suture was obliterated. The nasal bones may be absent or poorly developed (Fraser 1876, Clift 1922, Kisling 1966). The interorbital distance is often reduced (Gerald & Silverman 1965) and differences in the size and position of the orbits, compared to normal controls, have been observed (Kisling).

In some cases, the maxilla is underdeveloped and the angle of the mandible may be somewhat obtuse, but a fair degree of variability occurs. Benda (1960) has reported abnormalities in the body of the sphenoid bone, displacement of the cribriform plate and changes of certain measurable distances within the skull. He also reported the lack of development of frontal and sphenoidal sinuses and spheno-occipital and sphenoethmoidal synchondroses. While Spitzer *et al.* have confirmed some of these X-ray findings, they pointed out that some of the apparently abnormal features might be distortions caused by projection errors. Thinness of the cranial bones was a frequent finding in the 29 cases reported by Spitzer *et al.* Timme (1921) described abnormalities in the sella turcica, but these were not confirmed by Clift. Kisling noted differences in dimensions of the sella, as well as other changes in size and shape of the cranial base, in Down's syndrome adult males compared to controls. In a cephalometric X-ray study of the cranial base of 131 Down's syndrome children and adults of both sexes, Roche *et al.* (1972) also observed reduction in various cranial base lengths. The most marked reduction, at all ages, was in the distance between the nasion and the midpoint of the hypophyseal fossa.

VERTEBRAL COLUMN

Hill (1908) stated that spinal curvatures in Down's syndrome are rare and that they are due to muscular weakness when present. Mautner (1950) reported that 37.5 per cent of 80 cases of Down's syndrome studied by X-ray had incomplete fusion of the arches of the lower portion of the vertebral column. This was in contrast to minor abnormalities and incomplete fusions in the lower spine which occur at most in 5 per cent of the general population. Rabinowitz & Moseley (1964) noted anomalous configuration of the lumbar vertebrae in Down's syndrome infants. This consisted of increase in vertical, and decrease in anteroposterior, diameter when viewed in lateral projection. In addition, there was a greater tendency of the anterior border of the vertebral body to be straightened or concave posteriorly. Tishler & Martel (1965) examined cervical spine films of 18 cases of Down's syndrome, of varying ages, and found dislocation of the atlas in 4 of them. They speculated that this increased incidence might be due to congenital abnormality of the transverse portion of the cruciate ligament and that it might reflect generalized joint laxity. In a more extensive subsequent study, they (Martel & Tishler 1966) reported atlas dislocation in 14 out of 70 cases. In addition, in the young adults in their series, they often found asymptomatic cervical intervertebral disc lesions characterized by narrowing of the disc with associated irregularities of the adjacent end-plates. They regarded these as Schmorl's nodes. Though usually asymptomatic, subluxation of the atlas can be accompanied by spinal cord compression resulting in neurological manifestations of varying degrees of severity (Dzenitis 1966, Curtis *et al.* 1968, Martel *et al.* 1969, Gerard *et al.* 1971, Aung 1973). Apart from particular circumstances of such kinds, the spinal cord in Down's syndrome appears generally to be normal (Solitaire 1969).

RIBS

The absence of one pair of ribs was observed in 11 (9 female and 2 male) out of 36 Down's syndrome children studies by X-ray (Beber 1965); in some there was also a defect of a vertebral body. A more extensive X-ray survey of 12th rib anomalies in 251 cases, ranging in age from 3 to 51 years, was undertaken by Thuline & Islam (1966). Twenty six per cent of the females and 15 per cent of the males had such anomalies (see Table 17). An X-ray investigation by Murray *et al.* (1966) of 162 Down's

Table 17. 12th-rib anomalies in Down's Syndrome
(After Thuline & Islam 1966)

12th-rib	Females	Males	Combined
One normal; other not visible or rudimentary	7	6	13
Both rudimentary	7	3	10
One not visible; other rudimentary	6	3	9
Neither visible	9	9	18
Both normal	83	118	201
TOTALS	112	139	251

syndrome individuals showed 19 females and 4 males with both 12th ribs absent. Sixteen of the females and all 4 of the males had only 11 thoracic vertebrae Reasons for such apparent differences between the sexes are not clear.

PELVIS AND HIPS

Diagnostic changes in the pelvic bones of Down's syndrome infants were first noted by Caffey & Ross (1956, 1958), and similar findings were observed by Schultze-Jena (1959). The pelvic bones of affected infants show flattening of the inner edges of the ilium, widening of the iliac wings and bodies, smallness of the ischial rami and coxa valga of the femur. More recently. Andrén & Hall (1968) reported increased outward curvature of the posterior part of the ilium in Down's syndrome infants compared to controls, and regarded this as a useful radiological diagnostic sign.

An estimation of the flattening of the lower edges of the ilium is made by measuring the "acetabular angle". In making this measurement a horizontal Y—Y line is drawn through the two "Y" cartilages. A second line is then drawn on each side which connects the two ends of the caudal edge of the ilium. The angles, between the Y—Y line and these secondary lines, which measure the tilt of the lower iliac edge, are called the acetabular angles (see Fig. 16).

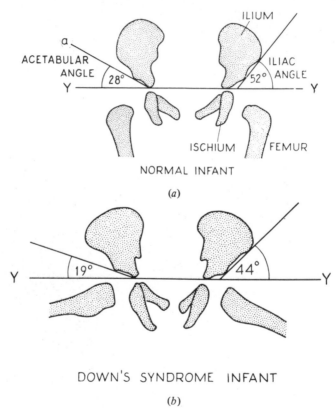

Fig. 16. Drawings from X-ray photographs showing the measurement of the acetabular and iliac angles in (a) normal and (b) Down's syndrome infants. In (b) note flattening of the lower edges of the ilium and the lateral flare of the iliac wings.

An estimation of the widening of the iliac wings and bodies is made by measuring the "iliac angle". For this purpose a similar Y—Y line is drawn through the "Y" cartilages and then a secondary line is drawn on each side; this second line connects the lateral end of the lower edge of the ilium with the outermost possible point of the lateral edge. The angles between the secondary lines and the Y—Y line are called the iliac angles.

As an aid to diagnosis an iliac index has been devised. This index is half the sum of both acetabular angles and both iliac angles. A comparison of these measurements with controls can be seen in Table 18. There is an

Table 18. Hip Angles in Down's Syndrome and Controls.
(After Caffey and Ross 1958)

Category	Acetabular Angles in Degrees		Iliac Angles in Degrees		Iliac Indices	
	Mean	Range	Mean	Range	Mean	Range
Birth to 3 months						
Down's syndrome	16	29−9	44	58−35	60	87−48
Controls	28	44−12	55	67−43	81	97−68
3 months to 12 months						
Down's syndrome	11	19−16	41	50−26	50	67−33
Controls	22	34−8 .	58	74−44	79	101−62

overlap in the measurements in Down's syndrome and normal pelves, but in general the X-ray findings are diagnostic in about 4 out of 5 cases of the syndrome, suggestive in about 4 out of 20, and uncertain or normal in less than 1 out of 20 (Caffey & Ross 1958). Rather similar findings were reported by Astley (1963) and by Mortensson & Hall (1972). The pelvic changes noted in Down's syndrome infants have also been reported in adults (Kaufmann & Taillard 1961); however, it should be remembered that calcification in the adult pelvis makes interpretation of this X-ray finding difficult. In a comparison between small groups of translocation and standard Down's syndrome individuals, Ong et al. (1967) found a tendency for the iliac index to be lower in the translocation cases. However, there was some overlap between the two groups and the overall differences were not substantial.

The Down's syndrome pelvis is small. Single characteristic signs are seen in normal infants and in association with other diseases, but the full combination is rarely noted except in the syndrome. Smallness of the ischial rami and coxa valga usually become apparent after 6 months of age and are thought to represent hypoplasia and disuse deformity. An increased incidence of dislocation of the hip has been observed in older patients (Kaufmann & Taillard). The cause is unknown but it is probably not related to the bony changes of the pelvis and may be of a secondary type such as that seen in patients with paraplegia. Hip dislocation of congenital origin was not observed more frequently in Down's syndrome children than among live births in general (Fabia & Drolett 1970b).

Nicolis & Sacchetti (1963) measured the hip angles of a group of 25 Down's syndrome and 45 normal control children all under the age of 1 year. They analysed their data in terms of discriminant functions (Fisher 1936, Welch 1939) to establish the combination of the measurement of the two angles that gave the best differentiation between Down's syndrome and normal children. This combination was found to be given by the linear function: $0.30a + 0.42i$, where a and i are the mean values in degrees of the two acetabular and of the two iliac angles respectively. The sum of values of the linear functions is called the "pelvic index". The critical value of this index was 25.2. Normal subjects generally showed a pelvic index greater than this and those with the syndrome a smaller value. Hall (1964) cautioned against the use of the pelvic index as an isolated diagnostic finding since a moderate transverse rotation of the pelvis during the X-ray examination can change the acetabular angles by as much as $10°$ and the iliac angles by $6°$. He noted that the Down's syndrome pelvis lacked a bony process along the medial border, corresponding to the posterior superior iliac spine.

HANDS AND FEET

Many unusual features of the hands in Down's syndrome have been reported. None of these findings is pathognomic since they also occur, albeit less frequently, in the general population. The hands are typically broad and stumpy. The metacarpal bones and the phalanges are shortened. In 1896, Telford Smith demonstrated by using X-rays that the second phalanx of the little finger is abnormally small. He also showed that the finger was usually incurved (clinodactyly), and he considered this deformity to be a distinguishing characteristic. West (1901), however, showed that this same finding also occurred in normal children. He examined 605 children and found that 18.5 per cent had little fingers which were straight; 28.9 per cent had fingers with a slight curve; in 32.9 per cent there was a distinct curve, and 19.6 per cent a marked curve. In an account of his clinical experience with Down's syndrome children, Thursfield (1921) reported clinodactyly of the little fingers in 13 out of 29 cases. Roche (1961) studied radiographs of the left hand, taken at

Table 19. Frequencies of Clinodactyly and Shortness of Digit V.
(After Beckman et al. 1962)

Sample	Clinodactyly		Shortness		Total
	Present	Absent	Present	Absent	
Down's syndrome males	33	26	28	31	59
Down's syndrome females	30	25	35	20	55
Severely retarded males	2	59	3	58	61
Severely retarded females	0	51	9	42	51
Moderately retarded males	1	36	6	31	37
Moderately retarded females	4	34	10	28	38
Normal male adults	4	96	2	98	100
Normal female adults	3	97	7	93	100
Normal children, male or female	3	97	2	98	100

regular intervals over a 4 year period, of 192 Down's syndrome children and 120 normal children; the incidence of clinodactyly of the little finger was found to be 55.2 per cent and 32.5 per cent respectively. Beckman *et al.* (1962) reported clinodactyly of the little finger in 55 per cent of Down's syndrome individuals and in 2–10 per cent of normal people and unspecified low grade defectives (see Table 19). These findings agreed well with Øster's who reported a 48 per cent incidence in Down's syndrome. No substantial sex or age variation has been noticed.

Beckman *et al.* classified the fifth finger as short if it did not reach the distal flexion furrow of the fourth finger. Using this classification they found that 55 per cent of Down's syndrome individuals had short fifth fingers. This occurred in 15 per cent of unspecified mentally defective patients and in 4.5 per cent of normal people. Other frequency data on this finding were reported by Øster (57 per cent) and Levinson *et al.* (1955) (66 per cent).

Smith (1896) noted that the fifth finger was considerably shorter than normal and that there was lateral displacement of the terminal phalanx. Hefke (1940) did X-ray studies on the hands of 100 persons with Down's syndrome and found no evidence of anomalies in 33 per cent, and evidence of some bony anomaly in 67 per cent. In 62 per cent the anomaly observed was the shortening or deformity of the middle phalanx of the fifth finger, which, when present, was always bilateral. Benda (1960) reported that 36 per cent of the Down's syndrome cases he studied had a similar anomaly (see Fig. 17).

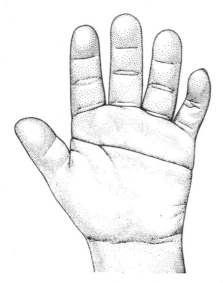

Fig. 17. Down's syndrome hand showing short, stubby fingers, single transverse palmar crease, and curved fifth finger with only one flexion crease.

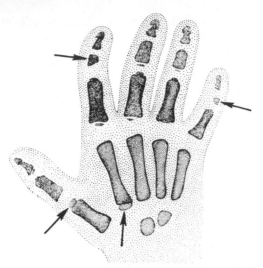

Fig. 18. Bones of Down's syndrome hand as seen in X-ray. In the fifth finger the bone of the second phalanx is small and there is slight displacement of the terminal bone. A proximal epiphysis is seen on the second, and a distal one on the first, metacarpal. The middle phalanx of the index finger is small.

Brachymesophalangia (i.e. shortness of the shaft of the middle phalanx) of the fifth finger was found by Roche (1961) in 27.1 per cent of 192 Down's syndrome children and in 3.3 per cent of 120 normal children. In nearly all children of both groups, brachymesophalangia was associated with clinodactyly. Furthermore, clinodactyly with a middle phalanx of normal length occurred with almost equal frequency in the Down's syndrome (25 per cent) and normal (29 per cent) children. Garn *et al.* (1972) reported incidences of brachymesophalangia of the fifth finger similar, though somewhat lower, to those observed by Roche in Down's syndrome and normal controls: 21 per cent and 1.4 per cent respectively. In affected juveniles, they noted absence of a cone-epiphysis, on the middle segment of the fifth digit, in those with Down's syndrome compared to a 47 per cent incidence of this trait in controls. Greulich (1973) also pointed out that dysplasia of the middle phalanx of the fifth fingers, which he found in 29 per cent of 324 Down's syndrome patients and fairly, though less, frequently in several normal populations, is different in the two groups. He observed that in Down's syndrome, the abnormal phalanx is typically shortened, disproportionately wide, frequently wedge-shaped and usually associated with clinodactyly; in the normal populations, the dysplastic phalanx is characterized by a concave defect in the base of its diaphysis, by a cone- or mushroom-shaped epiphysis, and the association with clinodactyly is inconstant. Moreover, in the Down's syndrome sample, slightly more males were affected whereas, in the normal individuals, more females showed the dysplasia.

Other X-ray anomalies of the hand occur much less frequently. The second metacarpal bone, which normally has a distal epiphysis, may also show a proximal epiphysis or notching of the bone. The first metacarpal bone normally has a proximal epiphysis and may also show a distal epiphysis. Occasionally the middle phalanx of the second finger is short and similar to that seen in the fifth finger (see Fig. 18). In practically all cases, the hands are from 10 to 30 per cent shorter than normal hands (Hefke). Presence of a short fifth finger is not as good a diagnostic discriminant in Down's syndrome as clinodactyly (see Table 19).

Hyperextensibility of the proximal thumb joint occurred in 77 per cent of Down's syndrome individuals and 25—30 per cent of controls (Beckman et al.). The incidence of generalized hyperflexibility of the joints has been reported as 47 per cent (Øster) and 88 per cent (Levinson et al.).

In some cases the two distal creases on the little finger are replaced by a single crease (Penrose 1931, Portius 1941, Øster). The new crease, usually double in character, takes the place of the distal and medial creases, and it lies between the distal and proximal interphalangeal joints (see Fig. 17). It was present in 16 out of 60 Down's syndrome patients studied by Penrose. In 8 the abnormality was present on one hand only. This anomaly and a single transverse palmar crease occurred together on the hands of patients with the syndrome with a greater frequency than would be expected by chance. This observation suggested that the two peculiarities were related to one another.

The characteristic transverse fold, also called the "four finger crease" or "simian line" as well as a "single transverse palmar crease", extends from the ulnar margin to the radial margin of the palm. It occurs in about 45 per cent of cases of Down's syndrome (Øster). This contrasts with an incidence of about 2 to 5 per cent in several newly born and older general population samples among whom the greatest frequency was in premature and malformed babies and those dying neonatally (Davies & Smallpeice 1963). Benda (1960) thought that the single transverse palmar crease in Down's syndrome differs somewhat from that seen in normal persons, since in normals the crease is usually bilateral, but in Down's syndrome a unilateral crease is almost twice as frequent as a bilateral one. However, Davies & Smallpeice found, among 80 unselected newly born infants with a single crease, that it was unilateral in 63 and bilateral in 17. Erne (1953) noted that the crease was more frequent in close relatives of Down's syndrome individuals than in a control population. According to Vrydagh-Laoureux (1967) and to Purvis-Smith (1972), an extention of the proximal transverse palmar crease towards the ulnar border of the hand (referred to by Purvis-Smith as the Sydney line) is substantially more frequent in Down's syndrome than in normal persons.

Würth (1937) stated that the furrows of the hand are not functional furrows, as they begin to develop in the second or third fetal month; the creases might therefore be reflections of the bony development of the hand. Popich & Smith (1970) regarded palmar and digital creases as secondary features consequent on early flexional folding in the skin of the developing hand. They provided evidence, from a study of normal and malformed hands, that this was determined by the form and function of the hand between the seventh and fourteenth weeks of development.

Syndactyly and polydactyly have been reported in Down's syndrome (Dignan 1973), but they are rare. Other rarities are perodactyly or synbrachydactyly (Schönenberg & Pfeiffer 1966), partial adactyly (Pueschel & O'Donnell 1974), complete absence of a hand, and severe malformations of forearm bones (Koivikko 1970); occasional occurrences of such kinds in individuals with Down's syndrome presumably are coincidental. Wolff & Rollin (1942) made a somewhat fanciful and unconvincing attempt to relate peculiarities of the hand in Down's syndrome to personality types.

The feet are short and broad. Brushfield (1925) emphasized the importance of the plantar furrow proceeding from the cleft between the first and second toe (see Fig. 19). A wide space between the first and

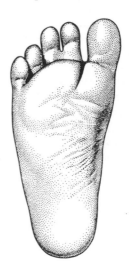

Fig. 19. Drawing of Down's syndrome foot showing short toes, furrow between the first and second and syndactyly of the second and third.

second toe is a well-known abnormality; however, the frequency with which this feature occurs varies greatly in different samples, from 47 per cent (Øster) to 90 per cent (Beckman et al.). According to Beckman et al. the anomaly occurs rather frequently in other types of mentally retarded individuals (24–37 per cent), but is rare in normal individuals.

Retroposition of the fourth toe has been reported by Hanhart (1960a) and Beckman et al., and this is observed in about 10 per cent of cases of Down's syndrome. The shortening of the fourth toe may be related to a shortening of the metatarsal bone (Steggerda 1942). Syndactylous toes occur with a frequency of 2.1 per cent (Hanhart) to 11.4 per cent (Beckman et al.). Syndactyly, moreover, of the second and third toes occurs both in Down's syndrome and in the general population. Syndactyly of the other toes has been found occasionally in the syndrome and also other malformations of the foot such as talipes planus, cavus (Sutherland 1899) and complete aplasia of the metatarsal bones and phalanges (Ingalls 1947), but these are rare and not particularly characteristic.

STATURE

There are considerable differences in stature between individuals with Down's syndrome matched for age and sex. Roche (1965) observed that stature is more variable in children with the syndrome of the same age and sex than in normal children. In general the newly born affected child is slightly shorter than normal although the linear growth during the first year of life seems close to the average. The over-all effect is for persons with Down's syndrome to be shorter than normal (Talbot 1924, Benda 1946). Adolescent spurts in stature occur in most cases (Roche). The average adult height of Down's syndrome males is approximately 151 cm. and of females approximately 141 cm. In the group of adults measured by Øster (1953) the height varied from 135 to 170 cm. in males and 127 to 158 cm. in females. According to Talbot the reduced stature in Down's syndrome is mainly influenced by the reduced length of the lower extremities; Thelander & Pryor (1966) reported similar findings. The length of the trunk closely approximates to the normal at least up till the age of 10 years (Talbot). The trunk length in adults is probably only slightly reduced as compared with the marked reduction in length of the lower extremities. The upper extremities are similarly reduced in length. There is a deficient growth at the distal ends of the long bones (Benda 1960, Engler); indeed, growth deficiency is pronounced towards the distal ends of all extremities, namely, the hands, fingers, feet and toes (Benda).

Dutton (1959a) reported that for a group of Down's syndrome boys (aged 6–18 years) none was within two standard deviations of normal boys of a similar age. Evaluated on a height quotient (height age multiplied by 100 and divided by chronological age) he found the affected boys to be 67.8 per cent of normal. He contrasted the markedly reduced height in Down's syndrome with the essentially normal skeletal development. Thelander & Pryor measured standing height in 83 Down's syndrome boys and 63 girls ranging in age from 6 months to 15 years. Both sexes were consistently short at all ages. Up to 4 years, the reduction averaged about one standard deviation below the norm, and from then till 15 years progressively fell further below the norm. From the age of 10 years, the boys showed a greater lag than the girls. At 15 years, on average, the boys attained a standing height of 8½ year old normal boys and the girls that of 10 year old normal girls. Weight curves were similar to those of height, with the Down's syndrome boys falling further below normal than the girls from 9 years of age. In a serial study, over a period of 12 years, of 68 Down's syndrome children, Rarick & Seefeldt (1974) found that the standing and sitting height means, at all ages from 7 to 18 years, were more than two standard deviations below the means in the control group.

MUSCULAR SYSTEM

Generalized hypotonia is characteristic of nearly all newly born and young children with Down's syndrome. This defect is partly manifested in the delayed ability to sit, stand and walk. With increasing age hypotonia becomes less pronounced. There seems to be a distinct tendency for extreme or marked hypotonicity to become more moderate within weeks or months of birth (Cowie 1970) and, in adulthood, mild hypertonia rather than hypotonia may be found (Owens *et al.* 1971). Normal muscle tone is lacking and stimuli responses are poor. There may be a poor Moro reflex and a weak response on stimulation of the patellar reflex, though there is some discrepancy between the observations of Hall (1964) and of Cowie in these respects. In addition to these considerations, Cowie found, in Down's syndrome infants, impaired resistance to traction on the arms, poor postural responses in a position of ventral suspension (Landau reaction), longer persistence of the palmar and plantar grasp reflexes and frequent absence of the placing reaction. About 50 per cent of Down's syndrome individuals show some abnormality of gait (Øster 1953). In adults the gait may be unsteady and the feet are kept wide apart. Patients may walk with a stoop and the head may hang forward. When they sit down they are accustomed to adopt a "tailorwise" posture. In general their movements are described as slow, clumsy and uncoordinated. Speculations about the cause of hypotonia and the associated manifestations have not yet separated the effects of abnormalities in muscle and connective tissue from those concerned with developmental errors in the nervous system.

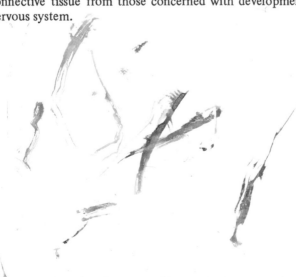

4. Mental Development

Of all the disabilities in Down's syndrome, the most crucial, from the point of view of the affected individual's capacity to cope with the environment, are those connected with mental development. Consideration is given to this subject in the present chapter.

CENTRAL NERVOUS SYSTEM

Observations on the brain began to be made fairly soon after Langdon Down's (1866) initial clinical account of the syndrome. Among the first reports was that by Fraser (1876). He noted that the brain was small and that the configuration was symmetrical and followed the outline of the skull. Some of the early authors who gave detailed descriptions of the brain are Wilmarth (1890), Phillippe & Oberthur (1901), Bourneville (1902, 1903), Tredgold (1908), Biach (1909), Apert (1914) and Comby (1917). A summary of the post-mortem findings as reported by many investigators was given by Apert (1914). He indicated that there were no well marked lesions visible to the naked eye. The brain is small and globular, like the skull, with the anterior part less well developed than the posterior and lateral parts. The convolutions are not sinuous and secondary fissures are shallow. Apert also summarized many of the microscopic lesions that were reported. He concluded that there was agenesis of the cellular elements of the cortex but he found it difficult to say whether or not the changes were primary or secondary to vascular or other meningeal reactions. These findings are somewhat similar to those reported, more recently, by Crome (1965) who noted that the neuropathological changes in Down's syndrome are usually diffuse and non-specific.

Lack of development of the brain-stem and cerebellum has been commented on by various authors (e.g. Davidoff 1928, Crome). In a statistical analysis, based on an examination of 19 Down's syndrome brains, Crome et al. (1966) reported a decrease of total brain weight to, on average, 76 per cent of normal and even greater reduction, to 66 per cent of normal, in the weight of the brain-stem and cerebellum taken together. Norman (1958) stated that the brain of a Down's syndrome adult seldom exceeds 1,200 gm. in weight and is usually nearer to 1,000 gm. Solitaire & Lamarche (1967), in a survey of brain weights of 18 Down's syndrome adults from their own material and another 18 from the literature, also noted that the brain is generally smaller than in other mentally retarded, as well as in normal, populations. Their data, however, showed a brain weight of more than 1,200 gm. in 11 of the 36 cases and a weight below 1,000 gm. in 7 instances. The range was fairly wide, from 850 gm. to 1,370 gm. According to Crome the simplification of the gyral pattern, which is frequently mentioned, is more difficult to evaluate since the observations depend too much on subjective evidence. Neurohistological defects, such as sparseness of cells, particularly in cortical layer III, or excessive neuronal density, are usually uncertain. Various other lesions of the brain have been noted, such as anomalous structure in the peduncles of the cerebellar flocculi (Jelgersma 1963) and fibrous gliosis in the white matter (Meyer & Jones 1939). Benda (1960) has also recorded many pathological findings in the brain and spinal cord in Down's syndrome. Many of the abnormalities reported by these authors have not been fully described and in some instances they have not been confirmed; therefore, at the present time, they have to be treated with reserve (Crome 1965).

With increased frequency of survival to adulthood of persons with Down's syndrome, pathological observations on the brains of older patients also became more frequent. In this context, the neuropathological features of Alzheimer's disease have been reported by numbers of investigators using both the light microscope (Jervis 1948, Jelgersma 1962, Solitaire & Lamarche 1966, Haberland 1969, Olson & Shaw 1969, Malamud 1972), and the electron microscope (Ohara 1972, Burger & Vogel 1973, Ellis et al. 1974). These features, which mainly include senile plaques, neurofibrillary tangles and granulovacuolar changes in an atrophic brain (Malamud), appear to be substantially more common, and more severe, in Down's syndrome than in similarly aged patients with other types of mental retardation, particularly after 40 years of age (see Table 20). The precise effects of such pathology on mental function in surviving

Table 20. Alzheimer's Disease in Adult Retarded Patients With and Without Down's Syndrome (After Malamud 1972)

	Below 40 years		Above 40 years	
	No. of cases	No. with Alzheimer's disease	No. of cases	No. with Alzheimer's disease
Down's syndrome	312	5(1.6%)	35	35(100%)
Other types of retardation	588	0	225	31(14%)

Down's syndrome patients remain to be fully evaluated. In some, dementia following slowly progressive intellectual and emotional deterioration is readily apparent (Jervis), whereas others seem less obviously affected (Solitaire & Lamarche, Owens et al. 1971). Precise tests, however, have shown significantly poorer performance in older, compared to younger, Down's syndrome patients in, for instance, object identification (Owens et al.) and visual retention capabilities (Dalton et al. 1974).

Electroencephalographic investigations have been made periodically and these have been reviewed by Ellingson *et al.* (1970). Various abnormalities have been reported, but no patterns specific for Down's syndrome have been identified. Ellingson *et al.* (1973) recently undertook the largest electroencephalographic study on Down's syndrome published to-date, involving the examination of 279 electroencephalograms from 202 karyotyped individuals with the syndrome ranging in age from one month to 63 years. Abnormalities found were asymmetry and/or asynchrony, diffuse slow activity and diffuse or focal "seizure activity". The overall rate of abnormality was 21 per cent compared to less than 10 per cent in healthy persons noted by the same observers. Most of the abnormalities were seen in children below 14 years. Abnormality rates in young adults were no higher than in the general population, but they appeared to increase in the fifth and sixth decades. Neither the rates nor types of abnormality found differed significantly in the few mosaic and D/G translocation cases from those in the standard trisomy 21 patients.

Other types of special investigation of the brain in Down's syndrome have not been extensive. A study of cerebral oxygen uptake by Lassen *et al.* (1966) showed no significant differences between Down's syndrome adults and normal controls. In an attempt to find possible neurochemical abnormalities in the syndrome, Stephens & Menkes (1969) examined the lipids in cerebral grey and white matter in 4 cases. No major abnormality in the composition of the principal lipids was detected.

Clinical findings, related to central nervous system involvement, which are regularly present in Down's syndrome, are mental retardation, muscular hypotonia, inco-ordination and reduced sensory responses. These abnormalities, which are discussed in other sections of this book, have not been correlated precisely with the pathology of the brain. Epilepsy is much less frequent with a reported incidence ranging from less than one per cent to nearly 10 per cent of cases (Kirman 1951, Walter *et al.* 1955, Schachter 1956, Macgillivray 1967, Seppäläinen & Kivalo 1967, Veall 1974). This variation is probably largely due to different diagnostic criteria and to different age ranges of patients studied. However, even a frequency of about 10 per cent is substantially lower than that usually found in general populations of persons with similar degrees of mental retardation (Malamud 1954, Berg & Kirman 1959). Epilepsy is often of the grand mal variety, but other types, including myoclonic seizures (Wolcott & Chun 1973) and petit mal, may occur. In some instances, the epilepsy is a consequence of a specific pathological event as, for example, in Kirman's case report of a Down's syndrome child whose fits and hemiplegia were a sequel of a cerebro-vascular catastrophe, and in Haberland's (1970) account of another child whose seizures and quadriparesis were due to subacute sclerosing panencephalitis. In Down's syndrome adults, epilepsy may be connected with the cerebral changes of Alzheimer's disease (Haberland 1969). Pareses and paralyses of the limbs are unusual in the syndrome (Gordon & Roberts 1938) except in the context of superimposed cerebral damage of the kinds mentioned above, and other causes of failure of ambulation (Paulson 1971) are also uncommon. Relatively slight neurological abnormalities, such as irregular pupils or ones with sluggish reaction to light, brisk mandibular reflex and facial muscle hyperreflexia, have been found in a substantial proportion of patients (Loesch-Mdzewska 1968).

SENSORY RESPONSES

Brousseau & Brainerd (1928) reported that in most cases of Down's syndrome there are no marked defects of the peripheral sense organs or of the sensory nerves. Defective sensation results from arrested or imperfect development of the sensory areas of the brain and of the centres for understanding impressions received. In many cases it is difficult to evaluate responses because of the short attention span of persons with the syndrome. Brousseau & Brainerd thought that the response to pain was usually normal, but in the low grade cases the response was reduced. Relatively good scores, compared to matched retarded controls, may be attained on visuomotor tests (Nakamura 1965). Sensibility to touch may be diminished, but this may be due to a lack of attention. A small group of Down's syndrome adults studied by Gordon (1944) tended to score less well on tactile than on visual discrimination tests, whereas the opposite tendency was found in normal controls matched for mental age. Rather similar results were obtained by O'Connor & Hermelin (1961) who found that Down's syndrome adults performed stereognostic shape recognition tasks much less well than other mentally retarded and normal controls. Down's syndrome individuals with I.Q. above 20 can usually distinguish substances that are hard, soft, rough or smooth. Irritating cutaneous stimuli can usually be easily localized. In general affected persons cannot discriminate between two different weights of equal size and shape; however, this disability may be due to lack of understanding of instructions rather than to faulty sensory mechanism. There tends to be hypersensitivity to extremes of heat and cold perhaps because of poor circulation or imperfect temperature control mechanism in the central nervous system. On the basis of a study of responses to different rates of metronome beats, Cantor & Girardeau (1959) called into question the widespread view that Down's syndrome individuals have a particularly good sense of rhythm. Sinson & Wetherick (1973) suggested that children with the syndrome show a specific deficit in short-term retention of colour information.

The sense of smell seems to be reduced; however, secondary changes of the mucous membrane, caused by chronic catarrh, make interpretation of this observation difficult. The fissured tongue, with hypertrophied papillae, does not seem to cause any abnormality in the sense of taste. Food preferences are shown, e.g. a liking for sweet and dislike of bitter substances. Hunger, thirst and nausea are normally present in affected individuals. They can usually be bowel and bladder trained during childhood. In severely retarded cases it may be difficult to diagnose visceral disease because of their reduced awareness of organic and somatic sensations. Sexual sensations are considered to be reduced in both Down's syndrome males and females. Adolescent males are able to have erection and ejaculation, but these responses are occasionally diminished and in some cases never attained (Stearns *et al.* 1960).

DEVELOPMENTAL PATTERNS

The age range over which developmental events occur is usually greater than that for a normal infant or child. The presence of a severe, or moderately severe, cardiac anomaly may delay development even in infants and children without central nervous system pathology. There is also evidence that environmental factors, such as good care at home and training, can improve the rate of development in Down's syndrome. The degree of change may be small but significant. Examples of environmental effects were demonstrated by Lyle (1959, 1960), Centerwall & Centerwall (1960), Kugel & Reque (1961), Stedman & Eichorn (1964) and by Carr (1970a). Persons with Down's syndrome brought up at home showed an increased rate of development over those brought up in an institution. In subsequent studies by Shotwell & Shipe (1964) and by Shipe & Shotwell (1965) similar results were found. They noted that home-reared Down's syndrome children were superior to those institutionalized at birth and that this superiority persisted. Their findings supported the conclusion that institutional placement during the earliest years of life adversely affected development. The adverse effects that retard development have not been clearly defined.

Some degree of poor head control and hypotonia may be present in normal newly born infants. However in the early months of infancy, the normal infant quickly develops good muscle tone and head control, while the Down's syndrome infant may remain hypotonic and show little evidence of being able to support its head. Levinson *et al.* (1955) reported on the developmental patterns of 50 infants with Down's syndrome and found that the ages at which they sat up, walked and used words were all late as compared with normal infants. For example, the usual sitting up age in Down's syndrome was 12 months or roughly 6 months later than that for the normal infant; however, some sat up as early as 6–8 months and others were delayed until 3 years. A normal infant begins to walk at about 12 months, but most children with Down's syndrome learn to walk after 2 years of age. Some, however, did walk at 12 months but others not until 4½ years, an age range close to that reported by Kučera (1969) for another series of cases. Language development was very variable, so that some used words at 12 months whereas others delayed until 6 years; the largest group of cases used words at approximately 2 years. In a study of 40 Down's syndrome children living at home, Strazzulla (1953) found that the average age at which words began to be used was about 34 months. Over the next 2 years, the majority started using phrases and, subsequently, sentences. The author noted wide individual differences in these respects. Aside from vocal defects speech development proceeds in the normal way, but it begins late and progresses much more slowly. These developmental patterns were similar to those noted by Erbs & Smith (1962) (see Table 21), Fishler *et al.* (1964) and by Melyn & White (1973). All these data show a wide range of variability between different individuals with Down's syndrome.

Table 21. Mean Ages and Age ranges at which Down's Syndrome Children reached the following Stages of Development.
(After Erbs & Smith 1962).

Event	Mean age in months	Range in months
Rolled over	7.7	1−36
Sat up	13.0	6−30
Stood (without support)	21.8	9−48
Walked	26.8	16−48
Bladder trained	35.2	24−48
Bowel trained	40.5	25−54

Physical independence of Down's syndrome youths and young adults was compared by Grotz *et al.* (1972) with that of patients from the same institutions whose mental retardation was due to phenylketonuria and to anoxia. The criteria used were performance in the acts of bathing, dressing, toileting, transferring (i.e. movements in and out of bed and chairs), continence and feeding. The Down's syndrome group were the most capable in these respects.

INTELLIGENCE

Opinions differ concerning the range of intelligence in Down's syndrome. Some of the early reports suggested that the majority had an I.Q. below 25; others maintained that most reached an I.Q. between 25 and 49 (Tredgold 1908, Shuttleworth 1909). It is of interest that the mean I.Q. of Down's syndrome patients in institutions has remained quite similar over a period of 30 years (see Table 22).

Many accounts of the intelligence levels in Down's syndrome have contained some bias because of selection of patients. For example, measuring the intelligence levels of patients institutionalized for long periods would favour low I.Q. scores. In other studies patients of high intelligence were selected by testing only those who were attending special schools (Pototzky & Grigg 1942, Wallin 1949, Dunsdon *et al.* 1960).

Table 22. Mean I.Q. of Down's Syndrome Patients in Institutions

Number	Mean	S.D.	Source
41	22.8	7.9	Penrose (1938b)
40	22.0	7.3	Murphy (1956)
64	23.2	6.9	Nakamura (1961)
64	25.6	9.1	Sternlicht & Wanderer (1962)
42	23.7	7.7	Shipe & Shotwell (1965)
2,606	28.6	—	Johnson & Abelson (1969b)

Pototzky & Grigg tested 21 such individuals and found that the mean I.Q. was 46. Two of them were considered to have border-line intelligence. Wallin reported on 49 pupils who attended special schools. In his group the mean I.Q. was higher for females (39.0) than for males (34.0) and the range was 19 to 63 in both groups. Dunsdon *et al.* studied 44 cases selected because they were considered to have relatively high grade intelligence. The majority of their patients were aged between 8 years and 15 years. All but 9 of the 44 (80 per cent) had I.Q.'s between 35 and 54, whereas 5 (11 per cent) had I.Q.'s over 55 and 4 had I.Q.'s between 19 and 34. The writers were interested in determining whether persons with Down's syndrome of high intelligence differed physically from others or not, and they found no such differences in *atd* angle measurements. Others also have attempted to ascertain possible differences in dermatoglyphic (Dicker 1972) and other physical features between Down's syndrome individuals with relatively high, and those with relatively low, intelligence. Gibson & Gibbins (1958), in a mainly non-metrical study of 32 cases, concluded that more physical stigmata of Down's syndrome occurred in those with highest tested intelligence. More extensive investigations of a similar kind (Johnson & Barnett 1961, Kääriäinen & Dingman 1961, Domino & Newman 1965, Shipe *et al.* 1968) did not indicate a distinct systematic relationship between intellectual level and physical findings. The subject has been reviewed by Baumeister & Williams (1967).

Brousseau & Brainerd (1928) reported on the intelligence levels of 206 institutional patients with Down's syndrome. Of these only 2 had I.Q.'s above 50 (54 and 66); 37.8 per cent had I.Q.s below 25 and 61.2 per cent between 25 and 49 (see Table 23). There were more females in the 25 to 49 I.Q. range than males. In this report a detailed description was given of mental responses at the various I.Q. levels. Malzberg (1950) examined the intelligence levels of 880 Down's syndrome cases in the New York State schools and found that 24.5 per cent had I.Q.s below 25, 71.6 per cent from 25 to 49, 3.8 per cent from 50 to 69 and in one case the intelligence level was not ascertained. There was no mention of the distribution of the level of intelligence by age.

During Øster's (1953) investigation in Denmark, he found that in 61 cases the records contained information on the intelligence quotient (Binet-Simon) or on the development quotient (Bühler-Hetzer). The

Table 23. Percentage of Down's Syndrome Cases in Various I.Q. Ranges

| | Brousseau & Brainerd (1928) | Malzberg (1950) | Øster (1953) | Loeffler & Smith (1964) | |
				3 years and under	3–9 years
Number of Cases	206*	880*	32	47†	34††
(0–24)	37.8	24.5	10	0	9
(25–49)	61.2	71.6	56	30	62
(50–69)	1.0	3.8	34	47	29
(over 70)	0.0	0.0	0	23	0
Undetermined	0.0	0.1	0	0	0
Total	100.0	100.0	100	100	100

*Institutional
† At home-Psyche-Cattell Infant Intelligence Scale.
†† At home—Stanford-Binet Intelligence Scale.

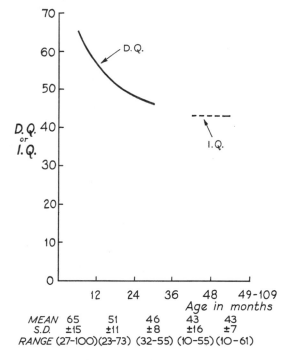

Fig. 20. D.Q. and I.Q. distributions according to age of Down's syndrome child. Patients aged 36 months or under were tested on the Psyche-Catell Intelligence Scale. Children of 37 months or over were tested on the Stanford-Binet Scale. (After Loeffler & Smith 1964).

intelligence quotients of 32 cases of 8 years of age, or older, showed that approximately 10 per cent had I.Q.s below 25, 34 per cent above 50 and the remaining 56 per cent between 25 and 49. He concluded that the results showed a tendency towards a falling I.Q. or D.Q. with increasing age and that a D.Q. over 75 in infants did not preclude the diagnosis of Down's syndrome.

Developmental quotients in Down's syndrome children under three years of age tend to be relatively high, and this is especially true during the first year of life (see Fig. 20). The result is that there are many more such children in this age group who have a D.Q. of over 70 than are found in the age groups 1 to 2 and 2 to 3 years. A number of patients under one year of age with D.Q. of 70 or above were found in the reports of Øster (1953) (6 out of 9), Koch et al. (1963) (12 out of 31), Loeffler & Smith (1964) (10 out of 20) and Dicks-Mireaux (1972). Dicks-Mireaux observed that Down's syndrome infants, as a group, showed a D.Q. significantly below normal by the age of 16 weeks.

There is relatively little information from longitudinal studies of intelligence levels in Down's syndrome. In the study by Koch et al., a group of young patients was tested, by using the Gesell development scale once a year over a three-year period. Thirty-one infants were tested, aged 2 to 48 months. The developmental quotients (D.Q.) and maturity ages (Mt.A.) were divided into four age groups (see Table 24).The highest Mt.A.

Table 24. Pearson Product-moment Correlation Coefficients between Gesell D.Q. and Mt.A. Scores: Infants with Down's Syndrome at Four Age Levels in Longitudinal Study. (After Koch et al. 1963)

Variable	Age groups in months	r	S.E.
*Mt.A.	2 to 13−14 to 24	0.86	0.05
Mt.A.	2 to 13−26 to 36	0.77	0.08
Mt.A.	14 to 24−26 to 36	0.87	0.04
Mt.A.	14 to 24−38 to 48	0.87	0.05
Mt.A.	26 to 36−38 to 48	0.93	0.03
†D.Q.	2 to 13−14 to 24	0.73	0.08
D.Q.	2 to 13−26 to 36	0.72	0.08
D.Q.	14 to 24−26 to 36	0.97	0.01
D.Q.	14 to 24−38 to 48	0.89	0.04
D.Q.	26 to 36−38 to 48	0.90	0.04

*Maturity age.
†Development quotient.

correlation coefficient (0.93) was that between Mt.A. for age group 26 to 36 months and Mt.A. for age group 38 to 48 months. For D.Q. the highest corresponding correlation coefficient (0.97) was that between the age groups 14 to 24 months and 26 to 36 months. A correlation coefficient of 0.78 was found between the D.Q. at 14 to 24 months and Stanford-Binet I.Q. at 5 years of age. Additional observations on the subject were subsequently reported by the same investigators (Share *et al.* 1964). More information is needed about the predictive value of the D.Q. scores and how they correlate at later ages with Stanford-Binet intelligence scores. The predictive value of the Gesell development scales has been criticized by some authors (Kirman 1953, Bayley 1958) while others have emphasized its usefulness (Illingworth 1960, Drillien 1961).

Koch *et al.* noted that during longitudinal testing of Down's syndrome infants the D.Q. decreased with age although the Mt.A. continued to increase. This same effect was noted by Loeffler & Smith (1964) (see Table 25). Koch *et al.* thought that since the Mt.A. continued to increase

Table 25. Longitudinal Intelligence Testing on Down's Syndrome Children at Various Age Levels. (After Loeffler & Smith 1964)

	Case	Sex	First Test C.A. yr	mo	M.A. yr	mo	Q.	Second Test C.A. yr	mo	M.A. yr	mo	Q.	Third Test C.A. yr	mo	M.A. yr	mo	Q.
(i)	1	♀	0	6	0	3	50	1	8	0	11	55					
	2	♂	0	8	0	6	71	1	1	0	8	62	2	1	0	11	44
(ii)	3	♂	0	8	0	4	50	1	8	0	9	45	3	1	1	8	54
	4	♂	0	8	0	6	75	1	10	0	10	45					
	5	♂	0	9	0	5	56	2	10	1	5	50					
	6	♂	0	10	0	5	50	2	0	0	11	46	4	0	1	8	42
	7	♂	0	10	0	7	70	1	11	0	11	48					
	8	♂	0	11	0	8	73	1	11	1	0	52	3	2	1	11	61
	9	♂	0	11	0	7	64	2	10	1	0	35					
	10	♂	0	11	0	3	27	2	1	0	8	32					
	11	♂	1	0	0	7	58	2	4	1	1	46	3	7	1	4	37
	12	♂	1	1	0	5	39	1	11	0	7	30					
(iii)	13	♂	1	3	0	9	60	4	1	2	0	49					
	14	♂	1	9	1	0	57	3	1	1	8	54	4	2	1	9	42
	15	♀	1	11	0	11	48	3	1	1	8	54	5	2	1	10	35
(iv)	16	♂	3	6	2	0	57	4	5	2	3	51					
	17	♀	4	0	1	8	42	5	3	2	0	38					
	18	♂	4	3	2	4	55	5	3	2	6	48					
	19	♂	4	7	1	9	38	5	11	2	2	37	7	0	2	0	29
	20	♀	5	0	2	0	40	6	3	2	8	43					
	21	♀	5	0	2	0	40	6	3	2	10	45					
	22	♀	5	11	2	3	38	6	11	2	5	35	8	1	3	1	38
	23	♀	6	9	3	8	54	8	3	4	10	49					
	24	♂	7	3	2	10	39	8	6	2	11	34					

C.A. = chronological age in years (yr) and months (mo).
M.A. = mental age in years (yr) and months (mo).
Q. = I.Q. or D.Q. Children 36 months (3 years) or under were tested using the Psyche-Cattell infant intelligence scale. Children 37 months and over were tested using the Stanford-Binet intelligence scale

		Testing Sequence:	1st Test	2nd Test	3rd Test
	Case Groups:	(i)	D.Q.	D.Q.	D.Q.
		(ii)	D.Q.	D.Q.	I.Q.
		(iii)	D.Q.	I.Q.	I.Q.
		(iv)	I.Q.	I.Q.	I.Q.

with age, the falling D.Q. was not a true sign of deterioration, as postulated by Masland *et al.* (1958), but an artefact derived from the formula D.Q. = (Mt.A ÷ C.A.) × 100, which assumes a linear relationship between maturity age and chronological age. It has been suggested that the I.Q. is relatively stable within the age range 5 to 19 years (Gibson & Frank

1961). In a study on institutional Down's syndrome patients, Durling & Benda (1952) found a peak development rate below 16 years in 16 per cent, between 16 and 19 years in 35 per cent and between 20 and 37 years in 48 per cent.

In an investigation of 97 institutional individuals with Down's syndrome, Zeaman & House (1962) did semi-longitudinal I.Q. studies using the Stanford-Binet test. Fifty of the patients were tested twice or more often with varying intervals of time between tests. Their ages varied from 6 to 51 years. From these studies it was found that the rate of progress in the mental age was proportional to the log. of the chronological age, and that the I.Q. declined a few points a year when the children were young and gradually stabilized as they became adults. The authors cautioned that the results might be only applicable to the Stanford-Binet test. It is of interest that Koch *et al.* also found a decreasing level of I.Q. with age; however, the two studies are not comparable since the quotient of Zeaman & House is not applicable below the age of 6 years, and Koch *et al.* studied young infants and children below 6 years of age. On the basis of a variety of tests (Stanford-Binet, Wechsler, Merrill-Palmer, Cattell and Leiter scales), Melyn & White (1973) also noted an overall tendency for the I.Q. to decrease with age over the years of childhood.

Most of the studies on the intelligence levels in Down's syndrome contain some element of bias or fail to be comprehensive. From the present data it is not possible to say with certainty at what age further development stops or whether or not deterioration in intellectual development occurs with ageing (Tennies 1943). A satisfactory under-standing of the capabilities of Down's syndrome individuals may be somewhat restricted by reliance on the Stanford-Binet tests. Durling & Benda emphasized that the use of the Stanford-Binet tests is not a proper method of appreciating the mind of the Down's syndrome child.

Social quotients in persons with the syndrome tend to be substantially ahead of their mental ages. Their ability to make certain social adjustments not infrequently causes them to appear more intelligent than they are. The mean social age for Down's syndrome children, determined on the Vineland tests, is 3 years 4 months above the mental age, while the mean social age for other types of mentally retarded children is 2 years 1 month above the mental age (Pototzky & Grigg 1942). In a study of 44 Down's syndrome individuals living at home, Cornwell & Birch (1969) found that the social quotient, on the Vineland scale, was consistently higher than the I.Q., on the Stanford-Binet scale, throughout the age period of 4 to 17 years.

There is evidence to suggest that the intelligence levels of mosaic cases of Down's syndrome is greater than that of non-mosaics (Penrose 1967, Rosecrans 1968). Penrose found that the intelligence range was roughly from I.Q. 35 to above normal average, with a mean at about I.Q. 70. The females were noticeably higher than the males (see Table 26). It is

Table 26. Intelligence Levels of Mosaic Individuals with Down's Syndrome
(Penrose 1967)

Approximate I.Q.	Sex		
	♂	♀	Total
122	0	1	1
100	1	3	4
78	0	4	4
56	3	1	4
34	2	2	4
Total	6	11	17
Mean I.Q.	56	78	70

of interest that four female mosaics were phenotypically normal and mothers of Down's syndrome children; one had superior, one had normal, one had border-line intelligence and the fourth was mildly retarded. Relatively little is known about the level of intelligence in relation to the degree of mosaicism that is present. The literature survey of Rosecrans, however, showed a correlation between intelligence level and the proportion of abnormal cells detected. He noted that intelligence tends to be higher with lower percentages of cells having 21 trisomy, though exceptions do occur. Different results were reported by Johnson & Abelson (1969a) in a study of 254 trisomic, 21 translocation and 18 mosaic patients with Down's syndrome. They found that, as groups, the translocation cases were highest, those with trisomy intermediate and the mosaics lowest in I.Q. scores. However, details of karyotyping procedures, such as number of cells and tissues examined, were not provided and the criteria for mosaicism were not specified.

PERSONALITY

Those with Down's syndrome are considered to have personality and behavioural traits which are in some respects stereotyped. The personality was described by the early authors. Langdon Down (1866) made the following observations: "They have considerable powers of imitation, even bordering on being mimics. They are humerous, and a lively sense of the ridiculous often colours their mimicry."

In a later report Down (1887) gave additional observations: "Several patients who have been under my care have been wont to convert their pillow-slips into surplices and to imitate, in tone and gesture, the clergyman or chaplain they have recently heard. Their power of imitation is, moreover, not limited to things clerical. I have known a ventriloquist to be convulsed with laughter between the first and second parts of his entertainment on seeing a mongolian patient mount the platform, and hearing him grotesquely imitate the performance with which the audience had been entertained. They have a strong sense of the ridiculous; this is indicated by their humourous remarks and the laughter with which they hail accidental falls, even of those to whom they are most attached. Another feature is their great obstinacy—they can only be guided by consummate tact. No amount of coercion will induce them to do that which they have made up their minds not to do. Sometimes they initiate a struggle for mastery, and the day previous will determine what they will or will not do on the next day. Often they will talk to themselves, and they may be heard rehearsing the disputes which they think will be the feature of the following day. They, in fact, go through a play in which the patient, doctor, governess, and nurses are the Dramatis Personae—a play in which the patient is represented as defying and contravening the wishes of those in authority. Whether it be the question of going to church, to school, or for a walk, discretion will often be the better part of valour, by not giving orders which will run counter to the intended disobedience, and thus maintaining the appearance of authority while being virtually beaten. They are always amiable both to their companions and to animals. They are not passionate nor strongly affectionate."

The newly born Down's syndrome infant not infrequently is described as being a "good baby", not easily disturbed and causing the mother very little trouble. It is doubtful whether or not these attributes in the very young infant are personality traits or merely reflections of reduced response to external stimuli and marked hypotonia. Later, the children are often described as happy and cheerful and are considered to be good-tempered and easily amused. Pogue (1917) referred to them as born optimists. They tend to mimic and may be mischievous. There are descriptions in the literature of patients who show other personality traits (Stickland 1954), and a minority are judged to be aggressive and hostile (Wunsch 1957) or to display other varieties of maladaptive behaviour (Moore *et al.* 1968).

Various methods have been used to describe the personality and behavioural traits in Down's syndrome (Blacketer-Simmonds 1953, Silverstein 1964, Domino *et al.* 1964, Domino 1965, Moore *et al.*, Johnson & Abelson 1969b, Francis 1970, Baron 1972). Silverstein tested Down's syndrome patients and matched mentally retarded controls using Peterson's Behaviour Rating Schedules. The Down's syndrome patients scored higher than the controls on the factor "General Adjustment" but for the factor "Introversion-Extroversion" there was no difference between the two groups. Those with the syndrome were rated higher than the controls on six variables; namely, well-mannered, responsible, cooperative, scrupulous, cheerful and gregarious. Using a rating and behavioural check list to evaluate a group of Down's syndrome females, Domino *et al.* found that the following descriptive terms were positively correlated with the diagnosis of the syndrome: unexcitable, content, relaxed, cheerful, good-natured, clownish, affectionate, friendly, stingy, warm, sociable, mild, open and playful. They concluded that these findings supported the clinical impression of a stereotyped personality. On the other hand, Baron, on the basis of a questionnaire to mothers of Down's syndrome children aged 6 to 18 months and living at home, found no evidence of sterotyped behaviour. The scores allocated to these children for such features as adaptability, mood, distractibility and persistence were comparable to those attained by normal infants of similar mental ages.

From census data on over 23,000 residents in United States institutions for the retarded, Johnson & Abelson (1969b) reported that the Down's syndrome patients showed a greater frequency of social competence (as measured by various forms of adaptive behaviour) but poorer communication ability than the other patients (see Table 27). These authors (Johnson

Table 27. Behavioural Competence of Down's Syndrome and other Mentally Retarded Patients (After Johnson & Abelson 1969b)

Behaviour exhibited	Down's syndrome (2,606 patients) %	Others (20,605 patients) %
Dresses self	44.8	38.6
Communicates to others understandably	18.8	35.2
Understands others	70.6	62.6
Brushes own teeth	48.9	42.2
Feeds self with knife, fork and spoon	49.6	40.3
Stays neat in grooming	27.9	26.2
Uses toilet independently	67.0	53.5
Never or infrequently wets bed	65.2	49.5
Candidate for ward helper	31.5	28.2
Candidate for work project	21.1	22.3
On work reward system	14.8	13.7

& Abelson 1969a) concluded that translocation cases of Down's syndrome in their study tended to be more active and aggressive than those with standard or mosaic trisomy. From the same census material, Moore et al. (1968) compared 536 Down's syndrome patients with an identical number of matched controls in regard to maladaptive behaviour. Of the 21 variables tested, the patients with Down's syndrome showed significantly less maladaptive behaviour in fourteen (see Table 28). The data in Tables 27 and 28 reinforce observations by others that Down's syndrome patients are more often better adjusted than populations of peers with other varieties of mental retardation. It may be added here that not all the variables in Moore et al.'s list are necessarily indicative of unreasonable behaviour. Furthermore, institutional populations of Down's syndrome tend to be less well-adjusted than those living at home, probably partly because the more behaviourally disturbed are more likely to be admitted to institutions and because large, and often overcrowded, institutional settings are certainly not always conducive to exemplary behavioural

Table 28. Maladaptive Behaviour of Down's Syndrome and other Mentally
Retarded Patients (After Moore *et al.* 1968)

Behaviour exhibited	Down's syndrome (536 patients) %	Others (536 patients) %
Hyperactive	31.7	44.6
Aggressive	36.9	46.6
Likely to escape	3.9	9.0
Self-destructive	9.0	17.7
Passive	33.6	32.3
Withdrawn	30.4	29.1
Homosexual activity	19.4	16.6
Heterosexual activity	6.3	5.2
Exposes self	12.7	14.2
Molests children	5.2	6.2
Refuses clothes	3.9	7.6
Smears faeces	7.5	9.5
Manifest psychotic behaviour	10.4	19.6
Attacks employees	2.6	11.4
Attacks patients	14.7	29.1
Destroys clothing	15.3	20.1
Destroys ward property	12.1	17.0
Breaks windows	5.2	11.6
Upsets furniture	11.4	21.6
Runs and paces	9.9	19.8
Bangs doors when secluded	6.0	13.6

patterns. Francis (1970, 1971) has documented the adverse behavioural
effects of some institutional environments.

MENTAL ILLNESS

In contrast to intellectual deficit, mental illness is generally not
considered to be a distinctive feature of Down's syndrome, though
evidence of such illness is sometimes reported. Menolascino (1965), in a
study of psychiatric problems, found that 11 of 86 Down's syndrome
children were emotionally disturbed. In these 11, absence of speech
development was common, as was a high incidence of abnormal
electroencephalograms. Disharmony in family relationships also seemed to
predispose to psychiatric disturbance.

In older patients, mental symptoms may develop as a consequence of the
changes of Alzheimer's disease in the brain (see page 62). Some reported
cases with mental illness could be explicable on this basis. Earl (1934)
described catatonia and waxy flexibility in certain instances of Down's
syndrome and considered that these symptoms were true indications of
psychosis. Similar observations were made by Rollin (1946). Other forms
of psychosis which have been noted occasionally are paranoid schizophrenia
(Neville 1959) and evidence of psychotic depression (Keegan *et al.* 1974).
Hysterical mutism also has been recorded (Bradway 1937).

5. Dermatoglyphs

The ridge patterns of the hands and feet are laid down permanently during the third month of fetal life and remain unchanged, except for an increase in size with physical growth. Normal variations of the patterns, which represent mainly hereditary differences, are found between separate populations, members of the same population and members of the same family. Differences are also found between males and females of the same population and between the hands and feet of the same individual. A comprehensive account of the genetics of dermal ridges has been published by Holt (1968).

The ridge patterns on the finger tips have been long used for personal identification (Cummins & Midlo 1943) and, based on a systematic classification proposed by Galton (1895), are still widely employed for identification purposes by police and other officials.

The examination of pattern type and detail of ridge formation, which can be undertaken separately, took on clinical and diagnostic significance when it became apparent that distinct dermatoglyphic features were associated with particular pathological conditions. Down's syndrome is the outstanding example in this regard. Cummins (1936, 1939) first demonstrated that the dermatoglyphic patterns in the syndrome were characteristic. The usefulness of such studies was also shown by Workman (1939), Holt (1951), Penrose (1954a) and Ford Walker (1957), and by many additional investigators in more recent years.

In Down's syndrome, and also in some other conditions where development is retarded, the dermal ridges are poorly formed. This is particularly noticeable at birth. Instead of ridges there appear to be irregular projections of the skin. These are often seen in the hypothenar region, but occur also in other areas of the palms and on the soles (Wolf *et al.* 1963). As the child gets older, ridges become visible in the irregular patches. The irregularities are largely concerned with the imperfectly formed pores of the sweat glands.

FINGER-TIPS

On the finger-tips the dermal ridges are arranged in patterns called arches, loops or whorls (see Fig. 21), and the classification of each pattern is based upon the number of triradii present (Penrose 1968). There is no triradius in a simple arch, only one in a loop and two in a whorl. A radial

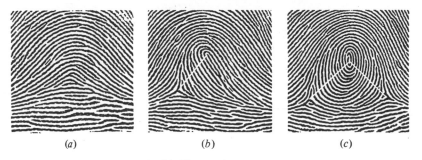

(a)   (b)   (c)

Fig. 21. Finger-print patterns.

(a) arch; no triradius and zero ridge-count;
(b) loop; one triradius and ridge-count of 10;
(c) whorl; two triradii, ridge-counts of 14 and 15.

loop opens towards the radial side of the hand and an ulnar loop towards the ulnar side. A triradius is formed at the meeting point of three fields of almost parallel ridges. The central point is sometimes represented by a dot. Theoretically, there are three radiant ridge-lines which make angles of 120° with one another. Unless the angle between radiant ridges is 90° or more, no triradius is deemed to exist. Various arrangements of ridges at triradii are shown in Fig. 22.

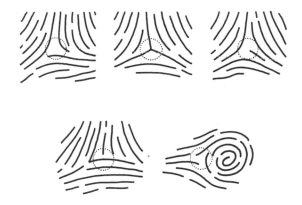

Fig. 22. Typical dermal ridge configurations. Triradial points occur at centres of the dotted circles.

Galton (1892) first attempted to evaluate the hereditary likeness in finger-print patterns and Bonnevie (1924) developed the method, quantifying the dermal patterns by counting ridges in a manner which had first been suggested by Galton. The basic mechanism for the control of finger print patterns is not known, but there is much evidence to suggest that they are determined by genes. By using the "total ridge-count" of the fingers to measure pattern size, Holt (1961) demonstrated hereditary likeness between family members (see Table 29). The correlation

Table 29. Correlation Coefficients with Standard Errors for Pairs of Relatives Normal (N) or Affected (M) with Respect to Three Dermatoglyphic Characters

Type of related pair	Total finger ridge-count (Holt 1961, 1964a)	Maximal *atd* angle (Penrose 1963b)	Third interdigital pattern (Fang 1950)
(N)–(N)			
Parent-child	0.49 ± 0.04	0.30 ± 0.04	0.43 ± 0.06
Mother-child	0.49 ± 0.04		0.26 ± 0.07
Father-child	0.50 ± 0.04		0.32 ± 0.07
Mid-parent-child	0.67 ± 0.03		
Sibs	0.50 ± 0.05	0.37 ± 0.04	0.27 ± 0.05
Like-sexed dizygotic twins	0.49 ± 0.08		
Monozygotic twins	0.95 ± 0.01	0.63 ± 0.09	0.78 ± 0.08
(N)–(M)			
Mother-child	0.49 ± 0.06	0.25 ± 0.04	
Father-child	0.41 ± 0.07	0.04 ± 0.07	
Sibs	0.46 ± 0.06	0.29 ± 0.05	
(M)–(M)			
Sibs	0.52 ± 0.14	0.22 ± 0.21	

coefficient of +0.95 for monozygotic twins, as opposed to +0.49 for dizygotic twins, is evidence of hereditary influence

The frequencies of the various dermal ridge patterns on the fingers in Down's syndrome differ from those in the general population. In the syndrome there are fewer whorls, and, contrary to the usual tendency for the frequency of arches to increase as whorls diminish, there are few arches. There is also a reduction in the frequency of radial loops and when they occur they are chiefly on digits IV and V, instead of on digit II. The deficiency of all these patterns is compensated by an increase in ulnar loops which tend to be high and L-shaped. These findings were first described by Cummins (1939) and later confirmed by Turpin & Caspar-Fonmarty (1945), Ford Walker (1957, 1958) and Holt (1961, 1964a).

The distribution of pattern types for Down's syndrome males and females is shown in Table 30. In the syndrome over 80 per cent of fingers have ulnar loops, which is nearly 20 per cent more than in the controls. Whorls, arches and radial loops are all greatly reduced in the syndrome. Nearly 70 per cent of the radial loops occur on digit IV on both hands. Of diagnostic significance is the high frequency of ulnar loops on all ten fingers. These were found in 31.1 per cent of Down's syndrome males and 38.5 per cent of Down's syndrome females. Comparable frequencies in

Table 30. Percentage Frequencies of Pattern-types on the Fingers in Down's Syndrome (D.S.) and Unrelated Controls. (After Holt 1964a)

| | Left | | | | | Right | | | | | All fingers |
	V	IV	III	II	I	I	II	III	IV	V	
D.S. MALES (167 cases)											
Whorls	11.98	21.56	7.78	3.59	10.18	13.17	2.40	4.79	26.95	18.56	12.10
Ulnar loops	86.83	72.46	88.62	86.83	80.84	83.23	93.41	94.01	67.66	79.64	83.35
Radial loops	0.60	4.19	1.20	4.19	0.00	0.60	0.60	0.60	4.19	1.80	1.80
Arches	0.06	1.80	2.40	5.39	8.98	2.99	3.59	0.60	1.20	0.00	2.75
CONTROL MALES (500 cases)											
Whorls	14.20	33.60	16.40	29.60	29.60	39.60	33.20	21.60	50.20	15.20	28.32
Ulnar Loops	84.40	63.80	72.80	38.00	66.60	58.60	30.60	69.20	47.00	84.00	61.50
Radial loops	0.00	0.00	4.20	23.00	0.40	0.20	26.60	3.40	0.80	0.40	5.90
Arches	1.40	2.60	6.60	9.40	3.40	1.60	9.60	5.80	2.00	0.40	4.28
D.S. FEMALES (143 cases)											
Whorls	16.08	22.38	6.29	8.39	14.69	12.59	6.29	4.20	28.67	13.99	13.36
Ulnar loops	81.12	68.53	90.91	86.01	74.13	84.62	90.91	94.41	65.73	85.31	82.17
Radial loops	2.10	6.29	0.70	1.40	0.70	0.00	0.00	0.70	4.90	0.70	1.75
Arches	0.70	2.80	2.10	4.20	10.49	2.80	2.80	0.70	0.70	0.00	2.73
CONTROL FEMALES (500 cases)											
Whorls	10.40	32.40	15.20	29.80	24.80	33.00	32.40	11.40	39.80	10.00	23.92
Ulnar loops	87.00	62.00	70.00	37.00	69.80	64.00	40.40	79.00	58.20	88.40	65.58
Radial loops	0.20	1.40	4.40	23.20	0.00	0.00	16.20	2.20	0.04	0.20	4.82
Arches	2.40	4.20	10.40	10.00	5.40	3.00	11.00	7.40	1.60	1.40	5.68

controls were 4.1 per cent in males and 6.9 per cent in females (Holt 1964b). Similar observations were reported by Lu (1968) and by Thompson & Bandler (1973). Combining the data from both sexes, Lu found ulnar loops on all 10 fingers in 116 of 363 Down's syndrome patients (32 per cent), 25 of 281 patients with other types of mental retardation (9 per cent) and 12 of 299 normals (4 per cent). In Thompson & Bandler's series, 39 out of 125 Down's syndrome children (31 per cent) had ulnar loops on all 10 fingers compared to 49 out of 592 normal controls (8 per cent).

In both normal and Down's syndrome sample populations, the frequency of the four basic patterns varies. The findings from different sources usually agree fairly well, and are exemplified by the results of Ford Walker (1958) and of Holt (1964a) shown in Table 31. The chief

Table 31. Pattern Frequencies in Down's Syndrome and Controls. (Holt 1964a)

	Down's Syndrome		Controls	
	N.America	U.K.	N.America	U.K.
Whorls	20.18	12.68	28.44	26.12
Ulnar loops	74.96	82.81	61.13	63.54
Radial loops	2.57	1.77	4.88	5.36
Arches	2.27	2.74	5.56	4.98
Totals	99.98	100.00	100.01	100.00

difference is in the proportions of whorls and ulnar loops in the two Down's syndrome samples, a difference which is also apparent, to a lesser extent, in the respective control groups. Results from two Oriental Down's syndrome populations (Matsui et al. 1966, Bryant et al. 1970) were similar to those given in Table 31, although the respective control groups showed a substantially higher proportion of whorls and lower proportion of ulnar loops than the controls in the Table.

The distribution of the total ridge-count on the fingers in Down's syndrome shows a marked difference from that in controls (see Table 32).

Table 32. Total Ridge-count. (After Holt 1964b)

Down's Syndrome

	Males (148)	Females (122)
Mean	130.29 ± 3.40	124.44 ± 3.01
σ	41.32	33.28

Control Population

	Males (825)	Females (825)
Mean	145.18 ± 1.76	126.97 ± 1.82
σ	50.49	52.33

The count might be determined by perfectly additive genes and the environmental effect on this character is small (Holt 1961). In the general population, mother–child, father–child and sib–sib correlations are all near to one-half. In Down's syndrome, the mother–syndrome correlation is higher than the father–syndrome correlation. This finding is similar to that shown by Penrose (1954a) for the maximal *atd* angle (see Table 29).

PALMS

The palmar dermatoglyphic configuration comprises four triradii, *a, b, c* and *d,* which can occur at the bases of the index, middle, ring and little fingers respectively. Another, known as the axial or *t* triradius, is also present. The configurational areas are the thenar, at the base of the thumb, four interdigital areas (usually numbered I to IV), the first (I) lying between the thumb and the index finger, the second (II) between the index and middle finger, and so on, and the hypothenar area (see Fig. 23).

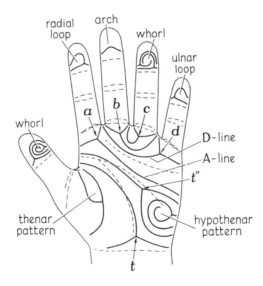

Fig. 23. Nomenclature of dermatoglyphs on palms and finger-tips. The thenar pattern as shown could be described as a loop in the first interdigital area.

The main lines are the radiants from the triradii and are indicated by corresponding capital letters; thus, the A-line corresponds to triradius *a,* and so on.

TRIRADIUS *t*

One of the most characteristic features of Down's syndrome is unusual dermal ridge markings on the palms, especially in the hypothenar region, as was first pointed out by Cummins (1939). Normally, the hypothenar ridges have a diagonal slant parallel to the A main line which originates from the *a* triradius located at the base of the second digit. The *t* triradius, in normal palms, is usually found near the flexion creases of the wrist. In Down's syndrome, however, the hypothenar ridges and the A main line tend to be transverse and a distal triradius (*t'* or *t''*) in the central area is common. Associated with *t'* or *t''* triradius in the hypothenar area is a large ulnar loop if *t* is also present (see Fig. 24). The presence or absence

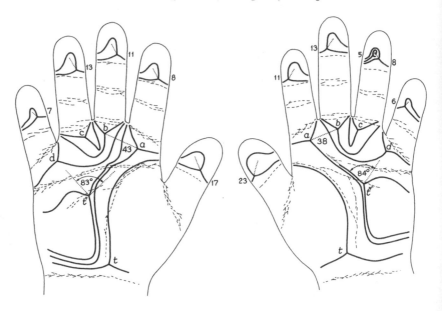

Fig. 24. Tracing of hands of Down's syndrome adult male showing finger pattern ridge-counts, maximal *atd* angles and *a−b* ridge-counts.

of pattern on the hypothenar area of the palm has been shown to be a familial trait (Weninger 1947).

Penrose (1949b, 1954a) used the *atd* angle to arrive at a quantity which could serve to replace the qualitative differentiation of a distal triradius, *t''*, from a proximal one, *t*, or from one in an intermediate position, *t'* (Cummins & Midlo 1943). The *atd* angle is that subtended at the most distal axial triradius by the most medial triradius (*d*) and the most lateral triradius (*a*) on each hand. The distribution of the *atd* angles is continuous.

The sum of the maximal *atd* angles can be compared in Down's syndrome and appropriate control series (see Table 33). It should be

Table 33. Comparison of Maximal *atd* Angles—Control Groups and Samples of Down's Syndrome

Sex	Age in years	Control population			Down's Syndrome			Index
		No.	Mean sum of R and L *atd* angles in degrees	Standard Deviation	No.	Mean sum of R and L *atd* angles in degrees	Standard Deviation	Difference of means ÷ mean S.D.
Male	0– 4	28	92.5	14.2	25	163.0	29.0	3.26
	5–14	483	88.2	15.9	75	142.2	27.9	2.47
	15–	510	85.0	15.3	32	137.3	27.5	2.44
Female	0– 4	32	97.5	19.6	16	162.0	33.5	2.43
	5–14	486	89.8	17.5	57	143.1	31.7	2.17
	15–	507	85.9	15.7	30	137.7	28.6	2.34

remembered that sex and age have to be taken into consideration when the *atd* angles are used for discriminative purposes. The distributions for this and other dermatoglyphic traits may, to some extent, vary also with ethnic background (Bryant *et al.* 1970). Penrose (1954a) found in his investigations that if the *atd* angles were the sole means of diagnosis, only 12 per cent of the Down's syndrome cases would be wrongly classified.

Family studies (Penrose 1949b, 1954a), using the measurement of the maximal *atd* angle on palms of parents and sibs of Down's syndrome individuals showed a slight but significant deviation in these relatives, as compared with controls, towards the syndrome type. The deviation is enhanced when there are two affected persons in the same sibship (see Fig. 25). The genetical factors which influence the width of the *atd* angle also

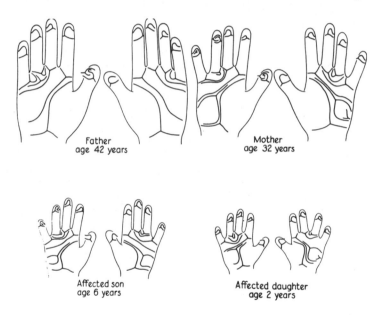

Fig. 25. Palmar main lines in familial Down's syndrome (after Penrose 1954a).

influence the susceptibility to Down's syndrome. The susceptibility appears to be increased when the predisposing genetical factors (e.g. mosaicism) are also present in the mother.

Penrose & Delhanty (1961a) noted, in their family study of the 13–15:21 translocation, that the three carriers of the chromosomal translocation had wide *atd* angles. A somewhat similar effect was observed in a family studied by Ford Walker *et al.* (1963). However, Sergovich *et al.* (1962) found no significant difference between the mean *atd* angles of eight 13–15:21 translocation carriers and thirteen non-carriers in a family that included one Down's syndrome child.

THIRD INTERDIGITAL PALMAR LOOP

The third interdigital area is located at the distal part of the palm between the bases of the middle and ring fingers. The pattern area is between the *b* and *c* triradii and the main lines B and C (see Fig. 23). Wilder (1930) described the types of configurations in this area. These can be seen in Fig. 26. The *b* triradius is nearly always present but the main

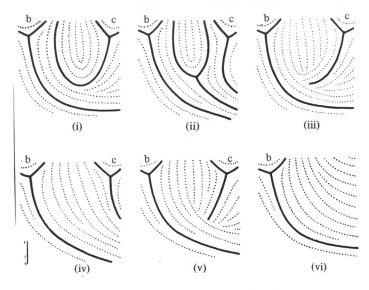

Fig. 26. Third interdigital patterns on the palm.

  (i) loop without accessory triradius (L);
  (ii) loop with accessory triradius (D);
  (iii) vestige with tendency towards loop (L^V);
  (iv) open field (O);
  (v) vestige without tendency towards loop (V);
  (vi) absence of triradius *c* (O).

line B very seldom takes part in the formation of the pattern. The type of configuration is, therefore, mainly controlled by the presence or absence of the triradius *c* and by the course of the main line C (Fang 1950).

Cummins (1939) found patterns, including vestiges, on 89.3 per cent of right and 70.2 per cent of left palms of Down's syndrome patients (see also Table 34). In a study by Snedeker (1948) it was found that 95.5 per cent of patients had a pattern in the third interdigital area of one or other palm as opposed to 40.8 per cent of the controls. She noted that the dermal patterns on the right hand tended to be well developed, whereas those on the left hand were more likely to be small loops or vestiges. The frequencies of the third interdigital pattern in Down's syndrome reported by Fang and Ford Walker are in fairly good agreement (see Table 35). The

Table 34. Percentage Incidence of Third Interdigital Configurations on the Palm

Source	Number and type of subject	Left palm			Right palm		
		True pattern	Vestige	Open field	True pattern	Vestige	Open field
Fang (1950)	205 Down's syndrome cases	52.2	26.3	21.5	83.9	8.8	7.3
Ford Walker (1957)	150 Down's syndrome cases	54.0	18.0	28.0	85.4	5.3	9.3
	1,000 controls	31.3	17.1	51.6	55.5	5.7	38.8

Table 35. Frequencies of Third Interdigital Pattern Types in Down's Syndrome and Controls

Third interdigital area of palm	Fang (1950)								Ford Walker (1957)							
	Left palm				Right palm				Left palm				Right palm			
	Down's syndrome (205)		Controls (926)		Down's syndrome (205)		Controls (926)		Down's syndrome (150)		Controls (1,000)		Down's syndrome (150)		Controls (1,000)	
	No.	%	No.	%	No.	%	No.	%	No.	%	No.	%	No.	%	No.	%
True patterns: Loop (L), Loop with accessory triradius (D), Whorl (W)	107	52.2	238	25.7	172	83.9	446	48.2	81	54.0	313	31.3	128	85.4	555	55.5
Not true patterns: Loop vestigial (L^v), Vestige (V), Open field (O)	98	47.8	688	74.3	33	16.1	480	51.8	69	46.0	687	68.7	22	14.6	445	44.5

slight deficit in the pattern frequencies in the series reported by Ford Walker is probably due to the fact that she classified loop vestigial (L^v), and vestige (V) (see Fig. 26) as "not true" patterns, whereas the other authors classified vestiges as true patterns. Although Japanese (Matsui *et al.* 1966) and Chinese (Bryant *et al.* 1970) series of Down's syndrome were found also to have a greater incidence of palmar third interdigital patterns than respective controls, the frequency of such patterns was reduced in both affected patients and controls compared to the frequencies shown in Tables 34 and 35.

Fang found the following correlation coefficients for third interdigital configurations: father—child 0.32, mother—child 0.26, total parent—child 0.43, sib-sib 0.27 and identical twins 0.78. The mode of inheritance could not be determined from these figures but there was evidence that presence or absence of pattern was influenced by environment.

OTHER PALMAR DERMATOGLYPHIC OBSERVATIONS

Palmar dermatoglyphic patterns, as well as those on the sole, have been reported in Down's syndrome by Penrose & Loesch (1970a, b) on the basis of a topological classification devised by them. The system involves a description of all loops and enumeration of all triradii. A study of the direction and termination of the C-line in the syndrome was made by Plato *et al.* (1973). Termination of the D-line on the radial border of the hand, which is rare in normal persons, occurred in 4.5 per cent of Down's syndrome patients studied by Holt (1970).

Thenar/first interdigital patterns (see Fig. 27) are unusual in Down's

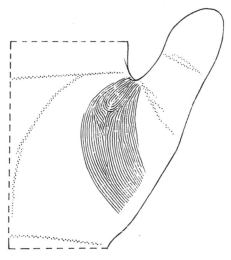

Fig. 27. Thenar/first interdigital pattern in a Down's syndrome patient (note loop with ridge-count of 4).

syndrome (Berg 1968a, Plato *et al.* 1973). They were about one-third as frequent in the syndrome as in normal controls in the series studied by Berg (see Table 36). The low incidence even in controls does not make such patterns a particularly useful discriminant for Down's syndrome. Berg reported that the intensity and size of the patterns in the syndrome were also reduced compared to controls.

Various ridge-counts have been undertaken on the palms in addition to those referred to in regard to the thenar/first interdigital area. Holt (1970) observed that there appears to be no significant difference in the a - b ridge count between Down's syndrome and normal individuals. However, ridges in the a - b interval were noted by Penrose & Loesch (1967) to be significantly narrower in Down's syndrome adults of both sexes compared to controls, a finding which was thought likely to be a reflection of the relatively short stature of persons with the syndrome. The counting of ridges between the t and d triradii provides a useful supplement, or alternative, to the *atd* angle, and was found by Berg (1968b) to discriminate well between Down's syndrome and normal persons. Some observations have also been made, in a small group of Down's syndrome patients and their parents, on the ridge-count between the point of termination of the A-line (A') and the d triradius (Glanville 1964).

Table 36. Frequencies of Thenar/First Interdigital Patterns in Down's Syndrome and Normal Controls (Berg 1968a)

	Individuals			Hands		
	No.	No. with patterns	% with patterns	No.	No. with patterns	% with patterns
Down's syndrome	300	13	4.3	600	14	2.3
Controls	300	35	11.7	600	46	7.7

TOES

Dermatoglyphic features of the toes have received much less attention than those of the finger-tips because the former are less conveniently accessible and more difficult to visualize and to print. On the feet, a fibular loop opens towards the fibular side and a tibial loop towards the tibial side, so that these loops are the counterparts, on the hand, of an ulnar and radial loop respectively. No such variations in terminology are required for whorls and arches.

Smith *et al.* (1966) examined pattern-types on the toes of Down's syndrome patients and normal controls. Differences between the two groups were apparent on comparing individual toes (see Table 37). In general, fibular loops, the most common pattern in both groups, were more frequent, and whorls less frequent, in those with Down's syndrome

Table 37. Percentage Frequencies of Pattern-types on the Toes in Down's Syndrome (D.S.) and Unrelated Controls (After Smith *et al.* 1966)

| | Left | | | | | Right | | | | | All toes |
	V	IV	III	II	I	I	II	III	IV	V	
D.S. MALES (88 cases)											
Whorls	0.0	1.2	11.5	0.0	26.4	21.6	1.2	9.1	0.0	0.0	7.1
Fibular loops	49.4	72.3	63.2	73.9	66.6	72.7	86.0	76.1	81.8	55.2	69.7
Tibial loops	2.3	4.8	2.3	.9.1	4.5	3.4	5.8	1.1	4.6	1.1	3.9
Arches	48.3	21.7	23.0	17.0	2.4	2.3	7.0	13.6	13.6	43.7	19.3
CONTROL MALES (78 cases)											
Whorls	0.0	12.8	60.0	20.5	14.0	10.0	25.7	62.5	17.9	0.0	22.3
Fibular loops	49.0	78.2	35.0	71.8	67.0	76.0	69.2	35.0	69.0	59.0	60.9
Tibial loops	5.0	0.0	0.0	1.3	14.0	6.0	0.0	0.0	1.5	0.0	2.8
Arches	46.0	9.0	5.0	6.4	5.0	8.0	5.1	2.5	11.6	41.0	14.0
D.S. FEMALES (41 cases)											
Whorls	0.0	0.0	12.2	0.0	31.7	29.2	4.8	14.6	0.0	0.0	9.2
Fibular loops	51.3	85.0	75.6	80.4	63.4	68.3	80.5	75.7	92.5	40.0	71.3
Tibial loops	0.0	2.5	9.8	9.8	4.9	2.5	2.4	2.4	2.5	0.0	3.7
Arches	48.7	12.5	2.4	9.8	0.0	0.0	12.2	7.3	5.0	60.0	15.8
CONTROL FEMALES (68 cases)											
Whorls	0.0	14.8	48.6	16.0	13.0	15.0	18.0	47.0	10.3	1.5	18.4
Fibular loops	38.0	60.2	45.5	73.5	72.0	82.0	79.0	49.0	75.0	39.7	61.4
Tibial loops	0.0	1.5	1.5	1.5	9.0	0.0	0.0	0.0	0.0	0.0	1.4
Arches	62.0	23.5	4.4	9.0	6.0	3.0	3.0	4.0	14.7	53.8	18.8

than in the controls. Less marked differences between the groups were noted for tibial loops and for arches.

SOLES

Eight configurational areas are specified on the sole (see Fig. 28). The first, I, combines the hallucal, the distal thenar and the first interdigital regions; II, III and IV are the second, third and fourth interdigital areas.

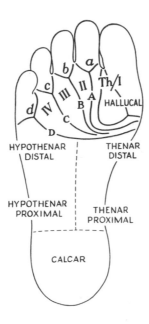

Fig. 28. Nomenclature of dermatoglyphs on sole.

These four areas usually may be distinguished not only through the presence of triradii and radiants (main lines) which limit them, but also by the fact that each often bears a discrete pattern. There are also the hypothenar distal, hypothenar proximal, thenar proximal and calcarine areas, which are usually devoid of pattern and which have not been greatly studied in Down's syndrome.

HALLUCAL AREA

The hallucal area shows seven main types of pattern: whorl, distal loop, tibial loop, fibular loop, and three types of open field pattern (see Figs. 29 to 35). Two open field patterns are associated with either an *e* or *f*

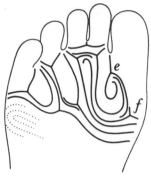

Fig. 29. Whorl pattern on hallucal area
with *e* and *f* triradii indicated (W).

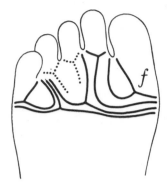

Fig. 30. Distal loop pattern on hallucal
area with *f* triradius (L).

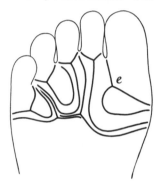

Fig. 31. Tibial loop pattern on hallucal
area with *e* triradius (T).

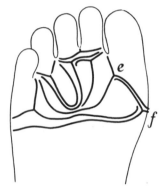

Fig. 32. Fibular loop on hallucal area
with *e* and *f* triradii (F).

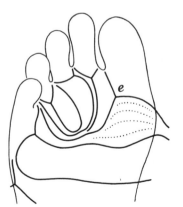

Fig. 33. Open field pat-
tern on hallucal area
with *e* triradius (O).

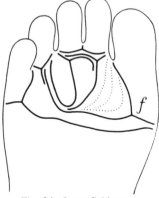

Fig. 34. Open field pat-
tern on hallucal area
with *f* triradius (O).

triradius, and the third, the tibial arch, with no specified triradius. These patterns show merging variation in the general population (Cummins & Midlo 1943, Cummins 1963).

Ford Walker (1957) pointed out the high incidence of the tibial arch (see Fig. 35) in Down's syndrome as compared with normal controls (see Table 38). In addition, she showed that persons with the syndrome could be distinguished from normal controls by the presence of a small distal

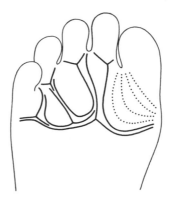

Fig. 35. Open field tibial arch pattern on hallucal area without associated *e* or *f* triradii (A).

loop, which contains 20 or less ridges. Similar findings have been noted by Smith (1964c). In his series, there were slight differences in frequencies of the patterns in males and females for both Down's syndrome and controls.

Table 38 shows that a tibial arch occurred on about half the right or left soles in Down's syndrome but on less than 0.5 per cent of normal soles. In a study of the foot prints of 750 male and female controls, a tibial arch was not found on both right and left feet of any (Smith 1964a). It should be noted, however, that a tibial arch occurs in a much higher frequency (about 5 to 6 per cent) in normal Oriental populations (Wagner 1962, Ford Walker & Johnson 1964, Matsui *et al.* 1966, Bryant *et al.* 1970) and in about 90 per cent of Oriental Down's syndrome series (Matsui *et al.*, Bryant *et al.*). Though a small distal loop is about three times as common in Down's syndrome as it is in controls (see Table 38), if the loop is considered without regard to size, its frequency is about equal in the syndrome as in controls. Whorls have a low frequency in Down's syndrome but a high frequency among controls.

A quantitative evaluation of the patterns in the hallucal area was made by Smith & Turral (1965). Ridge counts from the *f* triradius show separate distributions for Down's syndrome and controls. Males and females with the syndrome have very low counts with combined totals on both feet of 0–9 ridges The controls have much higher ridge-counts with the median total for both feet between 50 and 59 ridges. The ridge-count in the hallucal area was shown to be an inherited character. Parent–child correlations of 0.26 ± 0.09 and 0.45 ± 0.08 were found for the *e* and *f* triradii, respectively, and sib-sib correlations of 0.47 ± 0.07 and 0.40 ±

Table 38. Percentage Frequencies of Pattern Types in the Hallucal Area

Patterns	Ford Walker (1957) (Males and females combined)				Smith (1964)							
	Left sole		Right sole		(Males) Left sole		Right sole		(Females) Left sole		Right sole	
	D.S.* (116)	Controls (300)	D.S. (116)	Controls (300)	D.S. (92)	Controls (183)	D.S. (92)	Controls (183)	D.S. (53)	Controls (110)	D.S. (53)	Controls (110)
Arch tibial (A)	46.6	0.3	47.4	0.3	54.4	0.0	52.2	0.5	52.8	0.0	37.7	0.0
Small loop distal (1) (1–20 ridge counts)	33.8	10.0	31.2	13.3	30.4	10.4	28.3	12.0	30.2	9.1	43.4	12.7
Large loop distal (L) (21 or more ridge counts)	12.7	41.0	13.6	42.0	14.1	39.4	15.2	36.6	15.1	45.5	15.1	47.3
Loop tibial (T)	2.6	10.0	0.9	9.7	1.1	8.7	2.2	10.9	1.9	11.8	1.9	13.3
Whorl (W)	0.9	33.7	2.6	29.7	0.0	38.3	2.2	35.5	0.0	24.5	0.0	18.2
Others: Vestigial loop distal (L^v) Tented arch Arch fibular Loop fibular (F) Open-field (O)	3.4	5.6	4.3	5.4	0.0	2.7	0.0	4.3	0.0	9.1	1.9	8.2

*D.S. = Down's syndrome

0.08 (Smith 1964c). By using the ridge direction, Brismar (1965) also found a significant mother—child correlation for hallucal area patterns.

FOURTH INTERDIGITAL PLANTAR PATTERN

Ford Walker (1945) pointed out that a distal loop (see Fig. 36) in area IV occurs in 32 per cent of Down's syndrome soles and is about twice as

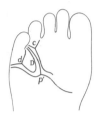

Fig. 36. Distal or digital loop (L) in the fourth interdigital area of the sole formed by main line D. Here the associated central triradius is called p '.

frequent as in controls. A similar effect was noted by Smith (1964b) who found that the loop occurred on one or both feet in 66 per cent of Down's syndrome males and 50 per cent of females. A similar loop occurred in 22 and 11 per cent of the male and female controls, respectively (see Table 39). The distal loop was shown to be an inherited dermal pattern. The parent—child correlation coefficient was + 0.20 ± 0.09.

Table 39. Percentage of Down's Syndrome Patients and Controls having a Digital Loop in the fourth Interdigital Area of the Sole on One or Both Feet, or on Neither Foot.

| | Males | | Females | |
	L present*	L absent†	L present	L absent
Down's syndrome	66	34	50	50
Controls	22	78	11	89

| | Down's syndrome | 94 males | 62 females |
| | Controls | 300 males | 250 females |

* Indicates a digital loop on one or both feet.
†Indicates the absence of a digital loop.

DERMATOGLYPHIC INDICES

On the basis of a variety of characters, which included dermatoglyphics, Turpin & Lejeune (1953) devised a quantitative measure of discrimination between Down's syndrome and normal persons. They applied this index also to the detection of a tendency towards Down's syndrome in close relatives of patients. Another system, using 8 different dermal traits, was proposed by Beckman et al. (1965). This system was based upon the sum of scores, weighted directly by the magnitude of the difference between patient and control.

More exact methods were employed by Ford Walker (1957, 1958) who made use of data on the frequencies of dermatoglyphic patterns in Down's syndrome and controls. Each finger was separately scored for whorl, arch, radial or ulnar loop. Third interdigital pattern and position of axial triradius was noted on each palm and hallucal pattern on each sole. For each feature, the relative frequency in Down's syndrome, as compared with the normal, was found. These values, treated as probabilities, were multiplied together to form an index. For convenience, the results were expressed as logarithms to the base 10 and a substantial degree of discrimination was achieved. The ratios as presented do not take into consideration that the sex difference is much greater in the control population than in the Down's syndrome population, nor do they allow for the fact that patterns on the right and left extremities are highly correlated (Holt 1959).

Indices using a combination of dermatoglyphic traits as a means of distinguishing Down's syndrome from unaffected persons, and based on discriminant analysis, have been devised by von Greyerz-Gloor et al. (1969b) and by Reed et al. (1970). Both these groups of investigators reported less overlap between Down's syndrome individuals and controls than in Ford Walker's series. To facilitate practical application of their system, Reed et al. presented a simple nomogram requiring examination of only 4 variables: the right hallucal pattern, the right atd angle and the patterns on both index fingers. Subsequent publications by Borgaonkar and his colleagues (Borgaonkar et al. 1971, 1973b, Bolling et al. 1971) described the development and testing of an index score derived from the evaluation of dermal patterns in Down's syndrome by predictive discrimination. The score was found to have a high degree of discriminative efficiency. Methods of diagnosis of Down's syndrome and of several other chromosomal disorders, by the application of discriminant function to patterns on the fingers, palms and toes, have also been elaborated by Penrose & Loesch (1971a, b). Use is made of the presence or absence of all possible loops and of certain triradii as constituent characters.

Several of the dermatoglyphic indices referred to here have recently been evaluated, on Down's syndrome and normal control populations, in a series of papers by Deckers et al. (1973 a, b, c) and in another by Oorthuys & Doesburg (1974).

EFFECT OF MOSAICISM

In an analysis of dermatoglyphic patterns in Down's syndrome mosaics Penrose (1965a, 1967) showed that for almost all traits the mosaic was intermediate between the normal and the fully affected individual. Details of dermatoglyphic patterns in 17 mosaics are given in Table 40. The Table

Table 40. Studies on Mosaicism in Down's Syndrome: Dermatoglyphic Patterns (Penrose 1967)

Serial No.	Finger-tips Left V	IV	III	II	I	Finger-tips Right I	II	III	IV	V	Palms Area III Left	Right	max atd angle Left	Right	% mongol L + R atd	Soles Hallucal area Left	Right	Area IV Left	Right
1	U	W	W	W	U	U	U	W	W	U	L	L	55	84	64	L	L	L	L
2	U	R	U	A	U	U	U	U	R	U	O	O	69	87	91	A	T	L	L
3	U	W	U	U	U	U	U	U	U	U	O	O	60	45	11	A	A	O	O
4	U	U	U	U	A	U	U	U	W	W	O	L	86	85	153	L	A	O	L
5*	U	U	U	U	U	W	U	U	W	U	O	O	43	55	23	L	A	L	O
6*	U	U	U	U	U	U	U	U	U	U	O	L	87	74	142	T	L	O	O
7	U	U	U	W	W	U	U	U	W	U	L	O	42	48	−11	A	A	O	O
8	U	U	U	R	U	W	U	U	U	U	V	L	84	79	136	A	W	O	O
9	U	W	U	U	W	U	W	U	U	U	L	L	67	64	76	W	L	O	O
10	U	U	U	W	U	U	U	U	U	W	O	L	53	46	9	L	A	O	O
11	U	W	W	U	U	U	U	U	U	U	L	L	82	82	138	A	A	L	L
12	U	U	U	U	U	U	U	U	R	U	L	L	80	80	144	T	W	O	O
13*	U	W	U	R	A	U	U	U	U	U	O	L	50	50	25	L	W	O	L
14*	U	U	U	U	W	U	U	U	U	U	L	O	48	47	3	A	A	O	O
15	U	U	U	U	U	U	U	U	U	U	O	O	52	55	20	L	L	O	O
16	U	U	U	U	U	U	U	U	U	U	O	O	51	73	41	L	L	O	O
17	U	U	U	A	U	U	U	U	U	U	O	O	62	66	39	A	A	L	L

Notes: * Indicates mother of a fully affected child
Pattern types: A, Arch; O, open field; U, ulnar loop; V, vestigial loop; L, digital loop; T, tibial loop; W, whorl; R, radial loop.

(See also Table 86)

shows the following pattern frequencies, which are between the average for normal and for standard trisomic persons. Ten ulnar loops occurred on the finger tips in 5 instances (29 per cent); a loop in the third interdigital area of the palm was present on 16 hands (47 per cent); the mean percentage deviation of the *atd* angle sum was 64 per cent towards the Down's syndrome average; a tibial arch or open field was found on the hallucal area on 16 feet (47 per cent); and a digital loop in area IV was noted on 10 feet (29 per cent).

As indicated, in mosaics the average deviation of the *atd* angles from the normal mean value is about 60 per cent of the way towards the mean position in standard Down's syndrome. Penrose (1954a) found that in a series of 223 mothers of Down's syndrome children the *atd* angles deviated by 7 per cent in the direction of the syndrome; this is consistent with the view that about 10 per cent of the mothers of Down's syndrome individuals were themselves Down's syndrome mosaics. In sibships with two affected sibs the mother's *atd* angles deviated 35 per cent towards the mean for the syndrome; thus about half of these mothers could be mosaics. On the basis of a study of parents of Down's syndrome individuals and controls, using the Walker dermatoglyphic index, Priest *et al.* (1973) tentatively estimated that the contribution of maternal and paternal mosaicism to all cases of the syndrome was about 11 per cent and 8 per cent respectively.

EFFECT OF TRANSLOCATION

Comparisons of dermatoglyphic patterns between translocation and standard trisomic cases of Down's syndrome have not shown significant differences on the fingers and palms (Soltan & Clearwater 1965, Dallapiccolo & Ricci 1967, Rosner & Ong 1967). However, Soltan & Clearwater found a substantial difference in the hallucal area, which would require confirmation in a bigger series to become well established. In particular, large distal loops were substantially more frequent in their 29 D/G translocation cases (31 per cent) than in the standard trisomics (8 per cent). The mean ridge count of the loops in the hallucal area were similar in the 2 groups. In general, dermatoglyphic examination has not proved helpful in distinguishing between translocation and standard trisomic patients.

TWINS

The dermatoglyphic patterns of monozygotic twin pairs, though individually specific in detail, are usually very similar to one another. On the corresponding hands of identical twins, the general configurations usually differ about as much from one another as do the left and right hands of an individual. One important exception was, as reported by de

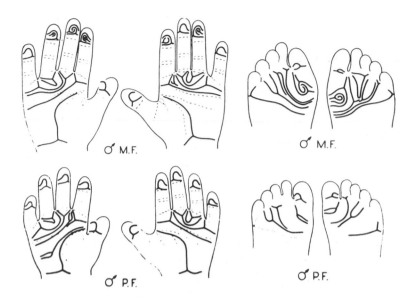

Fig. 37. Dermatoglyphic main lines on palms and soles of probably monozygotic twins; one was normal (M.F.) and the other a trisomic case of Down's syndrome (P.F.) (after Schärer 1962).

Wolff *et al.* (1962), a pair of monozygotic twins, one of whom was normal and the other a typical case of Down's syndrome. The latter's dermal patterns showed ten ulnar loops on the fingers, a distal *t* triradius on the left hand and a third interdigital loop on the right. The feet had small tibial loops in the hallucal areas. These findings were consistent with the diagnosis of Down's syndrome. The differences between the ridge patterns of the Down's syndrome twin and his normal twin, however, are less than those usually found between a person with the syndrome and a sib of the same sex (see Fig. 37).

6. Haematology

Considerable data, of varying significance, are now available on haematological aspects of Down's syndrome. The subject is considered in this chapter.

ERYTHROCYTES

While the early reports on red blood cell count, haemoglobin, cell volume and fragility test show normal variation in Down's syndrome (Benda 1960), that is to say, the distributions of the values are the same as for the normal population, later studies do not indicate that this is necessarily true. Naiman *et al.* (1965) have reported significant macrocytosis with increased packed-cell volume and mean corpuscular volume. Based upon the erythrocyte glutamic-oxaloacetic transaminase activity in the red cells, they considered macrocytosis to be the result of a young erythrocyte population. Eastham & Jancar (1969) also have shown evidence of macrocytosis; the mean cell volume for Down's syndrome adults was 102 compared with a normal range of 76-96. It has also been suggested that Down's syndrome individuals tend to have a lower haemoglobin level than normal (Kiossoglou *et al.* 1963a). In their study, the mean haemoglobin values for Down's syndrome males and females were 14.35 (S.D. 1.59) and 13.18 (S.D. 0.68) respectively; normal controls, male and female, had mean haemoglobin levels of 14.79 (S.D. 1.26) and 13.76 (S.D. 0.52) respectively.

The reticulocyte count is significantly higher in Down's syndrome adults compared to mentally retarded controls (see Table 41). Walker &

Table 41. Mean Reticulocyte and Haemoglobin Counts In Down's Syndrome and Controls (After Walker & Garrison 1966)

	Down's Syndrome		Controls	
	Male (16)	Female (15)	Male (35)	Female (35)
Reticulocyte Mean	2.24	2.26	1.68	1.65
Haemoglobin Mean	15.08	13.54	14.65	12.65

Garrison (1966) suggested that, with advancing age, the reticulocyte count in the syndrome decreases in males and increases in females.

Eastham *et al.* (1965) found plasma viscosity elevated in Down's syndrome. Plasma viscosity is probably related to the patient's age and the authors speculated that the abnormal protein found in the serum of patients with the syndrome results most probably from repeated undetected infections.

In a comprehensive study of neonatal polycythaemia, Down's syndrome was noted with a greater than expected frequency (Weinberger & Oleinick 1970). Nine of 402 polycythaemic infants (2.2 per cent) had the syndrome. Polycythaemia occurred nearly 19 times more frequently than expected, or, alternatively, nine of 61 (15 per cent) live born infants with Down's syndrome were polycythaemic compared with less than one per cent of live born infants without the syndrome. Normal haematocrits were considered to range from 50 to 65. The nine Down's syndrome infants had haematocrits ranging from 77 to 86 (see Table 42). Weinberger & Oleinick

Table 42. Haematocrits and Haemoglobins in Polycythaemic Down's Syndrome Newborns (After Weinberger & Oleinick 1970)

Sex	Birth Weight (gm.)	Haematocrit (%)	Haemoglobin (gm.%)
M	3,005	80	24
F	2,948	82	23
F	2,495	77	-
M	3,203	79	-
F	2,892	81	28
M	2,070	86	28
M	5,103	78	22
M	2,268	83	-
F	2,296	85	26

pointed out that their data support the previous suggestion of a congenital bone marrow defect in the syndrome (Ross *et al.* 1963, Behrman *et al.* 1966). Fetal erythroproliferative disorders in the syndrome have been observed by Eliachar *et al.* (1958). Examples of bone marrow dysfunction of all three cellular elements, alone or in combination, occur in the syndrome. Gruter *et al.* (1965) showed that newborn mice respond with lymphocytosis to an unidentified substance in the plasma of individuals with Down's syndrome. Associated with this there were also increased numbers of red blood cell precursors in the peripheral smears of these mice.

LEUCOCYTES

The total leucocyte count in Down's syndrome is within the normal

range (Shapiro 1949, Mittwoch 1958a, Benda 1960, Kiossoglou *et al.*
1963a). Mittwoch (1958a) found the mean leucocyte count in 50 Down's
syndrome and 50 other mentally retarded children to be 8,254 and 7,965
respectively per cm. (see Table 43). Kiossoglou *et al.* reported the mean

Table 43. The Leucocyte Count in Children (Mittwoch 1958a). Mean Number
of Cells per cm. of Blood in 50 Down's Syndrome Children and 50 Controls

Type of cell	Down's syndrome	Controls	Difference	*t* value
Total granulocytes	5,492	4,402	1,090	2.69*
Neutrophils	5,184	4,048	1,136	2.84*
Eosinophils	282	339	−57	1.00
Basophils	26	15	11	2.40*
Lymphocytes	2,102	2,888	−786	3.36*
Monocytes	660	674	−14	0.25
Total leucocytes	8,254	7,965	289	0.53

*Judged to be significant.

leucocyte count for Down's syndrome males and females to be 7,167 and
8,165 respectively and for controls, males and females, as 8,450 and 9,538
respectively. The conclusion to be drawn is that, when there is any
increased leucocytosis in Down's syndrome, it is probably associated with
infection (Mittwoch).

A low lymphocyte count has been found in Down's syndrome children
in the age group 3 to 6 years (Mittwoch 1958a, Benda 1960), and
this was associated with an increased neutrophil count. The relative
neutrophil counts were significantly increased; for example, 5,184 or 62.9
per cent for Down's syndrome and 4,048 or 50.9 per cent for controls.
Normally, infants have a relatively high lymphocyte count which falls with
increasing age. At the age of 4 years lymphocytes and neutrophils should
be present in about equal numbers (Kato 1935) and thereafter the
lymphocyte count continues to fall throughout childhood. This reduction
of lymphocytes is not obvious in young Down's syndrome children since
they have a constantly low lymphocyte count during this period. In
Down's syndrome adults, the percentages of neutrophils and lymphocytes
are about the same as those found in the normal population (Shapiro
1949, Kiossoglou *et al.*).

Evidence has accumulated that, in patients with Down's syndrome, the
nuclei of the polymorphonuclear neutrophil cells have fewer lobes than
normal. This peculiarity was first explored by Turpin & Bernyer (1947)
and has since been considered by others (Shapiro 1949, Ridler & Shapiro
1959, Mittwoch 1957). Polymorphonuclear leucocyte lobe counts for
Down's syndrome males are 2.11 and for females 2.19; for control
males and females the counts are 2.62 and 2.61 respectively (Mittwoch
1958b, 1964a). There was a statistically significant difference independent
of the absolute neutrophil count (see Fig. 38). No sex difference was noted

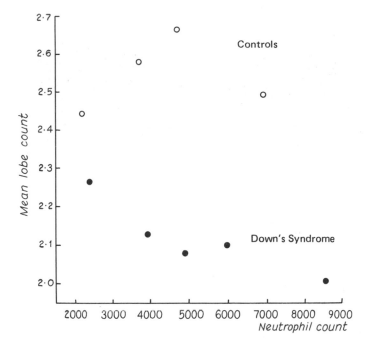

Fig. 38. Mean lobe count compared with neutrophil count in 50 Down's syndrome individuals and 50 controls. Each circle indicates the mean of 10 cases grouped by neutrophil count (after Mittwoch 1958b).

in these studies. Kiossoglou *et al.* have since called attention to the fact that normal adult females have a significantly lower total lobe count than males, and that normal males and females show a decrease in the total lobe count with increasing age. Kluge (1959) also recorded a lower total lobe count, considered to be a leucocyte shift to the left. He compared this with findings associated with the Pelger-Huët anomaly (Pelger 1928, Huët 1932).

Davidson & Robertson Smith (1954) made the discovery that a proportion of the polymorphonuclear neutrophil leucocytes of females carried a nuclear appendage which they called a drumstick (See Fig. 39). The average incidence of drumsticks in normal females is 14 for every 500 neutrophilic cells. In Down's syndrome females the incidence is very low with a mean of 3.8 per 500 cells. Mittwoch (1959, 1964b) showed that the low incidence of drumsticks observed in Down's syndrome was connected with the lowered lobe count; however, a comparison of cells with a constant lobe number suggested that the inhibition of drumstick formation was greater than the inhibition of lobe formation. The same phenomenon was also found in Klinefelter's syndrome and in triple X females.

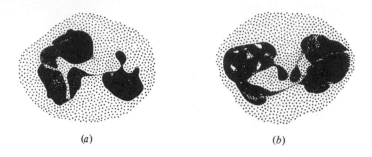

(a)   (b)

Fig. 39. Polymorphonuclear neutrophil leucocyte with (a) one and (b) two
drumsticks

PLATELETS

An increase in platelet number and size, in association with a myeloproliferative disorder in a case of Down's syndrome, was reported by Miller *et al.* (1967). The authors suggested that an ineffective regulation of production and maturation of the bone marrow elements was operative in the syndrome. Qualitative platelet abnormalities, including polycythaemia and disseminated intravascular coagulation, have been found in a Down's syndrome infant (Pochedly & Ente 1968).

Piussan *et al.* (1973) reported congenital thrombocytopenia with megakaryocytosis in the neonatal period of an infant with Down's syndrome. There was a partial regression of the condition by the time the child was 7 months of age. No other blood lines were affected. The authors attributed the thrombocytopenia to the trisomy 21, though the pathogenesis of the haematological disorder was not established.

NEONATAL JAUNDICE

Prolonged and occasionally marked neonatal jaundice (Zuelzer & Brown 1961), associated with an elevated haemoglobin and a high haematocrit reading, has been observed in newly born Down's syndrome infants. The significance of these observations is not clear. Panizon (1965) showed a significant elevation in the bilirubin levels of Down's syndrome infants when compared with matched controls. The mean of the highest levels of bilirubin (per 100 ml serum) reached in each case was 15.2 mg± 5.1 for the Down's syndrome group and 8.1 ± 4.2 for the control group. Additional haematological investigations were performed and the only other abnormal finding was that the mean haematocrit value was significantly higher in the Down's syndrome group. Naiman *et al.* (1965) proposed that the red-cell lifespan may be shortened in Down's syndrome. This could be an explanation for the neonatal hyperbilirubinaemia;

however, Panizon measured red-cell lifespan and found the red cells to be in the range of the normal newborn population. He argued that hyperbilirubinaemia must be considered to be metabolic rather than haemolytic in nature.

Renkonen et al. (1968) noted an increased incidence of erythroblastosis in Down's syndrome infants. ABO immunized mothers and mothers of hyperbilirubinaemic children had more children with Down's syndrome than expected. Two explanations were offered. Either children with Down's syndrome are often hyperbilirubinaemic or ABO-immunized mothers have a higher incidence of children with the syndrome. The authors found more cases of Down's syndrome among erythroblastotic (0.45 per cent) than among non-erythroblastotic children (0.14 per cent).

ABO BLOOD GROUPS

Early investigation on the distribution of antigens in the blood in Down's syndrome were justified on the grounds that they might shed light on the hypothesis that these persons have some genetical affinity to

Table 44. Distribution of the ABO Antigens in Down's Syndrome
(i) Observed numbers

Source	District	O	A	B	AB	Total
Orel (1927)	Vienna, Austria	15	21	7	1	44
Penrose (1932a)	Eastern Counties, England	66	83	14	3	166
Bixby (1939)	Massachusetts, U.S.A.	60	48	12	5	125
Lang-Brown et al. (1953)	London, England	81	53	9	5	148
	Total	222	205	42	14	483

(ii) Expected numbers based upon population surveys

Source	District	O	A	B	AB	Total
Routil (1933)	Vienna, Austria (4,170)	15.7	18.5	6.9	2.8	43.9
Penrose & Penrose (1933)	Eastern Counties, England (1,000)	71.7	79.2	10.6	4.5	166.0
Landsteiner & Levine (1929)	New York State, U.S.A. (1,708)	55.6	47.4	16.5	5.6	125.1
Ikin et al. (1939)	London, England (3,459)	64.3	66.1	12.7	4.8	147.9
	Total	207.3	211.2	46.7	17.7	482.9

Mongolian populations. The approach was of questionable value (Keynes 1932). Nevertheless, from these studies it was demonstrated that the distribution of the ABO antigens in samples of Down's syndrome did not differ appreciably from that in the general populations from which they were drawn (Orel 1927, Penrose 1932a).

More recent studies (Lang-Brown *et al.* 1953, Shaw & Gershowitz 1962, 1963, Kaplan *et al.* 1964) have shown that, although the distribution of the ABO antigens in Down's syndrome is similar to that in the general population, there are slight differences in frequency which may be of importance (see Table 44). In the survey by Lang-Brown *et al.* there was an excess of group O Down's syndrome individuals; this could have been due to an excess of group O mothers in the survey. However, it has also been shown that there is an increase of group O infants in older maternal age groups of mothers of normal children (Boorman 1950). Shaw & Gershowitz reported that there were too few group O Down's syndrome individuals and an excess in Group A (see Table 45). Attempts have been

Table 45. Comparison of ABO Blood Groups for Down's Syndrome and Controls (After Shaw & Gershowitz 1963)

	A No.	A %	B No.	B %	AB No.	AB %	O No.	O %	Total
Down's Syndrome	443	(44.3)	116	(11.6)	36	(3.6)	405	(40.5)	1,000
Controls	621	(41.2)	144	(9.6)	55	(3.6)	688	(45.6)	1,508

made to locate the ABO locus on chromosome 21, based upon segregation ratios in a family of translocation Down's syndrome (Shaw 1962a); there is, however, no serological evidence of the triplication of the ABO locus in standard trisomic Down's syndrome (Lawler 1962).

Theoretical formulae for gene frequencies under disomic and trisomic conditions have been worked out by Bateman (1960) and Kaplan *et al.* An extension of these formulae to cover crossing over during the first division of meiosis had been published by Penrose (1963a). The data of Kaplan *et*

Table 46. Observed O and AB Group Proportions in Down's Syndrome and Controls. (After Kaplan *et al.* 1964)

	Down's syndrome		Controls					
			Population		School children		Blood donors	
Blood group	No.	%	No.	%	No.	%	No.	%
O Group	123	42.2	1,586	41.0	609	38.6	840	42.9
AB Group	15	5.2	201	5.2	89	5.6	124	6.3
Total number tested	(290)		(3,871)		(1,578)		(1,959)	

al. on ABO group frequencies fits disomic gene frequencies rather than trisomic. From their data they concluded that the ABO locus was not on chromosome 21. There was good agreement between the AB and O blood groups for Down's syndrome and controls (see Table 46). The data suggested a slight increase in the number of group O Down's syndrome individuals over the controls, similar to that found by Lang-Brown *et al.*

Goodman & Thomas (1966) determined the ABO blood types of a large Down's syndrome group. They found a slight deficiency of types O and B and a slight excess of types A and AB. Their data did not support or contradict the hypothesis of linkage of the ABO locus to chromosome 21. They concluded that linkage of any locus exhibiting complete dominance will be difficult to establish using population gene frequencies analysis, unless the locus is absolutely linked to the kinetochore and trisomies arise largely or solely through first meiotic division by non-disjunction.

Penrose (1957) pointed out that, in the case of Down's syndrome, not only has it been impossible to demonstrate any unusual maternal—fetal incompatibility but the evidence tends in the other direction, namely towards an unusual degree of similarity in blood group phenotype. A possible explanation is the fact that Down's syndrome children are born, on the whole, at late maternal ages and thus tend to be at the end of large families. In such data, families showing examples of antigenic incompatibility are not likely to be represented.

OTHER BLOOD GROUP SYSTEMS AND HAEMOGLOBINS

Lang-Brown *et al.* presented blood type data on over 100 families, each selected by the presence of at least one case of Down's syndrome. No gross anomalies in the distribution of the antigens MNS, Rhesus, P, Lewis and Kell were observed either in the propositi or their sibs. Slight deficits of Rhesus D^+, Le(a—) and Kell$^+$ cases among Down's syndrome individuals were noted as compared with the general population estimates. They concluded that Down's syndrome cannot result from antigenic incompatibility between mother and fetus for any of the antigens studied. In most of these systems (see Table 47) maternal and fetal phenotypes are more similar than would be expected on the random mating hypothesis (Penrose 1957). Specific observations on Rhesus incompatibility have indicated that this is not a predisposing factor for Down's syndrome (Turpin *et al.* 1947, Pantin 1951). Weinstein & Rucknagel (1964) studied sickle and fetal haemoglobins in 91 Down's syndrome Negroes. The number with the sickle cell trait was similar to that in controls and there was no evidence that the beta or gamma haemoglobin loci were on chromosome 21. Seven Down's syndrome individuals had a significantly elevated fetal haemoglobin but it was thought that this was a non-specific response and not a trisomic gene effect.

Table 47. Degree of Significance in Similarity of Phenotype in Parent and Child. (Penrose 1957)

Antigen system	Values of χ^*	
	Mother	Father
ABO	+3.33	−1.18
MNS	+0.22	+0.11
CDE	+1.61	−0.60
P	+2.52	+1.22
Lewis	+0.97	−0.90
Kell	+1.86	+1.36
Total	+10.51	+0.01
S.E.	±2.46	±2.46

*The normal variate.

Price Evans *et al.* (1966) studied 82 Down's syndrome-normal sib pairs and their parents at Liverpool and a similar number of pairs at Buffalo, New York. The bloods were examined for A_1, A_2, BO, Lewis, MNSs, Rh, P_1, Duffy, Kell, Lutheran, Kidd, Vw, Ml^a and Di^a. Secretor salivas were tested for ABH secretor status. The results were added to the previous data of Lang-Brown *et al.* (1953) and showed no significant association between blood-group phenotype and Down's syndrome, except in the case of Kell, where a significant excess of Kell-positive cases were found. The investigators raised the possibility that the Kell locus may be on chromosome 21.

Weinstein *et al.* (1965) studied 91 black Down's syndrome patients and a similar group of matched controls. There was no significant difference in the level of Hb A_2 Between the two groups. Four of the Down's syndrome individuals with sickle cell trait had levels of Hb S comparable to those of otherwise normal Hb A-S heterozygotes. The finding of seven cases of Down's syndrome with elevated fetal haemoglobin was thought to be a result of the nonspecific developmental retardation of the trisomic individual.

Rittner & Schwinger (1973) found no association for Down's syndrome and the following: ABO, Rh(D), MNSs, K, P, Fy(a, b), JK(a, b), Gm(1, 2), InV(1), Ag(X), Lp(a), TF, C_3, acP, PGM_1, and GPT. None of these markers was associated with age or the presence or absence of the Au/SH antigen in Down's syndrome. Gm(+1) was more frequent in the syndrome than among normal controls.

Rittner & Rittner (1973) investigated the Xh serum factor in Down's syndrome. They concluded that affected persons have higher concentrations of this antigen than do other mentally retarded individuals and that the frequency of Xh positive reactions in the syndrome appears to be age-dependent.

GRANULOPOIESIS AND GRANULOCYTE KINETICS

Differences in the leucocyte population in Down's syndrome have been demonstrated morphologically and enzymatically. It has been suggested that the mean age of the granulocyte population is shortened (Mellman *et al.* 1967, 1970). This could be reflected in a higher enzyme activity which is frequently associated with immature cells (Hook & Engel 1964). Mellman *et al.* (1967) presented leucokinetic studies indicating a shortened mean circulating half-life in several adult males with Down's syndrome and significant increase in granulocyte turnover rate in these patients. In contrast to this, Galbraith & Valberg (1966) presented normal leucocyte survival curves in four adults with Down's syndrome. In addition, normal mean blood granulocyte mass and turnover rates were determined. Pearson (1967) noted normal mitotic and maturation granulocyte pools in the syndrome and these were evidenced by the finding of normal marrow cellularity and morphology. Endotoxin injections indicated a normal marrow granulocyte reserve. Normal levels of serum muramidase support the concept of a normal granulocyte turnover rate. Pearson considered it unlikely that the increases in leucocyte enzymes are due to a relatively immature granulocyte population. Rather, they may reflect some general effect of genetic imbalance.

CAPILLARY FRAGILITY

Abnormal capillary fragility was detected in 60 of 74 Down's syndrome patients by Dallapiccola *et al.* (1971). The authors speculated on factors involved in the production of capillary fragility in the syndrome. These included congenital abnormalities of the capillaries, connective tissue and platelets, as well as poor dietary intake of vitamin C and bioflavonids.

LIVER ABNORMALITIES

Mori & Koike (1971) studied the livers of 16 autopsy cases of Down's syndrome. They observed giant cell transformation of hepatic cells with fibrosis in a severe form in three cases and a milder form in an additional three cases. The authors considered the findings consistent with those in neonatal hepatitis and that the changes could have progressed to a cirrhotic liver condition.

LEUKAEMIA

A concurrence of Down's syndrome and acute leukaemia of childhood was first suggested in 1954 by Bernard *et al.* who described three cases in

France. Isolated examples of the association of the two conditions can be found in the literature before that time (Bernhard *et al.* 1951, Schunk & Lehman 1954). Additional reports, published by Krivit & Good (1956) and Merrit & Harris (1956), fostered a greater awareness of the association. This led Krivit & Good (1957) to send questionnaires to 300 hospitals in the United States concerning children under four years of age with Down's syndrome and leukaemia. Thirty-four cases of leukaemia associated with Down's syndrome for the years 1952-55 were reported. They estimated that, if chance alone were operating, 12.3 cases of combined leukaemia and Down's syndrome would be expected to occur. There was thus a three-fold increase in the association of the two conditions. Stewart *et al.* (1958) in Great Britain made a similar observation. They reported that 17 out of 677 childhood deaths from leukaemia during 1953-55 were associated with Down's syndrome. From their study, the risk of Down's syndrome children developing leukaemia was 20 times that of the normal population. Additional surveys have confirmed the original findings. Jackson *et al.* (1968) surveyed the incidence in California State hospitals and gave a risk figure of 12 times that for the normal population. Wald *et al.* (1961) in Pennsylvania gave the highest figure—61 times the normal population risk. In a Swiss survey (deWolff 1964), 5 out of 134 Down's syndrome children investigated had leukaemia. The frequency of leukaemia in the syndrome was eight to nine times higher than among normal children from the same locality. More recently, Evans and Steward (1972) in Manchester put the risk at 10 to 18 times that in the normal child population. With the widespread use of antibiotics and the repair of congenital heart abnormalities, leukaemia may become an important lethal factor in the syndrome (Fabia & Drolette 1970b).

Rosner & Lee (1972) produced evidence from several American hospitals that acute leukaemia in children with Down's syndrome may be no different in incidence or in distribution of cell types from leukaemia which occurs in normal children. Their observations on incidence figures are not in total agreement with those quoted above. Rosner & Lee had 43 patients (41 children and two adults) with Down's syndrome and leukaemia in their study group. Of these, 70 per cent had acute lymphoblastic and 30 per cent had acute myeloblastic leukaemia. There were nine newborns with a leukaemia-like picture. Seven of the newborns had myeloblastic, one lymphoblastic leukaemia and one had a leukaemoid-leukaemic reaction. Rosner & Lee reviewed the world literature and found 276 recorded cases of Down's syndrome and leukaemia (see Table 48). Forty-seven were new-borns, 227 were children below 20 years of age and two were adults. Of the 227 children, 30.9 per cent had acute myeloblastic leukaemia and 69.1 per cent had acute lymphoblastic leukaemia. Among the 47 newborns with Down's syndrome, 57.9 per cent had myeloblastic leukaemia and 42.1 per cent had lymphoblastic leukaemia (see Table 49). Chronic leukaemia, both myelogenous and lymphocytic, myelofibrosis and myeloid metaphasia are extremely rare in Down's syndrome. Acute

Table 48. 276 Reported Cases of Down's Syndrome and Leukaemia (After Rosner & Lee 1972)

	Children	Newborns
Acute leukaemia		
Granulocytic		
Acute myeloblastic leukaemia	41*	26†
Acute erythroleukaemia	2‡	1‡
Acute monocytic leukaemia	1	1‡
Acute promyelocytic leukaemia	2	0
Lymphocytic		
Acute lymphoblastic leukaemia	62	5
Acute stem cell leukaemia	32	4*
Acute hemocytoblastic leukaemia	2	1
Other		
Leukaemic reticuloendotheliosis	1	1
Acute leukoblastic leukaemia	3	0
Acute leukaemia, type NOT specified	77	6
Chronic leukaemia		
Chronic myelogenous leukaemia	4	2
Chronic lymphocytic leukaemia	2	0
Totals	229	47

*Two patients had "transient" leukaemia.
†Fifteen patients had "transient" leukaemia.
‡One patient had "transient" acute leukaemia.

Table 49. Morphologic Types of Acute Leukaemia in Down's Syndrome (After Rosner & Lee 1972)

	Acute Myeloblastic Leukaemia (%)	Acute Lymphoblastic Leukaemia (%)
Summary of Literature		
Down's syndrome children	30.9	69.1
Down's syndrome newborns	57.9	42.1
Current Data		
Down's syndrome children	30.2	69.8
Down's syndrome newborns	80.0	20.0

erythremic myelosis or DiGuglielon's leukaemia has been reported (Juberg & Jones 1970. Kung et al. 1970). Well documented reports of leukaemia and Down's syndrome have been published by Ross & Atkins (1962) and Vincent et al. (1963).

Lashof & Stewart (1965) first reported that the peak in leukaemia mortality in Down's syndrome occurs at one year of age, which is two to

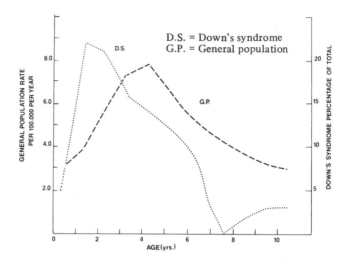

Fig. 40. Distribution of leukaemia mortality by age in Down's syndrome as compared with that in the general population in the United States 1950-59. (After Miller 1970)

three years earlier than in the general population (see Fig. 40). A peculiar geographic difference in the rates of leukaemia and Down's syndrome has been reported among institutionalized patients in Pennsylvania (Wald *et al.* 1961) where it was found to be much higher than in California (Jackson *et al.* 1968). The California investigators suggested that environmental factors accounted for the different results in the two States. These views were refuted by Miller (1970) who found no geographic difference in the incidence of the two conditions in the United States.

Information on leukaemia in mosaic and translocation forms of Down's syndrome are difficult to evaluate because of the relative rarity of these forms of the syndrome. However, a relationship possibly exists. Behrman *et al.* (1966) described two sibs with G/G translocation Down's syndrome with a leukaemoid reaction at birth. One sib recovered and the other died with a diagnosis of chronic myelocytic leukaemia. Acute lymphocytic leukaemia has been reported in a D/G translocation carrier (Whang-Peng *et al.* 1969).

Down's syndrome and leukaemia have been found in the same family (Buckton *et al.* 1961, Miller 1963). Miller reported 5 cases of Down's syndrome among 1,000 sibs of leukaemic patients. One Down's syndrome individual also had co-existent leukaemia. Buckton *et al.* described a sibship of three Down's syndrome children, one phenotypically normal child and one abortion. At the time of investigation two of the Down's syndrome children were dead and the third had 46 chromosomes with a (13–15) : 21 translocation. The mother had 45 chromosomes and a similar translocation, while the phenotypically normal child had died at 4 years of age with acute leukaemia. Stewart (1961) reported a sibship in which a Down's syndrome male had stem-cell leukaemia and a normal sister died of lymphatic leukaemia. Miller *et al.* (1961) described a family with an XXXXY male, a leukaemic male and two standard trisomic females, all closely related.

NEONATAL LEUKAEMIA (CONGENITAL)

There is an increased incidence of congenital leukaemia in Down's syndrome. It is among this group of infants that spontaneous remissions have been reported (De Carvalho 1963, Honda *et al.* 1964). A number of these infants in whom spontaneous remission has occurred were never given antileukaemic medications (Schunk & Lehman 1954, Ross *et al.* 1963, Lahey *et al.* 1963, Engel *et al.* 1964, Conen & Erkman 1966, Behrman *et al.* 1966, Nagao *et al.* 1970). Spontaneous remissions of congenital leukaemia in patients with normal karyotypes seem to be rare but have been reported (Stransky 1968, van Eys & Flexner 1969). Undoubtedly, some of the diagnoses of congenital leukaemia in Down's syndrome were mistakenly made for other haematological problems; however, what appear to be well authenticated cases have been reported. No adequate explanation has been put forward to account for the remissions in these cases. Some authors have speculated that the condition might be an abnormal leucocyte response to stress, e.g. severe infection or haemolytic disease.

TRANSIENT LEUKAEMIA

Evidence keeps accumulating which indicates that all the cells of the haematopoietic system are in some way abnormal in the syndrome. Many of the differences may be subtle and, on routine haematological studies, they may not be recognized. Turpin & Bernyer, as early as 1947, recognized that the nuclei of the polymorphonuclear cells in the syndrome have fewer than the normal number of lobes (see p. 102). In addition, it has been known for many years that certain leucocyte, lymphocyte and erythrocyte enzyme levels are abnormal (see p. 132). Probably the greatest liability of the haematopoietic system occurs during the newborn period and may be detected as an abnormal proliferation of the granulocytes, erythrocytes, platelets or all three. Certainly, the most unusual manifestation of an abnormality of the haematopoietic system is the "transient leukaemia" occurring in the newborn period of life.

Of interest are the cases of Down's syndrome with clinical and haematological signs resembling acute leukaemia in whom the abnormal haematological findings disappear without treatment. Rosner & Lee summarized 22 such cases reported in the literature (see Table 50). The

Table 50. Transient Acute Leukaemia in Patients with Down's Syndrome
(After Rosner & Lee 1972)

Case No.	Reference	Type of Leukaemia	Age at Diagnosis	Associated Conditions	Outcome
1	Schunk & Lehman, 1954	Acute monocytic	Newborn	Rh incompatibility	Died 6 yr of age; no evidence of leukaemia
2	Eliachar et al., 1958	Erythroleukaemia	1 yr	Severe pulmonary infection	No mention of leukaemia at autopsy
3	De Carvalho, 1963	Stem cell	Newborn	ABO incompatibility	Complete recovery; haematologically normal at age 4 yr
4	Lahey et al., 1963	Myeloblastic	3½ mo	None stated	Normal at 16 mo of age
5	Ross et al., 1963	Myeloblastic	Newborn	Facial rash	Complete recovery; no evidence of leukaemia at autopsy nearly 3 yr later
6	Engel et al., 1964 Case 1	Myeloblastic	Newborn	Rash	No leukaemia at age 3 yr when patient died
7	Case 2	Myeloblastic	Newborn	Otitis media	Haematologically normal at 3 yr of age
8	Case 3	Myeloblastic	Newborn	None stated	Haematologically normal at 9 mo of age
9	Mattelaer & Riley, 1964	Acute myeloblastic	Newborn	Pneumonia and icterus	No leukaemia found at autopsy
10	Conen & Erkman, 1966	Myeloblastic	Newborn	Fever and diarrhoea	No leukaemia found at autopsy at 8 mo of age
11	Behrman et al., 1966	Leukaemoid reaction	Newborn	None	Complete recovery; haematologically normal at 3 yr of age
12	Wegelius et al., 1967	Blastic	Newborn	None stated	Complete recovery; haematologically normal at 4 yr of age
13	Germain et al., 1967	Myeloblastic	39 days	Pulmonary infections	Haematologically normal at 17½ mo of age
14	Halikowski et al., 1968	Leukoerythroblastic	Newborn	None stated	Haematologically normal at 2 mo
15	Drescher et al., 1968	Erythroleukaemia	Newborn	Congenital heart disease and cirrhosis	Erythromyeloid hyperplasia of liver, spleen and lymph nodes found at autopsy but not leukaemia
16	Drescher et al., 1968	Leukaemoid reaction	Newborn	Jaundice and cirrhosis	No evidence of leukaemia at autopsy
17	Chan, 1969	Myeloblastic	Newborn	ABO incompatibility	Haematologically normal at 2 mo of age; died 4 wk later of sepsis. no evidence of leukaemia at autopsy
18	Tanaka & Okada, 1969	Leukaemoid reaction	Newborn	None stated	Died of sepsis at age 2 wk; no evidence of leukaemia but granulocytic hyperplasia at autopsy
19	Chaptal et al., 1970 Case 1	Myeloblastic	Newborn	Jaundice	Haematologically normal at 7 yr of age
20	Case 3	Lymphoblastic	3 yr	None stated	No evidence of leukaemia at autopsy; died of Candida sepsis
21	Case 4	Myeloblastic	Newborn	Congenital heart disease and 2° polycythaemia	Haematologically normal at 4 mo of age
22	Nagao et al., 1970	Myeloblastic	Newborn	None stated	Haematologically normal at 1½ yr of age

findings of leukaemia spontaneously disappeared over a period of weeks or months. Eighteen of the patients were newborns, one was a 39 day old infant, another was a three and one-half month old baby, and two others were one and three years old respectively. All 22 patients had complete clinical and haematological recovery. Of those who died, no evidence of leukaemia was found at postmortem examination. Death was usually caused by intercurrent infection. Three of the newborns with transient leukaemia had major blood group incompatibility (one Rh and two ABO). Jaundice without blood group incompatibility was present in three other newborns. Three patients had severe pulmonary infections after birth. Congenital cyanotic heart disease was present in at least two patients and cirrhosis in two others. In only seven of the 22 patients with Down's syndrome and transient leukaemia was an associated condition present that might explain the transient abnormal haematological findings. Ross *et al.* (1963) have referred to transient leukaemia as an ineffective regulation of granulopoiesis masquerading as congenital leukaemia in a Down's syndrome child. The important difference, according to Rosner & Lee, between children with Down's syndrome and normal children, is not in the incidence of leukaemia but in the incidence of transient leukaemoid reaction resembling leukaemia which occurs rarely in normal children but not infrequently in children with Down's syndrome.

RISK OF LEUKAEMIA IN FAMILY MEMBERS

There are some data indicating that autosomal and sex chromosomal aneuploidy are not randomly distributed in the population but tend to concentrate in some families (Hecht *et al.* 1964). There is also a suggestion that childhood leukaemia is part of this constellation of familial diseases (Miller 1964). Good epidemiologic information is equivocal in this regard, but Miller thinks that if there is an increased risk it is less than five times greater than the normal expectation. There does not seem to be an increased risk of leukaemia in the parents of Down's syndrome children, according to Holland *et al.* (1962), even though it was noted that three fathers of Down's syndrome children died of leukaemia.

OTHER MALIGNANCIES

Holland *et al* (1962) studied leukaemia in Down's syndrome in relation to other forms of cancer. In Down's syndrome with leukaemia they found that the death rate was 18 times that in the general population and, for other malignancies, the death rate was 2½ times that in the general population. The factor of 2½ was not considered statistically significant but the factor of 18, for leukaemia in Down's syndrome, was significant and in agreement with that in earlier reports. No specific type of cancer other than leukaemia was identified. The same authors also studied deaths from cancer in the parents of Down's syndrome individuals and the observed and expected numbers did not differ significantly. In general, the types of cancers were in the same proportions as in the general population. Turner (1963) and Miller (1970) also made large surveys.

At the present time there is no good evidence that any form of cancer other than leukaemia is associated with Down's syndrome. While other cancers have been found in Down's syndrome individuals (see Table 51), a relationship has not been established and may go unnoticed since other childhood cancers are far less common than leukaemia. As Miller (1970) has pointed out, recognition of a link of other forms of cancer with Down's syndrome may be difficult on anything less than a national scale unless the strength of the association is immense. As seen in Table 51,

Table 51. Cancers in Mortality Studies of Down's Syndrome (After Miller 1970)

Total Size of Samples	Leukaemia	Brain Cancer	Retino- blastoma	Testes Cancer	Other
Pooled Prospective Down's Syndrome Series					
5,607	17	2	1	2	8
Pooled Death-Certificate Surveys for Cancer					
43,137	189	3	1	0	5

brain tumours have been reported in the syndrome but probably occur no more often than would be expected by chance. This was also shown by Stewart *et al.* (1958) when only one case of brain tumour was found in a Down's syndrome individual. Only two instances of Hodgkin's disease occurring in Down's syndrome have been reported (McCormick *et al.* 1971); thus there seems to be no link between the two conditions even though G-group chromosome aberrations have been noted in lymph node cultures from Hodgkins disease patients. There have been individual case reports of retinoblastoma (Taktikos 1964), seminoma (Matsaniotis *et al.* 1967) and phaechromocytoma (Kuni 1973) in Down's sydrome.

Stoller *et al.* (1973) carried out two surveys to discover if there was an association between Down's syndrome and malignancy or congenital abnormalities. A questionnaire survey was conducted on the families of 341 Down's syndrome subjects. The results failed to show any variation in cancer and leukaemia morbidity compared with the normal population, nor was there any significant variation in the incidence of congenital malformations. A search of the cancer register in Victoria was made to assess the prevalence of cancer in mothers of Down's syndrome individuals. Forty-four mothers developed cancer as compared with an expected number of 47 based upon a similar age grouping.

CHROMOSOMES IN DOWN'S SYNDROME INDIVIDUALS WITH LEUKAEMIA

The results of peripheral blood chromosomal studies on Down's syndrome individuals with leukaemia have been varied. The first report (Tough *et al.* 1961) on 5 cases showed no abnormalities except standard trisomy. Later studies have described cell lines with 48 (Johnston 1961, Warkany *et al.* 1963), 49 (Ross *et al.* 1963, Vincent *et al.* 1963), 51 (Kiossoglou *et al.* 1963b) and 54 (Lejeune *et al.* 1963) chromosomes. Johnston reported a 3-year-old Down's syndrome boy with myelogenous leukaemia. Blood cultures before treatment showed that a major portion of the cells contained 47 chromosomes with trisomy in group 21–22; but a few cells contained 48 chromosomes (extra chromosome in group 7–12), a chromosomal fragment and chromosomal breaks. After treatment the chromosomal number was 47 and no additional chromosomes or fragments were seen. Two collateral adult male relatives had died of leukaemia. A Down's syndrome patient with acute myelogenous leukaemia, who had a blood chromosome count of 48 before treatment, was reported by Warkany *et al.* (1963). An extra medium-sized submetacentric chromosome (groups 6–12) was found in addition to trisomy of chromosome 21. After treatment the majority of cells showed a standard Down's syndrome karyotype.

Ross & Atkins (1962) reported a case of myelogenous leukaemia in a Down's syndrome individual who had an initial standard chromosome count of 47. A repeat culture, 3 weeks before death, showed that practically all the cells contained 49 chromosomes with seven acrocentrics in group 21–22. In two-day peripheral blood cultures, nearly all cells contained 49 chromosomes. In aliquots of the same sample, cultured for 3 days, 75 per cent of the cells contained 47 chromosomes and 25 per cent contained 49. This suggested a selective process in favour of the 47 chromosome cell line.

A different response was noted in another Down's syndrome individual with myelogenous leukaemia, namely, that the proportion of cells with 49 chromosomes was significantly greater in the 3-day and 4-day peripheral blood cultures than in the 2-day cultures (Vincent *et al.* 1963). The cells which contained 49 chromosomes showed an extra abnormal pair of large metacentrics and an extra chromosome in group 6–12, monosomy in group 19–20 and trisomy in group 21–22. Variations in the chromosome number, dependent upon the length of time in culture, have also been noted by Lejeune *et al.* (1963). A Down's syndrome male with leukaemia who had a modal chromosome count of 51 was reported by Kiossoglou *et al.* Multiple chromosomal aberrations were found in both the autosomes and sex chromosomes. It was of interest that his mother and older sister showed chromosomal aberrations in the blood even though they had no signs of leukaemia. The patient's twin sister was normal.

Most of the cases, so far reported, of Down's syndrome with leukaemia have been standard trisomics; however, examples of translocation Down's syndrome with leukaemia are known. German *et al.* (1962) reported a (13–15) : 21 translocation Down's syndrome male infant who died of leukaemia. His mother was found to be a translocation carrier. In another case, leukaemia was found in a Down's syndrome individual with a 21 : (21–22) type of translocation, but the parents' karyotypes were normal (Cooper & Hirschhorn 1962).

In the cases of leukaemia in Down's syndrome summarised in Table 52, there has been no constant chromosome abnormality (a possible exception is an extra chromosome in group 6–12). Some of the differences probably reflect the circumstances in which the blood chromosome cultures were obtained, i.e. before treatment or after, whether the disease was active or in a stage of spontaneous remission. It would seem that the length of time the peripheral blood remains in culture before harvesting the cells may influence the karyotype. Skin cultures have not shown any abnormality other than that usually found in the syndrome.

Table 52. Aberrant Cell Line Found in Blood Cultures from Down's Syndrome Individuals with Leukaemia

No. Cases	Chromosome No.	Author
5	47	Tough et al. (1961)
2*	47	Sandberg et al. (1961)
1	48	Johnston (1961)
1	48	Warkany et al. (1963)
1	49	Ross et al. (1963)
1	49	Vincent et al. (1963)
1	51	Kiossoglou et al. (1963b)
1†	54	Lejeune et al. (1963)
1‡	46	German et al. (1962)
1§	46	Cooper & Hirschhorn (1962)

*Both cases show increase in aneuploid cells.
†Leukoblastic abnormality.
‡15 : 21 translocation Down's syndrome.
§21 : (21—22) translocation Down's syndrome.

Buchanan & Becroft (1970) reported on a Down's syndrome patient with acute myeloblastic leukaemia who was a mosaic for the cell lines in culture. The karyotypes of the two cell lines were 47,XX,21+/49,XX,C+,G+,G+.

De Mayo et al. (1967) discovered in the bone marrow of a Down's syndrome patient a minor line of cells with a complement of 50 chromosomes. This cell line was found several weeks before overt leukaemia was detectable. The predominant cell in the marrow, however, had 47 chromosomes. They proposed that careful cytogenetic studies combined with serial clinical evaluation may disclose an important relationship between chromosomal mutation, aneuploid stemlines and the production and evolution of neoplasms.

Increased spontaneous chromosomal fragility in Down's syndrome was reported by Kahn & Abe (1969). The authors examined the chromosomes cultured from mothers and fathers of Down's syndrome children and found the number of chromatid breaks to be three times higher (1.25 per cent) than was found in parents of normal children. Schuler et al. (1972) reported that their study did not support the proposal of Stark & Mantel (1967) that advanced maternal age facilitated the development of leukaemia in children with Down's syndrome. Schuler et al. were unable to show an increase in spontaneous chromosomal fragility under normal culturing conditions but when an alkylating agent was added to the culture media, there was an increase in the number of chromosomal breaks in the lymphocytes of Down's syndrome patients compared to lymphocytes from control individuals. There was no accumulation of nicotinic acid amine dinucleotide (NAD) in the leucocytes of Down's syndrome children as had been found in the leucocytes of certain leukaemic individuals (Ehrhart et al. 1969). Todaro & Martin (1967) observed that the fibroblast cultures of Down's syndrome individuals showed an increased susceptibility to transformation by oncogenic virus SV 40.

7. Biochemistry

There are many reports of biochemical deviations in Down's syndrome, but none of these deviant biochemical changes provides an explanation of the basic pathology in the syndrome or offers an adequate basis for a rational therapeutic programme. Even when there is general agreement about an abnormal biochemical finding in Down's syndrome, there is usually controversy about its cause and significance. The biochemistry of certain metabolic disorders, determined by specific genes, is often fairly well understood, but a more complex situation is encountered in chromosomal disorders like Down's syndrome. With advances in biochemical technology, it may be expected that some resolution of such dilemmas will be forthcoming in due course.

SERUM CALCIUM AND INORGANIC PHOSPHATE

Low serum calcium levels in Down's syndrome have been reported (Sobel *et al.* 1958, Stern & Lewis 1958). Berg & Stern (1963) found that, in a series of 40 Down's syndrome children and 40 controls, the difference between the means was significant. None of the levels, however, was grossly abnormal, and nearly one-third of the Down's syndrome individuals had calcium levels that fell within two standard deviations of the mean for normals. Bixby (1939) and Benda (1960) considered the serum calcium level to be within normal limits (8—11.5 mg./100 ml.) for a group of Down's syndrome children and adults. Similar results were found by Maas (1964).

There has been no precise agreement concerning the level of inorganic phosphate in Down's syndrome. It has been reported as slightly increased (Stern & Lewis 1958) and as being within normal limits (Bixby 1939, Sobel *et al.* 1958, Benda 1960).

Stern & Lewis (1958) noted that the lowered calcium and raised phosphate in children with Down's syndrome (see Table 53) could not be satisfactorily explained by hypofunction of the pituitary or thyroid gland, nor was there any evidence of a defect in calcium absorption or impairment of renal function which could give rise to these findings. However, later studies suggest that there may be faulty absorption of calcium (Stern 1964). In hypoparathyroidism the calcium is low and the inorganic phosphate is high but the quantitative changes are much greater than those found in Down's syndrome.

119

Table 53. Serum of Children with Down's Syndrome and of other Mentally
Retarded Children as Controls. (After Stern & Lewis 1958)

	Children with Down's syndrome			Controls			Signifi-cance of differences
	No.	Mean	S.E.	No.	Mean	S.E.	P
Calcium (mg./100 ml.)	40	8.8	0.05	40	9.5	0.07	<0.001
Inorganic phosphorate (mg./100 ml.)	40	5.0	0.10	40	4.7	0.09	<0.05
Alkaline phosphatase (KA units)	26	18.1	0.89	26	17.3	1.16	>0.5
Acid phosphatase (KA units)	35	2.8	0.09	27	3.0	0.12	>0.1

SERUM SODIUM, POTASSIUM, MAGNESIUM, CHLORIDE AND BICARBONATE

No abnormalities have been detected in the serum level of sodium,
potassium, chloride or bicarbonate (Bixby 1940, Sobel et al. 1958, Benda
1960). Serum magnesium levels and the mean red cell magnesium content
have been reported as elevated in Down's syndrome and other mentally
retarded children (Stern & Lewis 1960). The mean serum magnesium level
in Down's syndrome is 2.23 mg./100 ml. (S.D. 0.17) and in normal
controls, 2.10 mg./100 ml. (S.D. 0.11).

SERUM PROTEINS

Serum proteins in Down's syndrome have been studied by a number of
authors (Donner 1954, Stern & Lewis 1957a, Sobel et al. 1958, Benda
1960, Pritham et al. 1963, Appleton & Pritham 1963). The results have
shown some consistent findings, but still leave many questions
unanswered.

The total serum proteins are considered to be in the lower normal
range; however, albumin is decreased and gamma globulin is increased (see
Table 54) (Donner 1954, Stern & Lewis 1957a, Sobel et al.). Stern &
Lewis (1957a) reported that lowering of the serum albumin level in
Down's syndrome was particularly noticeable in the 6–10 age group.
Pritham et al. found elevated gamma globulin levels in institutional
patients but reported no abnormality in the serum albumin and gamma
globulin levels for non-institutional cases. They postulated a faulty
structure of gamma globulin. Donner found that the gamma globulin,
though elevated in institutional patients, was normal in its ability to form
antibodies. She concluded that the Down's syndrome individuals'
increased susceptibility to infections was not the result of abnormalities in
gamma globulin.

Table 54. Serum Proteins in Down's Syndrome. (After Stern & Lewis 1957a) Fractions and total proteins in the sera of 36 Down's syndrome cases and 36 control children.

Protein fraction	Down's syndrome Percentage of total protein		Controls Percentage of total protein		Significance of differences between means
	Mean	S.E.	Mean	S.E.	P
Albumin	48.3	0.77	53.4	0.84	<0.001
α_1 globulin	6.1	0.34	6.2	0.23	>0.1
α_2 globulin	10.9	0.29	11.1	0.31	>0.1
β globulin	13.1	0.28	12.6	0.27	>0.1
γ globulin	21.7	0.75	16.7	0.53	<0.001
Total	100.1		100.0		
	Mean level	S.E.	Mean level	S.E.	P
Total proteins (g./100 ml.)	6.58	0.09	6.59	0.07	>0.1

Significant differences in the relative proportions of alpha 1 and alpha 2 globulins in Down's syndrome and controls have been reported by Appleton & Pritham. Stern & Lewis (1957a), however, found that the alpha 1 and 2, and beta globulin levels were lower in the age group 6–10 years than in the age group 2–6 years for both their Down's syndrome and control groups.

Haptoglobins and transferrins were studied in a group of 100 Down's

Table 55. Incidence of Haptoglobin Phenotypes in Down's Syndrome. (Hutton & Smith 1964)

Source of samples	Phenotypes				Total
	0.0	1.1	2.1	2.2	
Male Down's syndrome cases	3	11	30	24	68
Female Down's syndrome cases	0	7	18	7	32
Total Down's syndrome cases	3	18	48	31	100
General population (Harris *et al.* (1959))	0	33	88	58	179
General population (Allison *et al.* (1958))	6	22	121	69	218
Controls: Total	6	55	209	127	397
Percentage	1.5	13.9	52.6	30.0	100.0

syndrome patients (Hutton & Smith 1964). The frequencies of the haptoglobin patterns were statistically the same as those found in the general population (see Table 55). No sex difference was noted. All the Down's syndrome cases had a transferrin C pattern, in agreement with the prevailing type in the general population. Ball *et al.* (1972) studied the haptoglobin distribution in Victoria and found no difference in Hp types between Downs's syndrome and control individuals.

Rundle (1973) studied polymorphic enzymes and protein systems. He applied mathematical models to determine if any of the enzymes were located on the No. 21 chromosome. Haldane's log ratio tests (1956), involving the combining of the homozygous forms, was considered and applied to the phenotype data on serum haptoglobins of 254 Down's syndrome individuals.

CARBOHYDRATE METABOLISM

The fasting blood sugar has been considered to be normal in Down's syndrome (Bixby & Benda 1942, Benda 1960, Sobel *et al.* 1958.). Benda examined fasting blood sugar levels in 51 cases. The range for the group was from 69 to 113 mgm. per 100 ml. of capillary blood. However, Runge (1959) reported that over 10 per cent of her Down's syndrome sample had a fasting blood sugar under 60 mgm. per 100 ml. Excessive fasting before the test could account for some of the low values found.

Glucose tolerance curves in Down's syndrome have been found to be abnormal in the direction of high tolerance by Brousseau & Brainerd (1928),· O'Leary (1931) and Bixby (1939). Benda (1960) observed evidence of delayed glycaemic response, with low or late peaks and a relatively slow return to fasting levels. There was a suggestion that the glucose tolerance curve became more abnormal with age. Runge considered about half the tolerance curves to be abnormal. She found three different types of abnormality (see Fig. 41) Type I(2 cases) showed an abnormally high peak but with a return to fasting level within 60 minutes; Type II (15 cases) showed a high peak with a delayed drop to fasting level; Type III (41 cases) showed a delayed drop to fasting level without a high peak following the intravenous glucose. Despite the fact that she used intravenous, instead of oral, glucose, the majority of her abnormal curves were similar to those reported by Benda. In Runge's series of cases, the curves became more abnormal with increasing age. In addition, a high proportion of Down's syndrome individuals with abnormal glucose tolerance had abnormal galactose tolerance.

Runge considered the response to the insulin tolerance test to be abnormal in 8 cases. The initial decrease in the fasting blood sugar was greater than that usually considered normal and the return to fasting blood sugar level was slow. The results suggested increased sensitivity to insulin. Benda reported the initial drop in fasting blood sugar to be normal but the

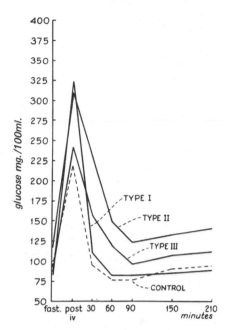

Fig. 41. Three types of intravenous glucose tolerance curves in Down's syndrome. Type I, high peak with return to normal levels similar to controls; Type II, high peak and delayed drop to fasting levels; Type III, showing delayed return to fasting levels (post iv = post intravenous) (after Runge 1959).

absolute blood sugar level after 2 hours was lower for Down's syndrome than for controls.

The response to adrenalin, in 9 Down's syndrome cases studied by Runge, showed a normal blood sugar elevation; however, there was delay in the return to fasting levels. The response to adrenalin was less marked in the older cases. Benda found decreased blood sugar response to adrenalin approximately the same whether the drug was given intravenously or intramuscularly.

There is no adequate explanation for these anomalies in carbohydrate metabolism. Runge thought that there might be an abnormality of liver enzyme function which affected deposition of glycogen or its mobilization from the liver. Benda suggested that the corticotropic hormone of the pituitary and the adrenal cortical hormone were at fault.

Down's syndrome persons with overt diabetes mellitus have been reported from time to time in the last few decades (Lawrence 1942, Jacobi & Rogatz 1949, Cone 1954, Pongiglione & Bezante 1965). Individual case reports left unresolved the question as to whether such occurrences were coincidental or not. However, more extensive data, derived from surveys, suggest an increased frequency of early onset diabetes mellitus in Down's syndrome individuals (Farquhar 1962, Milunsky & Neurath 1968). Milunsky and Neurath speculated about the possible role of autoimmunity in producing such an association (see Chapter 8).

Plasma immunoreactive insulin (IRI) levels were measured by a double antibody method at critical times after a glucose load. Tolerance to oral glucose in Down's syndrome was found to be normal though a flat, late peaked glycaemic response was characteristic of the group IRI and insulin levels did not significantly differ from those in the normal control group. The study did not support a significant relationship between diabetes mellitus and trisomy 21 through an alteration in insulin secretion (Serrano Rios *et al.* 1973a).

The intermediates of the glycolytic pathway in erythrocytes of children with Down's syndrome were investigated by Kedziora *et al.* (1972). There was a decrease in adenosine 5'-triphosphate (ATP) and 2,3-diphospho-glyceric acid (2,3-DPG) and an increase in the levels of adenosine 5'-monophosphate (AMP), guanosine 5'-triphosphate (GTP), nicotinamide adenine dinucleotide (NAD), nicotinamide adenine dinucleotide phosphate (NADP), inorganic phosphate (Pi) and hexose diphosphate (HDP). The authors speculated that the levels of the glycolytic pathway intermediates in erythrocytes of children with Down's syndrome may reflect disturbances of enzymatic activity. It is also possible that these differences are a result of nutritional disturbances or are caused by the incidence of a population of atypical erythrocytes.

LIPIDS

Cholesterol. Normal levels of serum cholesterol have been found by some authors (Bixby 1940, Sobel *et al.,* Benda 1960), while others (Stern & Lewis 1957b) observed that there was a significant difference in cholesterol levels between Down's syndrome persons and controls. Higher

Table 56. Serum Cholesterol Levels of Down's syndrome and other Mentally Retarded Children. (After Stern & Lewis 1957b)

| Cholesterol (mg./100 ml.) | Children with Down's syndrome | | | |
	Age 2–6 years	Age 6–12 years	Age 2–6 years	Age 6–12 years
<100	–	1	–	3
100–124	2	8	–	2
125–149	5	16	6	9
150–174	4	11	14	7
175–199	11	11	10	8
200–224	7	3	1	1
>224	2	–	4	1
	31	50	35	31
Mean cholesterol level (mg./100 ml.)	181.7	154.0	176.5	156.1
Median cholesterol level (mg./100 ml.)	183.5	150.0	169.0	156.0

levels were found more frequently in the younger age group (2–6 years) in both Down's syndrome and controls although there was more variability in the Down's syndrome group (see Table 56). Simon et al. (1954) reported that Down's syndrome and other retarded children had significantly higher serum cholesterol levels than normals.

Serum cholesterol has attracted attention in Down's syndrome because of the possibility of its reflecting abnormality of thyroid function. Stern & Lewis (1957b) pointed out that the abnormalities in serum lipids (cholesterol, phospholipids, and Sf 12–20 lipoprotein) suggest that the neuroendocrine control of lipid metabolism is impaired rather than that there is an abnormality in thyroid function.

Phospholipids. The phospholipids in Down's syndrome are increased in the age group 2–6 years (Stern & Lewis 1957b).

Lipoproteins. Simon et al., using an ultra-centrifuge method, reported that the lipoprotein (Sf 12–20) level of Down's syndrome individuals was significantly increased when compared with other mentally retarded and normal controls. Stern & Lewis (1959), using paper electrophoresis, reported an abnormally high ratio of β-lipoprotein to α-lipoprotein in Down's syndrome and also in other mentally retarded children. Nelson (1961) found an increase in the lipoprotein fraction in Down's syndrome children in the age group 2–11½ years. In contrast with these reports, Benda & Mann (1955) found no characteristic serum lipid pattern among 54 affected persons.

Cephalin. In general, liver function tests are considered to give normal results in Down's syndrome cases, except for an occasional individual who shows a 3 to 4 plus elevation in the cephalin flocculation test (Nelson). Abnormal cephalin flocculation tests are probably related to the elevated gamma globulin levels found in Down's syndrome (Stern 1964). Griffiths et al. (1965), in searching for effects of post-hepatitic liver damage, failed to demonstrate any kynurenine or 3-hydroxykynurenine in the urine.

AMINO ACIDS

Tryptophan. Abnormalities of tryptophan metabolism (see Fig. 42) have been reported several times (Gershoff et al. 1958, Jérôme et al. 1960, O'Brien & Groshek 1962, Jérôme 1962). Decreased urinary excretion of xanthurenic acid and indoleacetic acid were noted following oral tryptophan load and, to account for this, abnormality of a transaminase was proposed. However, it might be that the reduced amount of urinary metabolites of tryptophan found in Down's syndrome is caused by diminished or delayed intestinal absorption (O'Brien et al. 1962). Contrasting with these observations, McCoy & Chung (1964) found no difference between Down's syndrome persons and controls in the excretion of urinary metabolites before or after an oral load of tryptophan. In another experiment, when they inhibited the vitamin

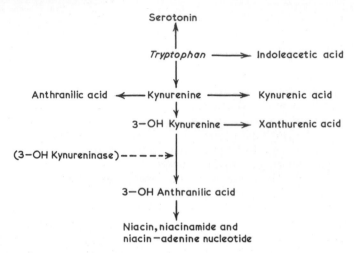

Fig. 42. Abbreviated outline of some pathways of normal tryptophan metabolism.

B_6-dependent enzyme, 3-OH-kynureninase, with deoxypyridoxine, there were exceptional increases in the excretion of xanthurenic acid and 3-OH-kynurenine, in Down's syndrome, after an oral tryptophan load. It was thought that these findings indicated that the 3-OH-kynureninase was specially sensitive to vitamin B_6 in Down's syndrome individuals as compared to controls.

Significantly lowered serotonic activity in the blood was found in 10 trisomic Down's syndrome individuals, as compared with 16 controls, by Rosner *et al.* (1965). The measurement in 7 translocation cases was normal.

Because of the decreased serotonin levels reported by Rosner *et al.*, 5-hydroxytryptophan was tried as a treatment in young Down's syndrome patients (Coleman 1971, Airaksinen 1971). Since 5-hydroxytryptophan is a precursor of serotonin, it was used to elevate the blood serotonin levels. Muscle tone was increased with 5-hydroxytryptophan and occasionally convulsions were produced if too high blood levels were attained. In general, the infants on 5-hydroxytryptophan did worse in their development than the Down's syndrome patients who did not receive the compound (Coleman 1973, Airaksinen 1973). Andersson *et al.* (1973) thought that they could demonstrate the existence of a defect in the metabolism of serotonin in the central nervous system in Down's syndrome. The nature of the defect was not determined.

Low platelet concentration of serotonin 5-hydroxytryptamine has been observed in the syndrome with a decrease of the platelet binding capacity for serotonin (Jérôme & Kamoun 1970). Boullin & O'Brien (1973) tried to determine if decreased 5-hydroxytryptamine binding by blood platelets in the syndrome involved changes in platelet monoamine oxidase. They concluded that it was not possible to relate a defect of platelet monoamine oxidase to 5-hydroxytryptamine decrease until the enzyme has been characterized.

Priscu *et al.* (1974) determined the amino acid levels of cerebrospinal fluid in 22 babies with Down's syndrome. Elevated levels of dicarboxylic acid were found, as well as modifications of the levels of lysine, histidine, valine and methionine. Differences in the phenylalanine/tyrosine and glycine/alanine ratios were also observed.

β-aminoisobutyric acid. In Down's syndrome increased amounts of urinary β-aminoisobutyric acid have been found (Lundin & Gustavson 1962). Using paper chromatography, Wright & Fink (1957) reported an increased incidence of high excretors in Down's syndrome (43 per cent) compared with normal controls (7 per cent) and unclassified mentally defective patients (17 per cent). In contrast, Perry *et al.* (1959), also using paper chromatography, found no significant difference in the number of high excretors in the three groups (Down's syndrome cases, 6 per cent; normal controls, 10 per cent; mentally defective patients, 5 per cent). Lundin & Gustavson suggested that the observed increase of β-aminoiso-butyric acid excretion might be interpreted as a physiological deviation characteristic of generally disturbed metabolism rather than as a specific genetical difference.

RNA POLYRIBOSOME PROTEIN SYNTHESIS

Typical profiles are shown in Fig. 43. Unstimulated lymphocytes do

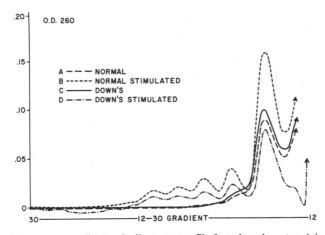

Fig. 43. Sucrose gradient polyribosome profile from lymphocytes. A indicates base line for normal adult; B, normal adult 60 hours after phytohemagglutin stimulation; C, base line for adolescent with Down's syndrome; and D, Down's syndrome 60 hours after phytohemagglutinin stimulation. OD indicates optical density.

not carry on much protein synthesis. It is not surprising that mainly single ribosomes were found on the profiles of both Down's syndrome and normal persons and polyribosomes were practically undetectable. In unstimulated lymphocytes the peak for single ribosomes was always slightly higher in Down's syndrome than in the normal controls. After phytohemagglutinin stimulation, the profiles showed an increase in the total number of ribosomes, and polyribosomes in appreciable numbers were found. The polyribosomes showed clear peaks of dimers, trimers, tetramers, pentamers and hexamers. In the phytohemagglutinin stimulated lymphocytes the total concentration of ribosomes and polyribosomes was greater in the normal controls than in the Down's syndrome patients (Hsia et al. 1971).

THYROID METABOLISM

The use of thyroid gland treatment has a long history in Down's syndrome. On the basis of autopsy studies, abnormalities have been reported in the thyroid gland (Benda 1946, 1960). Much of the early use of thyroid therapy was based upon supposed similarities between Down's syndrome individuals and cretins, upon abnormalities found after pathological sectioning of the gland (Bourneville & Royer 1906) and physical and mental responses in treated cases (Smith 1896, Bourneville 1903b).

During the past two decades more sophisticated techniques have been developed to measure thyroid gland function. Most Down's syndrome cases have normal protein-bound iodine levels; butanol-extractable iodine levels, according to Dodge et al. (1967), are often low. Sometimes an affected person is found with low levels and with other signs of hypothyroidism. Benda considered that, although most cases have a normal protein-bound iodine value, the globulin fraction itself is not normal.

In general, I^{131} uptake in Down's syndrome is within the normal range (Kearns & Hutson 1951, Friedman 1955, Kurland et al. 1957, Fisher et al. 1964), but low levels have been reported (Lowrey et al. 1949, Hoffman-Credner & Zweymüller 1957). Friedman found no difference in the I^{131} uptake in 61 Down's syndrome children and 68 euthyroid children with mental retardation. Twenty-one Down's syndrome cases were studied by Kurland et al., and the 24-hour thyroidal uptake ranged from 12.0 to 44.0 per cent with an average of 25.0 per cent (S.E. 1.5; S.D. 6.7). The mean thyroidal I^{131} uptake in Down's syndrome was not significantly different from that found in 23 euthyroid subjects of a comparable age. Hoffman-Credner & Zweymüller reported that, in 6 Down's syndrome children, the I^{131} uptake was lower than that in a group of normal children or those with cerebral palsy.

The average 24-hour urinary excretion of I^{131} in Down's syndrome is 46 per cent and not significantly different from euthyroid controls, and conversion ratios range from 13 to 15 per cent and are considered normal (Kurland *et al.*).

In Down's syndrome, the effective half-life of I^{131} is shorter than in normals, 5.4 days, and euthyroid controls have an average of 7.1 days. Kurland *et al.* thought that the discrepancy between the rapid thyroidal I^{131} turnover rate and normal serum protein-bound iodine concentration had not been resolved. They also stated that their findings were consistent with the hypothesis that thyroid function in Down's syndrome resided in only a small portion of the gland. That portion worked at an increased rate, and consequently the total iodine uptake was normal; there was a rapid turnover and a normal level of serum hormone was maintained. This was consistent with autopsy findings on the thyroid gland. The increased peripheral utilization of thyroid hormone in Down's syndrome still requires clarification.

Filter-paper electrophoresis, carried out on plasma of two affected persons to which I^{131} thyroxine was added (Kurland *et al.*) showed a single peak of radioactivity migrating with the alpha-2-globulin which is similar to that in normal controls.

Uptake of labelled triiodothyronine by red blood cells *in vitro* is increased (Hamolsky *et al.* 1957, Jackim *et al.* 1961, Pearse *et al.* 1963). Kurland *et al.* showed that the increased uptake was due to a plasma factor, since erythrocytes from controls had a normal uptake in plasma taken from Down's syndrome patients. Intravenous infusion of I^{131} labelled thyroxine showed that the plasma radioactivity decreased at a normal rate. Mosier (1967) measured one and two hour neck/thigh ratios of 131 Down's syndrome cases and mentally retarded controls. He showed that the ratio was significantly lower in the syndrome (see Table 57). Measurement of free thyroxine, PBI, thyroxine-binding globulin capacity

Table 57. Neck/Thigh Ratios in Down's Syndrome and Controls
(After Mosier 1967)

	Neck/thigh ratio* 1 hr	2 hr
Down's syndrome		
males	4.2±0.21(10)	5.7±0.32(10)
females	5.1±0.78 (7)	6.5±1.33 (7)
all	4.6±0.36(17)	6.1±0.59(17)
Controls		
males	6.1±0.84(10)	9.0±0.85(10)
females	6.1±0.75 (7)	9.7±1.54 (7)
all	6.3±0.59(17)	9.3±1.06(17)

Data expressed as mean ± SE (number of subjects)
*t test all Down's syndrome cases : all controls 1 hr $p \leqq .02$
2 hr $p \leqq .02$

and the 20—40 hour excretion of I^{131} showed no differences between the two groups.

Spinelli-Ressi & Bergonzi (1963) noted the mean I^{131}-triiodothyronine uptake of red blood cells to be elevated but, since 11 out of 25 Down's syndrome individuals had values within the normal range, they could not consider their finding to be characteristic. In an experiment, similar to that done by Kurland et al., they found that Down's syndrome red blood cells in normal plasma had a normal I^{131}-triiodothyronine uptake. Since it is known that abnormalities of the plasma proteins influence the red cell I^{131}-triiodothyronine uptake, they suggested that some plasma change was responsible for the increases found in the syndrome. They found no evidence to support the suggestion of Jackim et al. that the increased erythrocyte I^{131}-triiodothyronine uptake in the syndrome was due to enzyme anomalies of red blood cells.

Even though the majority of Down's syndrome individuals are euthyroid clinically, abnormalities in thyroid gland function and structure have been reported. Mosier (1965) demonstrated the presence of long-acting thyroid stimulator (LATS) in five Down's syndrome patients without hyperthyroidism. Spontaneous hypothyroidism occurs in the syndrome but is considered to be uncommon by Hayles et al. (1965). However, hyperthyroidism with a goitre (classic Grave's disease) seems to occur more frequently (Jagiello & Taylor 1965, Ruvalcaba et al. 1969). Despite the claim of efficacy of thyroid treatment for euthyroid Down's syndrome patients, treatment with thyroid hormone fails to improve linear growth, developmental quotient or general clinical status of these individuals, according to Koch et al. (1965).

Thyroid autoantibodies (see Chapter 8) were found in 5 Down's syndrome individuals out of 35 tested (Mellon et al. 1963). Four out of these five had normal protein-bound iodine levels. The fifth had a low protein-bound iodine level and obvious signs of myxoedema. Thirty-five non-Down's syndrome mentally retarded patients were also tested but no thyroid autoantibodies were detected. In a similar type of study using Steffen's antiglobulin consumption (A.G.C.) test with lyophilized thyroid tissue, Burgio et al. (1965) observed that 7 of 12 children with Down's syndrome had a positive test. Six mothers of Down's syndrome children, out of 12, also had positive tests, whereas in 48 controls only 3 children and 5 mothers had positive tests. Thyroid autoimmune antibodies have also been reported in other aneuploid conditions (Sparkes & Motulsky 1963). Fialkow (1970) and Fialkow et al. (1971) found significant increases in the frequency of thyroid antibodies in subjects with Down's syndrome and in their mothers but not their fathers (see Tables 58 and 59).

ADRENAL HORMONES

Adrenal deficiency was reported in 50 per cent of Down's syndrome

Table 58. Thyroid Antibodies in Down's Syndrome and Controls (Fialkow 1970)

	Positive	Negative
Down's Syndrome (314)	28%	72%
Controls	6%	94%

individuals on the basis of 24-hour urinary output of 11-oxycorticoids, 17-ketosteroids and the eosinophil response to corticotropin and epinephrine (Sandrucci & Piccotti 1958). Dutton (1959b) examined the steroids in a group of Down's syndrome and other mentally defective boys and found that there was no significant difference in the level of excretion of 17-ketosteroids and 17-ketogenic steroids. In a group of 32 cases, O'Sullivan et al. (1961) found the mean urinary 17-hydroxycorticoids to be within normal limits (for females 3.72, and for males 3.89). There was an increase of urinary 17-hydroxycorticoids in Down's syndrome adults as compared with adolescents. O'Sullivan et al. concluded that adrenal function in Down's syndrome was adequate.

CATECHOLAMINE METABOLISM

Low dopamine-β-hydroxylase (DBH) in plasma of Down's syndrome children has been reported by Wetterberg et al. (1972). It was felt that this indicated a possible disturbance in catecholamine metabolism. This observation stimulated the study of catechol-O-methyltransferase (COMT) in erythrocytes from children with Down's syndrome, since COMT is involved in the inactivation of catecholamines. Gustavson et al. (1973) reported an increase in COMT activity in the erythrocytes (see Table 60). It was thought that a low urinary excretion of epinephrine in Down's syndrome may also reflect an abnormality in the metabolic pathway of

Table 59. Thyroid Antibodies in Families of Subjects With Down's Syndrome and Controls (After Fialkow et al. 1971)

	Positive	Negative	Per Cent	Significance
Down's syndrome (106)	36	70	34	$<.001$
Controls (105)	6	99	6	
Mothers of Down's syndrome children (106)	32	74	30	$<.005$
Controls (105)	15	90	14	
Fathers of Down's syndrome children (77)	7	70	9	NSD
Controls (71)	5	67	7	

NSD = No significant difference.

Table 60. Catechol-O-methyltransferase (COMT) activity in erythrocytes and dopamine-β-hydroxylase (DBH) activity in plasma in children with Down's syndrome and controls. (After Gustavson *et al.* 1973)

No. of cases	Diagnosis	COMT activity* in erythro- cytes	DBH activity** in plasma
19	Down's syndrome	1.90±0.10	16±5
17	Retarded controls	1.56±0.17	84±14
16	Normal controls	1.35±0.17	158±16

The enzymic activity is mean ± SEM
*COMT is expressed as nmol normetanephrine formed from noradrenaline per hour per ml erythrocytes.
**DBH is expressed as nanomoles of octopamine formed from tyramine per ml plasma per 20 min incubation time.

biogenic amines (Keele *et al.* 1969). Significant erythrocyte macrocytosis (Naiman *et al.* 1965) may explain some of the increased COMT activity; however, based upon the work of Assicot & Bohvon (1971) who showed two types of COMT in rat erythrocytes, the possibility of a difference in COMT isoenzyme has to be considered.

TESTICULAR HORMONES

Benda's (1960) data indicate that in Down's syndrome adolescents there is diminished 17-ketosteroid production. Rundle *et al.* (1959) studied the urinary 17-ketosteroids of male and female Down's syndrome individuals and used other retarded males as controls. Both male groups showed an increase between the ages of 15 and 23 years and both approached steroidal maturity at the same rate. The maximal excretion rate in both groups was at 23 years of age. Examination of the fractionation patterns of the 17-ketosteroids (beta, alpha and II-oxo-fractions) showed no significant difference between the two male groups. Rundle *et al.* pointed out that the retarded development of pubic hair and external genitalia in Down's syndrome could not be accounted for in terms of steroid levels.

ENZYMES

In 1960, patients with chronic myelogenous leukaemia were shown to have an abnormally small acrocentric chromosome, the Philadelphia chromosome (Nowell & Hungerford 1960), and it was shown that the alkaline phosphatase activity of the polymorphonuclear leucocytes in such patients is diminished (Valentine & Beck 1951). From this it was argued that the Down's syndrome individual, who is trisomic for chromosome 21, should show an increase of leucocyte alkaline phosphatase. This difference was observed by using both histochemical (Alter *et al.* 1962), Lennox *et al.* 1962, Trubowitz *et al.* 1962, King *et al.* 1962, O'Sullivan & Pryles 1963, Phillips *et al.* 1967) and biochemical (Trubowitz *et al.*, Phillips *et al.*, Rosner *et al.* 1965) methods. The suggestion was made that the gene locus for alkaline phosphatase might reside on chromosome 21 and that the results of a triple gene dosage effect were being observed. It is now known that the Philadelphia chromosome is number 22 and that it is not deleted but that the missing portion is translocated to another chromosome (Rowley 1973).

Brandt (1962) and Brandt *et al.* (1963) found increased galactose-l-phosphate uridyl transferase in the whole blood of Down's syndrome cases and suggested that the locus for the gene that determines galactosaemia might also be located on chromosome 21. Working with erythrocytes, Ng *et al.* (1964) showed only a slight and not statistically significant difference between galactose-l-phosphate uridyl transferase levels in Down's syndrome as compared with controls. By separating leucocytes from erythrocytes, Hsia *et al.* (1964) were able to show that the difference of galactose-l-phosphate uridyl transferase was predominantly in the leucocyte fraction and not in the erythrocyte fraction, as shown in Table 61. This suggested that the main disturbance involved white blood cells and not red blood cells.

In the meantime, Krone *et al.* (1964) measured both the galactokinase and galactose-1-phosphate uridyl transferase in the erythrocytes and showed that the ratio of Down's syndrome to controls was approximately 1.5 to 1. They suggested that the enhancement of the galactokinase activity was a gene dosage effect. Donnell *et al.* (1965) showed that the ratio of galactokinase and galactose-1-phosphate uridyl transferase activity in Down's syndrome compared to controls was 1.2 to 1 (Table 61), and did not correspond to the 0.5 to 1 seen among heterozygotes for galactosaemia and persons normal for the latter enzyme.

Mellman *et al.* (1964) then found an increase not only of leucocyte galactose-1-phosphate uridyl transferase but also acid phosphatase and glucose-l-phosphate dehydrogenase (Table 61). Since the locus for the latter enzyme is located on the X chromosome, it appeared improbable .that the increase of leucocyte enzyme activity could reflect solely a gene dosage effect resulting from a trisomic state of an autosome (chromosome 21).

Enzymes in other tissues. Since several enzymes were found to be increased in leucocytes from patients with Down's syndrome, other studies on enzyme activity were carried out in erythrocytes, platelets and fibroblasts.

In erythrocytes, there is general agreement that patients with Down's syndrome show an increase of phosphohexokinase (Baikie *et al.* 1965,

Table 61. Blood and Leucocyte Enzymes Among Controls and Down's Syndrome Patients[*]
(After Hsia et al. 1971)

Author	Source	Method	Control Mean	Control ±SD	Down's Mean	Down's ±SD
Galactose-1-phosphate uridyl transferase						
Brandt et al (1963)	W	UDPG consumption (micromol/hr/gm Hb)	26.4	±3.6	36.9	±5.1
Ng et al (1964)	E	Galactose-1-phosphates-^{14}C (micromol/hr/ml)	1.89	±1.25	1.98	±1.03
Hsia et al (1964)	W	UDPG consumption (micromol/hr/gm Hb)	29.8	±9.3	41.8	±7.5
	E	UDPG consumption (micromol/hr/gm Hb)	33.3	±2.3	35.6	±7.5
	E	Galactose-1-^{14}C (cpm/1.5 hr/gm Hb)	50,980.0	±12,610.0	49,030.0	±10,690.0
	L	Galactose-1-^{14}C (cpm/1.5 hr/2 x 10^7 WBC)	2,490.0	±1,320.0	4,510.0	±1,780.0
Mellman et al (1964)	L	UDPG consumption (micromol/hr/10^9 WBC)	15.5	±4.9	26.4	±12.4
Rosner et al (1965)	W	UDPG consumption (micromol/hr/gm Hb)	33.1	...	57.2	...
	E	UDPG consumption (micromol/hr/gm Hb)	26.3	...	41.7	...
	L	UDPG consumption (micromol/hr/gm RNA)	10.0	...	25.5	...
Galactokinase						
Donnell et al (1965)	E	Galactose-1-C (micromol/hr/ml)	0.30	±0.065	0.36	±0.069
Glucose-6-phosphate dehydrogenase						
Mellman et al (1964)	L	NADPH (micromol/hr/10 WBC)	9.4	±2.6	14.4	±3.5
Shih et al (1965)	L	NADPH (micromol/hr/10 WBC)	1.24	±0.13	1.72	±0.28
Acid phosphatase						
Mellman et al (1964)	L	μg/hr/10 WBC	16.6	±4.0	23.6	±7.8
Rosner et al (1965)	L	Units/mμg protein	0.44	...	0.82	...

[*]W indicates whole blood; E, erythrocyte; L, leucocyte; Hb, haemoglobin.

Bartels *et al.* 1968, Pantelakis *et al.* 1970) and serum glutamic oxaloacetic transaminase (SGOT) (Bartels *et al.,* Naiman *et al.* 1965); an equivocal increase of glucose-6-phosphate dehydrogenase (Phillips *et al.,* Rosner *et al.,* Shih *et al.* 1965, Baikie *et al.,* Pantelakis *et al.*) and 6-phosphogluconate dehydrogenase (Pantelakis *et al.*); and no alterations in hexokinase (Baikie *et al.,* Pantelakis *et al.*), phosphohexose isomerase (Hsia *et al.,* Baikie *et al.*), adolase (Hsia *et al.,* Baikie *et al.,*), triose phosphate isomerase (Baikie *et al.*), glyceraldehyde phosphate dehydrogenase (Baikie *et al.*), phosphoglycerate kinase (Baikie *et al.*), phosphoglycerate mutase (Baikie *et al.*), enolase (Baikie *et al.*), pyruvate kinase (Hsia *et al.,* Baikie *et al.,* Pantelakis *et al.*), lactic acid dehydrogenase (Shih *et al.,* Baikie *et al.,* Pantelakis *et al.*), glutathione reductase (Hsia *et al.,* Baikie *et al.*), catalase (Pantelakis *et al.*) and dihydronicotinamine-adenine dinucleotide phosphate (NADPH) methaemoglobin reductase (Pantelakis *et al.*). Unlike Schwarzmeier *et al.* (1973), Layzer & Epstein (1972) observed increased red cell phosphofructokinase (PFK) acticity. Fibroblast, white cell and platelet PFK activity were not increased. They argued that it was unlikely that structural genes for PFK are located on chromosome 21.

In platelets, there is no alteration between controls and Down's syndrome cases for alkaline phosphatase (Shih & Hsia 1966), glucose-6-phosphate dehydrogenase (Shih & Hsia) and phosphohexokinase (Doery *et al.* 1968).

In fibroblasts there is no difference between controls and Down's syndrome patients for alkaline phosphatase (Doery *et al.,* Cox 1965, Walker & DeMars 1966, Nadler *et al.* 1967a), acid phosphatase (Nadler *et al.,* DeMars 1964), glucose-6-phosphate dehydrogenase (Nadler *et al.*), galactose-1-phosphate uridyl transferase (Nadler *et al.*), β-glucuronidase (DeMars) and uridine diphosphate glucose (UDPH)-4-epimerase (Krone & Brunschede 1965).

In general, it appears that patients with Down's syndrome show an increase of several leucocyte enzymes including alkaline phosphatase, acid phosphatase, galactose-1-phosphate uridyl transferase and glucose-6-phosphate dehydrogenase—and of two erythrocyte enzymes, phosphohexokinase and SGOT—and that all other enzymes tested in erythrocytes, platelets and fibroblasts seem to be unaltered.

Other enzyme studies. In 1965, Rosner *et al.* observed that the cellular biochemical changes in patients with Down's syndrome could be divided into two groups. Those with trisomy 21 showed the increase of enzymes and decrease of serotonin which had previously been reported, but those with translocations did not show these changes and their values were similar to controls. These observations have not been confirmed by others. For example, Berman *et al.* (1967) found the blood serotonin (expressed as micrograms per millilitre) to be 181.7±79.8 for 19 controls, 119.1±114.8 for nine patients with translocation Down's syndrome, and 100.3±36.2 for 14 patients with trisomic Down's syndrome. Herring *et al.* (1967) analyzed the variance for leucocyte alkaline phosphatase and erythrocyte glucose-6-phosphate dehydrogenase and found the overlap sufficiently great to preclude the use of these enzymes for differentiating Down's syndrome cases with translocations from those with standard trisomy.

Nadler *et al.* (1966) investigated the activity of leucocyte alkaline phosphatase, leucocyte acid phosphatase, leucocyte glucose-6-phosphate dehydrogenase, and erythrocyte galactose-1-phosphate uridyl transferase in nine patients with trisomy 18. There was an increase in alkaline phosphatase and a slight increase in acid phosphatase in these patients. Weber *et al.* (1965) carried out histochemical studies for alkaline phosphatase in patients with Klinefelter's syndrome and found no difference from controls.

Nadler *et al.* (1967b) separated leucocytes into lymphocytes and granulocytes using the glass bead columns described by Rabinowitz (1964). Patients with Down's syndrome showed a significant elevation of alkaline phosphatase, acid phosphatase and glucose-6-phosphate dehydrogenase in both the lymphocyte and granulocyte fractions, indicating that the alteration of leucocyte enzyme activity is not localized to any particular fraction.

Monteleone *et al.* (1967) next examined the isoenzyme patterns for alkaline phosphatase, acid phosphatase, and glucose-6-phosphate dehydrogenase in separated lymphocytes and granulocytes. They were unable to find any significant difference in the banding pattern of these enzymes between patients with Down's syndrome and controls. Subsequently, Weaver & Lyons (1968) confirmed these observations for leucocyte alkaline phosphatase, and Benson & deJong (1968) reported no differences in hexokinase isoenzymes between patients with Down's syndrome and controls.

Nadler *et al.* (1967b) also measured the changes in acid phosphatase and glucose-6-phosphate dehydrogenase during lymphocyte stimulation with phytohaemagglutinin. As shown in Table 62, there was no significant difference in the ratio of enzyme activity for Down's syndrome to controls during the cell cycle.

Table 62. Lymphocyte Acid Phosphatase and Glucose-6-Phosphate Dehydrogenase Activity During Stimulation With Phytohaemagglutinin in Controls and Down's Syndrome Patients (After Hsia *et al.* 1971)

Time (hr)	Acid Phosphatase (Millimolar para nitro phenol/hr/10^6 Cells)		Glucose-6-Phosphate Dehydrogenase (Micromol NADPH/hr/10^6 Cells)	
	Controls	Down's	Controls	Down's
24	11.70	23.00	0.22	0.33
48	4.20	8.00	0.17	0.24
72	4.80	10.30	0.13	0.18
120	10.50	20.10	0.22	0.31

Hook & Engel (1964) pointed out that the decrease of leucocyte alkaline phosphatase in chronic myelogenous leukaemia may be related to the increased life span of the leukaemic leucocyte and that the increase of leucocyte alkaline phosphatase in Down's syndrome may be related to the shorter life span of the leucocyte in the syndrome. Rosen & Nishiyama (1965) did not believe that the increase of leucocyte alkaline phosphatase could be explained on the basis of the life span of the leucocyte alone and suggested that there may be more than one population of leucocytes in humans. Additional observations were made by Pegg (1964).

Raab et al. (1966) performed leucokinetic studies employing an in vitro isofluorophate tagged with phosphorus 32 granulocyte labeling technique. They found that the granulocyte half-life was 3.7 hours in seven patients with trisomy 21 as compared with 6.6 hours in 100 normal adults. They proposed that leucocyte regulation may be related to the trisomic state of chromosome 21. These observations could not be confirmed by Galbraith & Valberg (1966) who found that the rate of disappearance of granulocytes labelled with isofluorophate P was the same in controls as in patients with Down's syndrome. Leucocyte kinetic studies by Pearson (1967) also failed to confirm the reduced half-life of these cells in Down's syndrome (see Chapter 6). Attempts to use changes of enzyme activity, in cells of aneuploid individuals, to establish linkage of genes have led to the observation that aneuploidy can affect the physiology of cells so that enzyme activities are altered, regardless of gene dosage or of the particular chromosome involved.

McCoy et al. (1966) examined the induction of leucocyte alkaline phosphatase with progesterone. This induction is actinomycin—and puromycin-sensitive and thus dependent upon RNA and protein synthesis. Patients with Down's syndrome had an average leucocyte alkaline phosphatase activity of 1.5 at zero hours, 4.7 at three hours and 6.3 at six hours after prednisolone administration, as compared with 1.1 at zero hours, 2.8 at three hours and 3.2 at six hours for transcription units operating in Down's syndrome compared to two units in controls.

Tada et al. (1972) found no indication that the enzymes hypoxanthine guanine phosphoribosyltransferase (HGPRT) and adenine-phosphoribosyltransferase (APRT) are controlled by genes on the number 21 chromosome. Smith et al. (1975) investigated enzyme levels of long term lymphocyte cultures (transformed lymphocytes) from Down's syndrome individuals. The enzymes glucose-6-phosphate dehydrogenase (G-6-PD), lactic acid dehydrogenase (LDH), β-glucuronidase, and acid and alkaline phosphatase were serially studied over a six week period. All the enzyme levels were increased in the Down's syndrome lymphocytes, except LDH, when compared with control lymphocytes.

GENES ON CHROMOSOME 21

While there has been no conclusive evidence for an assignment of a gene or genes on chromosome 21, the work of Tan *et al.* (1973, 1974) suggests that antiviral protein gene and indophenol oxidase gene (super-oxide dismutase) are both on this chromosome (see p. 230). Sinet *et al.* (1974, 1975) have demonstrated that superoxide dismutase activity (S.O.D.A.) is increased in the erythrocytes of children with Down's syndrome. The S.O.D.A. activity was found to be 1.4 times higher in the syndrome than in controls. Benson (1975), however, has questioned whether the enhancement of enzyme activity in erythrocytes is sufficient evidence of a gene dosage effect in Down's syndrome.

VITAMINS

The possibility of vitamin A deficiency has been of interest to some researchers because of defective skin and hair development in Down's syndrome. Reduced absorption of vitamin A in oil by Down's syndrome children has been reported by Sobel *et al.* (1958). Similar findings were also noted when vitamin A was given in aqueous solution (Auld *et al.* 1959).

The metabolism of the water-soluble vitamins, thiamine, riboflavin and vitamin C, was studied in a group of Down's syndrome and other mentally defective children. In studies of excretion no important differences were found (Gershoff *et al.* 1958).

Gershoff *et al.* administered oral nicotinamide to a group of Down's syndrome individuals and found low N-methyl nicotinamide and creatinine levels in the urine. This suggested a defect of the methylating ability in the syndrome. Careddu *et al.* (1963), however, reported that there was no significant anomaly in the urinary excretion of N-methyl nicotinamide before or after intramuscular injection of nicotinic acid. Before nicotinic acid was given, however, the Down's syndrome children excreted a greater amount of N_1-methyl-6-pyridone-5-carboxamide than the controls. After nicotinic acid was given this difference disappeared.

SERUM URIC ACID

Sobel *et al.* (1958) examined the serum uric acid levels in Down's syndrome individuals and controls and found no difference; however, in later reports, by Fuller *et al.* (1962) and Mertz *et al.* (1963), there was an elevation in the serum uric acid levels in the syndrome as compared with a group of undifferentiated mentally defective patients. Serum uric acid levels are also raised in conditions such as in myeloid leukaemia where increased nucleo-protein breakdown occurs (Nugent *et al.* 1962). In Down's syndrome there is an increased proportion of immature polymorphonuclear neutrophil leucocytes and an increased incidence of leukaemia. For this reason there has been speculation about the relationship of these abnormalities to the raised serum uric acid levels. In a study by Chapman & Stern (1964) raised serum uric acid levels were found; however, the levels for both the Down's syndrome patients and the controls were lower than those published by Fuller *et al.* and by Mertz *et al.* (see Table 63). It was suggested that the different serum uric acid levels

Table 63. Serum Uric Acid Levels

	Fuller *et al.*, 1962[†] Average*	Range*	Mertz *et al.*, 1963[‡] Average*	Range*	Chapman & Stern 1964[‡] Average*	Range*
Males:						
Down's syndrome	6.48	4.12–8.72	5.15	3.07–6.82	–	–
Controls	5.27	2.60–8.35	3.91	1.71–6.07	–	–
Females:						
Down's syndrome	6.24	4.81–9.16	5.93	4.06–9.62	–	–
Controls	4.85	3.68–7.70	3.61	2.06–5.04	–	–
Males and Females:						
Down's syndrome	6.36	4.12–9.16	5.42	3.07–9.62	3.8	1.88–6.04
Controls	5.06	2.60–8.35	3.87	1.71–6.07	3.1	1.50–5.38

*Values in mg/100 ml.
†Mainly adults.
‡Children.

reported may have been due to differences in methodology. Chapman & Stern noted that the increased serum uric acid levels found were mainly in Down's syndrome children below the age of 10 years. In addition, the urinary uric acid levels in Down's syndrome individuals were normal. Estimation of the urine uric acid/creatinine ratio, concurrently measured with the serum uric acid level, produced no evidence of over-production of uric acid and suggested that the raised serum levels might have been due to relatively decreased urinary excretion.

Table 64. Uric Acid Levels in Sweat (After Danton & Nyhan 1966)

	Uric Acid (mg/100 ml)
Down's syndrome (13)	0.637± 0.156
Controls (16)	0.202 ± 0.029

Danton & Nyhan (1966) detected an increase of uric acid in the sweat of Down's syndrome patients (see Table 64). The authors used an enzymatic spectrophotometric method to determine the uric acid levels. The significance of the elevated uric acid concentration in sweat of Down's syndrome patients is not certain, but probably is a reflection of the increased serum uric acid levels. Data on the incorporation of C^{14}-glycine into urinary uric acid in a Down's syndrome child did not reveal a difference from those of control children (Lesch & Nyhan 1964). Saliva and serum were examined for total protein, creatinine, amylase and uric acid concentrations in Down's syndrome and compared with controls. Slight differences in concentrations for the various constituents were found in Down's syndrome saliva. In serum, only the uric acid level was increased in the syndrome (Winer & Feller 1972).

DRUG SUSCEPTIBILITY

Berg *et al.* (1959) noted a rapid and sustained dilatation of the pupils in Down's syndrome when atropine was applied locally to the eye. A similar response was found by O'Brien *et al.* (1960), but they were unable to relate the pupillary response to decreased serotonin as previously suggested. No similar sensitivity to homatropine was demonstrated. More rapid onset of mydriasis in Down's syndrome patients was observed also by Mir & Cumming (1971) after topical application of atropine.

Priest (1960) noted a weak pupillary response to hydroxyamphetamine hydrobromide (paredrine hydrobromide). She concluded that the atropine itself was not responsible for the observed pupillary response, and she speculated on physical abnormalities in the pupil as a possible cause.

Variable results have been obtained in studies of the effects of intravenous atropine on heart-rate in Down's syndrome. Harris & Goodman (1968) noted a markedly increased sensitivity to the cardio-acceleratory effect of this drug, whereas Mir & Cumming found no such difference in comparison with controls. The reasons for this discrepancy are not clear.

CEREBRAL OXYGEN CONSUMPTION

Himwich *et al* (1940) pointed out that the normal adult brain has an oxygen consumption of 7.43 vol. per cent, but that in Down's syndrome there is a reduction to 5.62 vol. per cent. The normal brain usually removes 14.6 mg. per cent of the carbohydrate from the blood during each circulation; however, the amount of carbohydrate utilized by the brain of Down's syndrome persons was reduced to 8.0 mg. An interpretation of these findings in relationship to brain pathology was given by Himwich & Fazekas (1940).

8. Immunology

A defective immune system has been suspected in Down's syndrome because of the high incidence of upper respiratory infections and deaths caused by infections (see p. 245). While abnormalities involving both the cellular and humoral immune system have been reported, there is, as yet, no defect which has been demonstrated in the immune system that adequately explains why so many of these individuals are susceptible to certain infections.

IMMUNOGLOBULINS

Serum gamma globulin levels have been studied by Donner (1954), Stern & Lewis (1957a), Sobel et al. (1958), Benda (1960), Nelson (1961), Pritham et al. (1963), Appleton & Pritham (1963), and Appleton et al. (1966, 1967). Though the results of these studies vary, there appears to be a consensus that there is an increased level of gamma globulin in institutionalized Down's syndrome patients, while no such elevation is found in Down's syndrome individuals living at home. Pritham et al. postulated a faulty structure of gamma globulin while Donner concluded that affected individuals were normal in their ability to form antibodies and that the increased susceptibility to infections was not the result of an abnormality in their gamma globulin. Woodford & Bearn (1970) have criticized much of the work in many of these studies.

The IgG concentration in the serum of newborn infants with Down's syndrome is lower than that found in the normal infant and lower than that of the mother's serum at the time of delivery (Miller et al. 1967, 1969). To further substantiate their finding, these authors showed in a pair of dizygotic twins—one with Down's syndrome and the other normal—that the IgG level in the Down's syndrome twin was reduced when compared with the normal twin and the mother's IgG level at the time of birth.

An elevation of the three main immunoglobulin classes reveals that, while IgG concentration is regularly raised in adults, IgM may be normal or low, IgA normal or high, and IgD high (Stiehm & Fudenberg 1966, Adinolfi et al. 1967, Greene et al. 1968, Rundle et al. 1971). Agarwal et al. (1970) found no significant differences in total serum proteins, gamma globulins, IgA and IgG levels between Down's syndrome individuals and controls. However, the IgM levels were significantly lower in patients with

141

the syndrome compared with other mentally retarded patients. Low IgM levels were also reported by Lopez *et al.* (1973).

Differences have been found between the physical properties of the gamma globulin of Down's syndrome and normal individuals. Changes in electrophoretic mobility were shown by Pritham *et al.* (1963), Rowe *et al.* (1966), and Miller *et al.* (1969, 1970). Miller *et al.* suggested that IgG from Down's syndrome newborns had a more rapid migration upon electrophoretic analysis. From their studies, it would seem that the Fc piece was the apparent portion of the IgG molecule responsible for the difference in mobility. Fluck & Pritham (1964) showed a change in the peptide pattern and Appleton *et al.* a difference in the polarographic behaviour and diffusion coefficient. Thom & McKay (1972) showed that titres of GM4, 5, 10 and 11 were higher than would be expected from the rise in total IgG concentration in Down's syndrome. Their findings suggest that in the syndrome an uneven increase occurs in the H chain subgroups and allotypes of IgG.

Rosner & Kozinn (1972) found increased IgG levels in Down's syndrome. IgA levels were elevated only in affected adults over 18 years of age. The authors postulated that the abnormalities in immunoglobulin levels in the syndrome are the result, rather than the cause, of the increased susceptibility to infection.

Lopez (1974) studied the serum IgE levels in 16 patients with Down's syndrome and found the levels reduced, compared with controls. In two of the patients, no IgE levels could be detected. The author speculated that a defect in immunoglobulin synthesis may be present and noted that the low serum IgE was of interest in the light of a decreased incidence of atopic disease in the syndrome.

ANTIBODY FORMATION

Early attempts to measure the antibody response in Down's syndrome were made by Leibovitz & Yannet (1942). Later, Siegel (1948) measured the antibody response to tetanus toxoid and typhoid vaccine. In his study, the antibody response to primary as well as secondary antigenic stimulation was observed. Siegel found a poorer antibody response among Down's syndrome individuals than among controls. Those with the syndrome took somewhat longer for detectable antibodies to appear in the circulation, following primary inoculation, and the antibodies were of lower titre and disappeared more quickly from the circulation. Following reinoculation, both groups responded with an accelerated antibody response and there was a wide range of individual differences in the titres depending upon the specific antigen used (see Fig. 44). Siegel suggested that there was probably some defect in the mechanism by which specific antibodies are either formed in response to antigenic stimulation or released into the circulation. He concluded that the antibody defect may

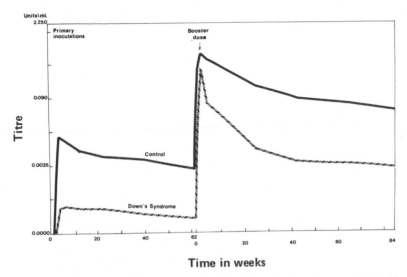

Fig. 44. Average antitoxin titre following primary and secondary inoculation of tetanus toxoid. (After Siegel 1948)

be due to an abnormal defence mechanism and to hormonal deficiencies. A normal antibody response to the same antigens was found by Leibovitz & Yannet and Griffiths & Sylvester (1967).

Donner measured the antibody response to B.C.G. in Down's syndrome patients and found it to be normal. Adinolfi *et al.* demonstrated normal anti-A and anti-B agglutinins and antibodies to Escherichia coli in the syndrome. More recently, a reduced response to influenza vaccine has been reported in older patients (Gordon *et al.* 1971) and Epstein-Barr virus antibodies have been found to be higher in affected children than in a normal control population (Osato *et al.* 1969). Antinuclear antibodies were not detected in Down's syndrome individuals in a study done by Rosner & Kozinn.

The antibody responses to Bacteriophage Øx 174 were studied in a group of 17 Down's syndrome individuals (Lopez *et al.* 1973, 1975). Primary antibody response was significantly impaired in 11 of them. Secondary immune response was normal in one, moderately impaired in seven and very low in nine patients. The group was further subdivided into two categories by the response to tertiary immunization. Those with moderately impaired secondary immune responses developed normal titres of IgG antibody. Individuals with low secondary immune responses had extremely impaired tertiary immune responses consisting mainly of IgM antibodies. Lopez *et al.* believed that premature aging of individuals with Down's syndrome would not account for their observations, since variability of the expression of the immunodeficiency and a quantitative, rather than an absolute, defect would be expected under these circumstances. This is not what was found in their patients. Half the patients were able to develop a normal antibody response on repeated immunization. The fact that the remainder failed to develop a normal immune response on repeated immunization raises the question of the optimal time of immunization for children with Down's syndrome.

The possibility of autoantibodies to the islets of Langerhans has been considered because an occasional Down's syndrome case of carbohydrate intolerance has been reported. Serrano Rios et al. (1973b) examined the serum of Down's syndrome individuals for IgG class insulin antibodies. Their results did not indicate evidence of autoimmune disease to account for the development of diabetes mellitus in certain individuals with the syndrome.

LYMPHOCYTE TRANSFORMATION

It has been suggested that peripheral lymphocytes from patients with Down's syndrome seem to be easier to culture and show more mitoses than those from normal subjects (Lejeune 1966). From this observation, a number of studies were done to measure the response of peripheral lymphocytes of Down's syndrome individuals to phytohaemagglutinin (PHA) and other mitogens. Interest has now centred on whether or not there is an abnormal response of peripheral lymphocytes in the syndrome which can be related to impaired cellular immune (delayed hypersensitivity) response (Rigas et al. 1970, Fowler & Hollingsworth 1973).

Hayakawa et al. (1968) observed an increased blastoid transformation of Down's syndrome lymphocytes to low doses of PHA. When the usual dilution of PHA was added to the cultures, there was no difference in the percentage of blastoid cells found between the lymphocytes from Down's syndrome patients and those from control subjects. Sasaki & Obara (1969) observed an increased hyperblastic response for Down's syndrome lymphocytes stimulated in mixed leucocyte cultures. On the other hand, Mellman et al. (1970) found that a decreased tritiated thymidine uptake for Down's syndrome lymphocytes was present but only when large amounts of PHA were used. Agarwal et al. also showed a significantly decreased tritiated thymidine incorporation by cultured lymphocytes of Down's syndrome patients compared with age and sex matched retarded controls and normal healthy volunteers. The impairment in response to PHA did not seem to be related to the presence of Australia antigen in the patients with Down's syndrome or to institutionalization itself. In contrast to the decreased tritiated thymidine activity, there was no significant difference in the percentage of blast transformation in the three groups studies. Fowler & Hollingsworth attempted to assess cellular immunity in patients with Down's syndrome by evaluating the response of peripheral lymphocytes to antigenic stimulation (PHA, PPD) and measuring ^{3}H-thymidine incorporation. They found that, in response to stimulation by specific antigens, tuberculin (PPD) or by PHA, the lymphocytes of Down's syndrome patients were not significantly different from those of other retarded or normal individuals.

DNA POLYMERASE ACTIVITY

Normal lymphocytes, when cultured with PHA, show increased DNA polymerase activity in 24 hours. This precedes the onset of DNA synthesis. Further large increases in enzyme activity occur in the next day or two of culture accompanying blast-cell formation and the start of mitosis. Agarwal *et al.* have shown a decrease in DNA polymerase production in stimulated lymphocytes of individuals with Down's syndrome. This correlated with their study showing a decrease in PHA stimulated Down's syndrome lymphocytes as measured by tritiated thymidine incorporation. They have attempted to relate these two findings to an impairment of cellular immune functions in the syndrome which may be one of the factors contributing to the vulnerability of these patients to repeated or persistent infections.

AUTOANTIBODIES

Other antibody systems have also been shown to be abnormal in Down's syndrome. There is an increased incidence of patients who have a positive test for thyroid auto-antibodies (see p. 130). Thyroid auto-antibodies have been studied in detail by Fialkow (1970) in Down's syndrome patients and their families (see also Chapters 7 and 12). The initial observation of an increased frequency of thyroid antibodies in the syndrome was made by Mellon *et al.* (1963). Similar findings were also reported by Fialkow (1964) and Burgio *et al.* (1965). Fialkow (1970) reported on a large group of Down's syndrome individuals and found that 28 per cent of them had thyroid autoantibodies as compared to 6 per cent of his control population. The mothers and sibs of affected individuals, but not the fathers, also had an increased incidence of thyroid auto-antibodies. While Fialkow favoured the hypothesis that a factor reflected by thyroid autoimmunity in mothers predisposes them to having children with Down's syndrome, he recognized the possibility that thyroid antibodies themselves may induce chromosomal abnormalities or that these antibodies may mask the presence of some other factor which causes chromosomal aberrations.

Vitiligo (skin depigmentation) occasionally has been observed in young teenaged and adult Down's syndrome individuals (Smith 1973). Since vitiligo is considered to be an autoimmune disease (Grunnet *et al.* 1970), it could be regarded as additional evidence of an abnormal immune system in these individuals.

AUSTRALIA ANTIGEN AND ANTIBODIES

Blumberg and his colleagues (Blumberg 1966, Blumberg *et al.* 1967, 1970, Sutnick *et al.* 1969) showed an unusual response to the Australia antigen (Au(1)) in Down's syndrome. They found that, in large institutions, the frequency of Au(1) antigen was 10 times higher in Down's syndrome than in other mentally retarded patients. A similar finding has been reported by Melartin & Panelius (1967). The evidence is that Down's syndrome individuals with Au(1) have a chronic anicteric type of hepatitis. Even though they show no presence of jaundice, their liver chemistries tend to be abnormal. One of the most important features of hepatitis in Down's syndrome is the persistence of the antigen which can be detected in the blood for many years. Blumberg *et al.* (1970) have interpreted their findings in two ways, both of which argue for an impaired immune system in the syndrome. First, that the persistence of Au(1) is a consequence of impaired immunity and, secondly, that affected individuals may be prone to repeated hepatitis because their immune system is faulty. In a much more complex way, Blumberg *et al.* (1967) have attempted to relate the susceptibility to chronic hepatitis in the syndrome to the propensity to develop leukaemia.

OTHER AUTOIMMUNE DISEASES

In the study by Fialkow *et al.* (1971), 11 maternal relatives were reported to have pernicious anaemia as compared with two control relatives. However, the diagnosis of pernicious anaemia could only be confirmed in four of the 11 family members. Multiple sclerosis was present in one Down's syndrome mother and six maternal relatives, compared with no cases in the control maternal relatives. No other examples of autoimmune diseases in relatives were noted.

MILK ANTIBODIES

In 1962, Heiner *et al.* demonstrated a relationship between chronic upper respiratory disease and bovine milk antibodies in normal children. Based upon these observations, Nelson (1964) decided to measure the incidence of bovine milk antigens in Down's syndrome individuals, because of the high frequency of upper respiratory infections in this group. Nelson found a higher incidence of bovine milk antibodies in the Down's syndrome group. McCrea *et al.* (1968) also found a high incidence of milk antibodies in Down's syndrome individuals (34 per cent positive) but they were unable to relate upper respiratory infections in these individuals to a positive bovine milk antibody response. Lange *et al.* (1974) examined the serum of 2,218 cases for precipitins to milk proteins. Of the 2,000 normal sera

Table 65. Response to Bovine Milk Precipitins (After Lange *et al.* 1974)

		+	−	Total	Percentage
A.	Normals	100	1600	1700	5.8
B.	Newborns	0	300	300	0
C.	Retarded Controls	6	121	127	4.7
D.	Down's Syndrome	17	74	91	18.6

tested, 5.8 per cent showed positive precipitins, whereas the incidence was 18.7 per cent in Down's syndrome and 4.7 per cent in other retarded individuals (see Table 65). Only antibodies against albumin, gamma globulin or both were detected in positive sera. These findings seem to strengthen the proposition of a generalized increase in immune sensitivity in Down's syndrome.

LEUCOCYTE FUNCTION

A defect in NBT (nitrobluetetrazolium) reducing capacity (Tan *et al.* 1973, Kretschmer *et al.* 1974) and a decrease in the staphylococcal bactericidal abilities (Gregory *et al.* 1972, Kretschmer *et al.*) were found in the leucocytes of approximately 50 per cent of individuals with Down's syndrome. Bactericidal activity against streptococci is normal. The results are similar to those found in heterozygous carriers of chronic granulomatous disease (Gregory *et al.*) suggesting a common disarray in the peroxidase-iodination bactericidal mechanism. However, the peroxidase and periodic-acid/Schiff activity in Down's syndrome leucocytes was found to be normal by Rosner & Kozinn (1972). These authors studied the in-vitro phagocytic ability of peripheral blood neutrophils to ingest live *Candida albicans* and they also investigated neutrophil adhesiveness in the syndrome. The results of both these tests were considered to be abnormal (see Table 66). According to Rosner & Kozinn, it is not clear whether abnormalities in leucocyte function are related to the increased incidence of infection in Down's syndrome. They were unable to demonstrate any antinuclear antibodies but had two Down's syndrome patients with high rheumatoid factor titres.

Table 66. Neutrophil Phagocytic and Adhesiveness Indices for Down's Syndrome and Normal Controls (After Rosner & Kozinn 1972)

	Phagocytic Index		Adhesiveness Index	
	Controls	Down's	Controls	Down's
Number of Cases	20	30	17	31
Mean Index	2.64	2.06	9.51	3.69
Range	0.97-3.68	0.46-3.49	1.5-30.9	1.4-20.8
Standard Error	0.14	0.14	2.51	0.64

ALLERGIC MANIFESTATIONS

In an investigation of several hundred children with Down's syndrome, Coghlan & Evans (1964) found that asthma, hay fever and eczema were less common in those with the syndrome than in their sibs. In addition, these same allergic conditions occurred less frequently in the syndrome than in other retarded individuals and their sibs. It was shown that, in Down's syndrome, the skin is capable of reacting to histamine and that a "Prausnitz-Kustner" reaction was present suggesting that the skin is capable of producing a histamine-like substance.

HL–A PHENOTYPES

Hirsch *et al.* (1974) described a pair of Down's syndrome twins who were discordant in morphological characteristics and HL–A phenotypes but concordant for trisomy of chromosome 21 and blood group markers. The authors speculated whether or not the boys might represent intermediates between dizygotic and monozygotic twins. Post-cleavage fertilization was excluded on the basis that the twins had different maternal HL–A haplotypes.

Harris *et al.* (1969) did HL–A typing on Down's syndrome patients but they found no patient with more than two LA alleles. They took this as evidence against the HL–A genes being on chromosome 21.

Boxer & Yokoyama (1972) studied lymphocyte surface antigenicity in Down's syndrome, as it is a reflection of diminished protein synthesis in response to stimulators of cellular immunity. Leucocyte typing was carried out on lymphocytes from 23 Caucasian children and 13 Japanese children with the syndrome. These children reacted less frequently than the children in the control group to the microcytotoxicity test. Six families of patients with Down's syndrome showed marked deletions of the expected HL–A haplotype.

9. Clinical Diagnosis

The importance of clinical recognition and delineation of Down's syndrome by no means has been abrogated as a result of the relative ease with which the syndrome can now be diagnosed by chromosomal examination. Clinical appraisal continues to be a major requirement for a number of reasons. In the first place, chromosomal tests are not always readily available and, when they are, the initial referral is dependent on a clinical judgement. Secondly, patients with the same standard trisomic condition vary greatly in their symptoms, their capabilities and disabilities, and their prognosis. Thirdly, there are numerous degrees of mosaicism, which give rise to all manner of incomplete types of Down's syndrome; and the connection between the proportion of trisomic cells in different tissues and the extent of clinical manifestation is still far from clear. Finally, there are many known instances where apparent trisomy or partial trisomy of a small acrocentric chromosome does not lead to a clinical state identifiable as Down's syndrome. Thus, clinical and cytological investigations have to complement each other in order to reach as exact an assessment as possible.

GENERAL PRINCIPLES OF DIAGNOSIS

The clinical diagnosis of Down's syndrome is made by deliberately or unwittingly adding up the points in its favour (Penrose 1933b). The number of observations required to establish the diagnosis depends on the tests available and on their discriminative efficiency. Some characters, like abnormal facial appearance, are easy to observe and highly characteristic but extremely difficult to define. Others, like dermatoglyphic patterns, are definite, but they occur also in other conditions and in normal members of the population. Furthermore, measurable characteristics, like head size, stature and birth weight, though they have different mean values in Down's syndrome and normals, have overlapping distributions.

The presence of any given sign or measurement, which is characteristic of the syndrome, increases the probability of the diagnosis and the absence of any such sign decreases the probability. Some signs, like radial loop on the fourth digit, are uncommon, strongly in favour of the diagnosis if present but with little effect on the judgment if they are absent. Other signs, like short anteroposterior head measurement, are present in almost every case so that their absence militates strongly against the diagnosis. In ordinary clinical practice, probabilities of this kind are weighed without being specified and, when an overwhelming impression is made by taking them all together, there is usually no further argument. It is interesting to note that, since the incidence of Down's syndrome at birth is about 0.015 per cent, the infant starts with a chance of about 650 to 1 of not being affected; the combined probabilities of all the relevant observations must be at least as strongly in favour of the diagnosis before it need be seriously considered. Thus, a particularly significant initial item of information is the age of the patient's mother. In the age range below 30 years the general population risk is less than 1/1,000 but, after the age of 45, the risk is of the order of 1/40. Other data from the history, for example of a familial incidence of the syndrome, can substantially modify these figures.

DIAGNOSIS IN INFANCY

Early diagnosis of Down's syndrome (see Fig. 45), or exclusion, is critical because of the implication that it holds for the infant and the anxiety that it creates for the parents. Furthermore, estimates of the incidence of the syndrome are intimately related to prompt, accurate diagnosis. More often than not, the diagnosis can be made fairly easily at birth by experienced observers. However, it must be remembered that mental retardation, which is a crucial finding in older patients, cannot be accurately assessed during the neonatal period.

The age at which the diagnosis was made in 226 Down's syndrome children was studied by Zappella & Cowie (1962). They found that the condition was recognized during the first six monthe of life in 168 cases (74 per cent). They also noted that the proportion of cases diagnosed at birth was much higher among those born in hospital (92 out of 141—65 per cent) than among those born at home and delivered by nurses or midwives (5 out of 43—12 per cent). In doubtful instances, chromosomal examination is of the utmost importance. Once a diagnosis has been made, parents usually prefer to be informed promptly or, at any rate, without undue delay (Fortune 1962, Drillien & Wilkinson 1964a, Cowie 1966, Berg *et al.* 1969, Carr 1970b, Gayton & Walker 1974).

Some of the more useful diagnostic physical findings, selected by Øster (1953), Levinson *et al.* (1955), Domino & Newman (1965) and Hall (1964) are shown in Table 67. The ten most characteristic signs selected by Øster for children and adults differ somewhat from those for the newly born given by Hall; the choice of signs depends upon the age group studied. There is fair agreement, between the data of Øster, Levinson *et al.* and Domino & Newman on the percentages of Down's syndrome children and adults having a particular abnormal physical finding. These data are derived almost exclusively from patients of European origin. However, Emanuel *et al.*'s (1968) clinical findings in Chinese cases of Down's syndrome are generally quite similar, as they appear also to be in patients

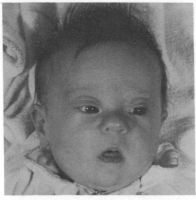
(i) Newly born.

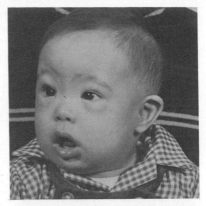
(ii) Aged six months

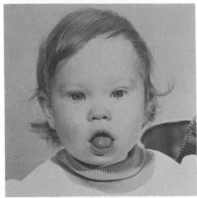
(iii) Aged 12 months

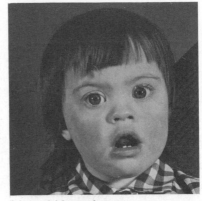
(iv) Aged 18 months

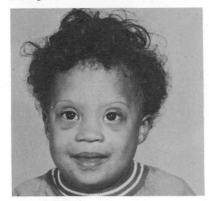
(v) Aged 2 years

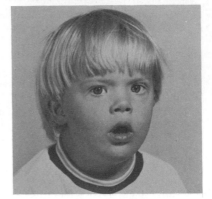
(vi) Aged 3 years

Fig. 45. Typical examples of Down's syndrome infants and children. All have standard trisomy 21, except (i) and (iii) who show 46,XX/47,XX,21+ mosaicism.

Table 67. Frequencies of Physical Signs in Down's Syndrome Expressed as Percentages

Sign	Øster (1953) Children or adults	Levinson et al. (1955) Children or adults	Domino & Newman (1965) Children or adults	Hall (1964) Newly born
Mouth:				
Habitually open	67	62	53	–
Fissured lips	–	56	–	–
*Small teeth	71	56	–	–
Irregular alignment	71	68	73	–
Large tongue	57	30	41	–
Protruding tongue	49	32	45	68
*Furrowed tongue	59	44	80	–
*Seemingly high-arched palate	67	74	59	–
Eyes:				
*†Oblique palpebral fissures	75	88	75	80
*Epicanthic folds	28	50	67	–
Speckled iris	70	30	58	42
Strabismus	23	14	28	–
Nystagmus	12	14	6	–
Ears:				
Prominent	47	50	51	–
Malformed	49	48	63	–
Small or absent lobes	82	80	48	57
Folded helix	–	–	–	53
†Dysplastic	–	–	–	62
Neck:				
Broad and short	39	50	71	–
†Abundant skin	–	–	–	81
Abdomen:				
Diastasis recti	–	76	87	–
Umbilical hernia	–	4	6	–
Genitalia:				
Small penis	98	50	61	–
Cryptorchism	27	20	16	–
Small scrotum	–	42	32	–
Head:				
*Flat occiput	74	82	73	–
Round shape	–	–	48	77
†Flat facial profile	–	–	–	89
Flat nasal bridge	59	62	–	79
Open fontanelle (after the age of 6 months)	–	16	–	–

Table 67 continued

Sign	Øster (1953) Children or adults	Levinson et al. (1955) Children or adults	Domino & Newman (1965) Children or adults	Hall (1964) Newly born
Chest:				
Funnel type	5	12	14	–
Pigeon breasted	5	14	6	–
Flat nipples	–	56	–	–
Dorsolumbar kyphosis	–	14	7	–
Hands:				
*Short broad hands	69	74	66	–
Short fingers	–	70	63	–
Short 5th finger	57	66	53	–
*Curved 5th finger	48	68	61	32
One flexion crease on 5th finger	31	10	19	14
*†Four-finger crease	43	48	64	54
†Dysplastic middle phalanx 5th finger	–	–	–	58
Feet:				
Excessive space between 1 and 2 toes	47	44	58	46
Plantar furrow	–	28	34	–
Joints and Muscles:				
*†Hyperextensibility or hyperflexibility	47	–	77	77
Hyperabduction of hip joints	–	–	–	84
†Muscular hypotonia	21	–	40	77
Weak patella reflexes	–	–	–	84
†Dysplastic pelvis	–	–	–	67
†Lack of Moro reflex	–	–	–	82

*Ten most characteristic signs selected by Øster (1953).
†Ten best diagnostic signs in newly born (Hall 1964).

of other ethnic backgrounds. The diagnostic significance of the traits is limited by the fact that they are usually not clearly definable and depend upon clinical impressions. Moreover, it is essential to have information about their frequencies of occurrence in control groups of normal infants or those affected by other diseases. Hall (1964) gave frequencies (Table 68) which show that some signs, like flattened features and excessive skin at the back of the neck, would be of very high diagnostic value indeed if they were clearly defined.

Table 68. Comparative Frequencies of Ten Critical Signs in the Newly Born.
(Hall 1964)

Character	Down's syndrome	Control
Oblique palpebral fissures	46/57	2/86
Dysplastic ears	23/37	2/40
Excessive skin on back of neck	46/57	1/86
Flattened features	50/56	1/85
Four-finger palmar crease (either hand)	30/56	8/86
Dysplastic middle phalanx on digit V (either hand)	25/43	2/37
Hyperflexibility	43/56	14/86
Muscular hypotonia	43/56	3/86
Dysplastic pelvis	25/37	–/–
Absence of Moro reflex	44/54	6/85

Table 69. Comparison of Birth Weight Distributions for Down's Syndrome and
Controls (Sex not Specified). (Smith & McKeown 1955)

Weight in lbs.	Down's Syndrome (103) %	Controls (4,931) %
Under 4	–	2.6
4–	2.9	1.3
4½–	7.8	2.5
5–	7.8	4.1
5½–	19.4	6.3
6–	14.6	11.3
6½–	15.5	14.0
7–	15.5	17.3
7½–	6.8	15.1
8–	6.8	11.3
8½–	2.9	7.4
9 and over	–	6.8
All	100.0	100.0

Table 70. Birth weight in Standard Trisomic and Translocation Down's
Syndrome Children (After Matsunaga & Tonomura 1972)

Subjects	Males		Females	
	Nos.	Mean birth weight (g.)	Nos.	Mean birth weight (g.)
Standard trisomy 21 Down's syndrome	40	2,843	42	2,805
Translocation Down's syndrome	40	2,711	42	2,810
All Japan–1969	–	3,214	–	3,131

The mean birth weight of Down's syndrome infants (see Table 69) is approximately 1 lb below that of normal infants (Smith & McKeown 1955). Data from Japan, reported by Matsunaga & Tonomura (1972), showed similar results and, moreover, revealed no significant differences between translocation and matched standard trisomic cases of Down's syndrome (see Table 70). In the series of Down's syndrome infants studied by Cowie (1970), birth weights tended to be low irrespective of length of gestation. The gestation period is often considered to be normal or only slightly shortened. However, Gustavson (1964) found the duration of pregnancy to be 269 days for males and 272 for females with Down's syndrome, whereas for a control group it was 280 days. In Cowie's sample, the mean gestation period was 267 days with a standard deviation of 16 days. Only one baby was born on the expected date of delivery, 56 were born sooner and 15 later. Burns (1973) observed that in Down's syndrome, as in normal infants, timing of parturition in the vast majority of cases is from 39 to 42 weeks. Since Down's syndrome babies tend to weigh less than the normal newly born, the incidence of "prematurity" is high and it has been reported as between 20 and 40 per cent. In a study by Parker (1950) it was found that 10 out of 32 children with Down's syndrome (31 per cent) were "premature" while in the control group the incidence was 12 per cent. The incidence of the syndrome, in a prematurity nursery, was found to be 1 in 354(10/3,543). Chen et al. (1969) noted a birth weight of under 5½ lbs. in 36 out of 174 (21 per cent) Down's syndrome babies and an increased infant mortality in these cases. Smith & McKeown (1955) found that 52 per cent of Down's syndrome infants had a birth weight of under 6 lbs; this proportion was nearly twice that found for the controls (28 per cent). They believed that the reduced birth weight could not be fully explained by the shortened period of gestation (average 38 weeks) and, therefore, it was attributed, in part, to a reduced rate of prenatal growth. Birth length also tends to be slightly reduced in Down's syndrome: the mean length of males was 48.3 cm. and of females 49.0 cm. whereas, in the control groups, the means were 51.2 cm., and 50.5 cm. respectively (Gustavson 1964). By contrast, Kouvalainen & Österlund (1967) found a tendency for placentas to be relatively large in Down's syndrome and they suggested that this might reflect an immunologic reaction of the mother against an incompatible fetus.

Such terms as "reduced rate of growth" and "retarded differentiation" (during the prenatal period) are used to explain some of the abnormalities seen at birth, but they add little to the knowledge of the embryological errors that have occurred. The study of abnormal embryonic development in the mouse has been helpful in explaining some of the complex abnormalities found in both newly born and adult mice (Grüneberg 1963). The results of these studies indicate the difficulty of understanding the basic embryological defects in Down's syndrome without following the early stages of embryonic development.

SUMMARY OF TRAITS FOR DIAGNOSIS IN THE NEWLY BORN

Face. The face lacks expression and the features are flattened. The abnormalities tend to be exaggerated when the infant cries because of the unusual wrinkling of the forehead and eyelids.

Head. The shape of the head is round with flattening of the occiput. The circumference is almost within normal limits but the cephalic index is increased because of a decrease in the head length. The fontanelles are large and the sutures widely separated. The so-called third fontanelle may be palpated. The frontal suture is sometimes patent down to the glabella and the sagittal suture may have an abnormal ridge formation.

Eyes. The palpebral fissures are oblique with an upward outward slant and epicanthic folds are frequently present. Speckling of the irides is noticeable, except in very dark eyes, but this must not be confused with white spots in the irides of normal infants.

Nose. The nose is short and has flattening of the bridge.

Mouth. The tongue is usually smooth and normal in size but it may protrude between the lips. The hard palate may seem highly arched.

Ears. The external ears are round and small. An angular over-lapping helix is frequently present. Attachment of ear lobes may be difficult to evaluate at this age.

Hips. Abnormalities of the pelvic bones may be seen by X-ray.

Hands and Feet. The hands and feet may be noticeably short and broad as compared with the normal and the fingers and toes tend to be stubby. The little finger may show a characteristic incurving with a short second phalanx and one flexion crease instead of two. A single transverse palmar crease is frequently seen on one or both hands. There is often an increased space between the first and second toes. The highly significant diagnostic dermal patterns on the hands and feet can be seen with a lens (e.g. +13 dioptres) but they may be difficult to print at this age.

Genitalia. In the male the penis and scrotum may be small and immature and, in females, there may be underdeveloped labia minora and pouchy labia majora.

Neuromuscular systems. Generalized muscular hypotonia is very characteristic; so also is hyperflexibility. Responses to stimuli are reduced. There may be a weak Moro reflex and a weak response on stimulation of the patellar reflex.

Skin. Skin elasticity is usually decreased and excessive looseness of the skin at the back of the neck is typical though webbing is rare. Acrocyanosis of the hands and feet is common.

Associated anomalies. Among the associated complications during the neonatal period are congenital heart disease, leukaemia and duodenal obstruction. These abnormalities aid in diagnosis and should be kept in mind when an infant is "doing poorly".

Behaviour. The newly born Down's syndrome baby usually presents no special difficulties in the nursery unless there is a severe associated anomaly. The infant tends to sleep most of the time. Feeding, on the whole, presents no undue problems though the infant is sometimes described as being lazy or a slow feeder. In general, mothers say that their affected babies are "good" and that they make very few demands. Some of the "good" behaviour is probably a consequence of the infant's reduced responses to both internal (hunger) and external (soiling) stimuli.

DISCRIMINATIVE VALUE OF A SINGLE TRAIT

If a single character, like head size or transverse palmar flexion crease, is used as a diagnostic criterion, the significance of the observation depends upon its relative frequency of occurrence in patients and controls. The character may be metrically or qualitatively determined. In either case the discriminative efficiency of the trait can be quantitatively expressed as an index in terms of the probability that diagnosis, based upon this trait alone, is correct. It is convenient to be able to compare the values of a great variety of such traits and to enable metrical and qualitative characters to be used on the same scale. For this, some formal analysis is necessary. A scheme suitable for metrical characters will first be set out.

METRICAL CHARACTERS

Assume two overlapping Gaussian distributions which contain equal numbers and have equal standard deviations, S. In practice, the equality of numbers in the two distributions is obtained by expressing them both as fractions of unity or as percentages. The standard deviations of two observed distributions are never exactly equal so the practical measurement to use is the average of the S-values of the two distributions, M and N; thus $S = (S_M + S_N)/2$. The means are $\overline{M}$ and $\overline{N}$, respectively, and $D = \overline{N} - \overline{M}$ as shown in Fig. 46.

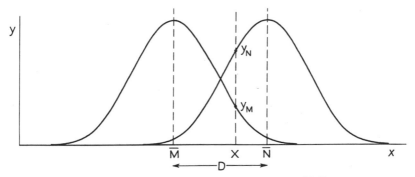

Fig. 46. Two overlapping Gaussian distributions with means $\overline{M}$, $\overline{N}$ and standard deviations S.

The relative probability, or odds, that a person with a given measurement, X, belongs to distribution M rather than to N is given by P where $P = y_M/y_N$. The values y_M and y_N are the ordinates of the two corresponding distribution curves at the point where the variable measurement, x, is equal to X. It follows formally that

(i) . . . . . . $\log_e P = \dfrac{D}{S}\left[\dfrac{\overline{M} + \overline{N} - 2X}{2S}\right]$

Further, when x has the value $\overline{M}, \overline{N}$ or $(\overline{M} + \overline{N})/2$, there are special cases as indicated in Table 71.

Table 71. Log_e Probability Ratios for Mean Values of Two Theoretical Distributions

Value of x	$\overline{N}$	$(\overline{N}+\overline{M})/2$	$\overline{M}$
Value of $\log_e P$	$-D^2/2S^2$	0	$+D^2/2S^2$

The discriminative efficiency, I, of the metrical trait concerned is measured by the distance between the means, $\overline{M}$, for affected, and $\overline{N}$, for controls, expressed in terms of S. The equivalent natural logarithm of the probability P is the index required. Thus, $I = D^2/S^2$. Examples of metrical characters, useful in the diagnosis of Down's syndrome, are shown in Table 72.

As an example, head length in adult males can be considered. For controls, $\overline{N} = 193$ mm. and, for Down's syndrome, $\overline{M} = 177$ mm.; thus D = 16 mm. For both distributions, S = 6.7 mm. It follows that $I = D^2/S^2 = 5.7$, which indicates a very high discriminative value for this trait.

The diagnostic value of any particular measurement, X, is found as in the following example.

If a particular male patient has head length 168 mm., the use of formula (i) will lead to the score of + 3.9 for $\log_e P$. The odds in favour of this patient having Down's syndrome on the result of this test alone is given by P which is equal to 49 to 1 (see Table 73).

QUALITATIVE TRAITS

Non-metrical characters are scored by their presence or absence in a given subject. The typical situation is that in which two populations, one of patients and the other of controls, are contrasted by the incidence of a particular trait in each of them as shown in Table 74. The relative probability, P, of Down's syndrome, as compared with normality when the trait is present, is m/n and $(1 - m)/(1 - n)$ when it is absent. In order to combine probabilities obtained for different independent traits, either metrical or qualitative, the logarithm of the probability is used. The index of discriminative efficiency, I, for a given qualitative trait is the difference

Table 72. Discriminative Efficiency of Some Metrical Characters

Character	Unit	Age	Sex	Down's syndrome $\bar{M}$	Controls $\bar{N}$	Difference D	Average Standard Deviation $\bar{S}$	Index of discrimination $(D/S)^2$	Source
Birth weight	lb.	0	♂ or ♀	6.44	7.13	0.69	1.18	0.34	(a)
				6.39	7.24	0.85	1.14	0.56	(b)
Gestation time	days	0	♂ or ♀	269.8	281.6	11.8	17.7	0.44	(b)
Acetabular angle	degrees	0–2 months	♂ or ♀	16	28	12	4.6	6.7	(c)
		3–11 months		11	22	11	4.2	6.7	
Maximal *atd* angle (sum, R + L)	degrees	0–4 years	♂	163.0	92.5	−70.5	21.6	10.6	(d)
			♀	162.0	97.5	−64.5	26.6	5.8	
Intelligence	Binet I.Q.	3–9 years	♂ or ♀	48.4	100.0	51.6	15.5	11.1	(e)
Segmentation of polymorph leucocytes	nuclear lobes	6–12 years	♂ or ♀	2.34	2.84	0.50	0.35	2.04	(f)
Head length	mm.	Adult	♂	177	193	16	6.7	5.7	(g)
			♀	168	183	15	5.7	6.8	
Head breadth	mm.	Adult	♂	149	156	7	5.9	1.4	(g)
			♀	142	149	7	4.8	2.6	
Standing height	mm.	Adult	♂	1,540	1,696	156	67.0	5.3	(g)
			♀	1,436	1,572	136	59.0	5.3	
Arm length	mm.	Adult	♂	630	778	148	37	16.0	(g)
			♀	576	706	170	37	12.2	
Interpupillary distance	mm.	Adult	♂	54.6	64.3	9.7	3.3	8.4	(h)
			♀	55.4	60.6	5.2	3.0	2.9	

Sources: (a) Smith & McKeown (1955)   (e) Loeffler & Smith (1964)
(b) Penrose (1954c)   (f) Turpin & Bernyer (1947)
(c) Caffey & Ross (1958)   (g) Øster (1953)
(d) Penrose (1954a)   (h) Kerwood et al. (1954)

Table 73. Natural Logarithms and Probability Ratio Equivalents

$\log_e P$	P	$\log_e P$	P	$\log_e P$	P	$\log_e P$	P
0.0	1.00	2.5	12.2	5.0	148	7.5	1,808
0.1	1.11	2.6	13.5	5.1	164	7.6	1,998
0.2	1.22	2.7	14.9	5.2	181	7.7	2,208
0.3	1.35	2.8	16.4	5.3	200	7.8	2,441
0.4	1.49	2.9	18.2	5.4	221	7.9	2,697
0.5	1.65	3.0	20.1	5.5	245	8.0	2,981
0.6	1.82	3.1	22.2	5.6	270	8.1	3,294
0.7	2.01	3.2	24.5	5.7	299	8.2	3,640
0.8	2.23	3.3	27.1	5.8	330	8.3	4,024
0.9	2.46	3.4	30.0	5.9	365	8.4	4,447
1.0	2.72	3.5	33.1	6.0	403	8.5	4,915
1.1	3.00	3.6	36.6	6.1	446	8.6	5,432
1.2	3.32	3.7	40.4	6.2	493	8.7	6,003
1.3	3.67	3.8	44.7	6.3	545	8.8	6,634
1.4	4.06	3.9	49.4	6.4	602	8.9	7,332
1.5	4.48	4.0	54.6	6.5	665	9.0	8,103
1.6	4.95	4.1	60.3	6.6	735	9.1	8,955
1.7	5.47	4.2	66.7	6.7	812	9.2	9,897
1.8	6.05	4.3	73.7	6.8	898	9.3	10,938
1.9	6.69	4.4	81.5	6.9	992	9.4	12,088
2.0	7.39	4.5	90.0	7.0	1,096	9.5	13,360
2.1	8.17	4.6	99.5	7.1	1,212	9.6	14,765
2.2	9.03	4.7	110	7.2	1,339	9.7	16,318
2.3	9.97	4.8	122	7.3	1,480	9.8	18,034
2.4	11.0	4.9	134	7.4	1,636	9.9	19,930
2.5	12.2	5.0	148	7.5	1,808	10.0	22,026

Table 74. Incidence of Presence (+) or Absence (−) of a Trait in Two Populations

Classification	(+)	(−)	Total
Population M	m	1 − m	1
Population N	n	1 − n	1
Relative probability, P	m/n	(1 − m)/(1 − n)	1

between the mean values of $\log_e y_M/y_N$ for Down's syndrome individuals and controls, thus

(ii) . . . . $I = (m - n) \log_e [m(1 - n)/n(1 - m)]$.

As an example, the presence or absence of tibial arch pattern on the hallucal area of the right sole may be considered. The presence of the arch pattern is positively scored as shown in Table 75.

The discriminative efficiency of this trait, based upon the formula $(m - n) \log_e [m(1 - n)/n(1 - m)]$, is 2.67. Thus the character, head length, is about twice as valuable, for diagnostic purposes, as hallucal pattern on one foot. Metrical characters are generally much more efficient discriminators

Table 75. Incidence of Presence (+) or Absence (−) of Tibial Arch Pattern on
the Hallucal Area of the Right Foot.

Classification	(+)	(−)	Total
Down's syndrome (M)	0.474	0.526	1.000
Controls (N)	0.003	0.997	1.000
Relative probability, P	158	0.543	1.000
$\text{Log}_e P$	5.06	−0.61	0.000

than qualitative traits (see Table 76) because they can take a greater number of different values and so give more information. Some traits give very high probabilities in favour of the diagnosis of Down's syndrome when they are present, but their discriminative index is low because they are uncommon even in the syndrome. An example is the presence of a radial loop on the fourth or fifth finger. Hallucal tibial arch is the best single physical sign of Down's syndrome so far described and analysed. The transverse flexion crease is theoretically one of the best qualitative traits for discrimination, but definition is less precise than in dermatoglyphic patterns.

COMBINATION OF CHARACTERS

The recognition of several coexisting signs, which point to a particular diagnosis, is of more significance than noting a single sign. This is of special importance if a condition is to be distinguished not only from the normal, but from other abnormal states. In clinically defining Down's syndrome, numerous attempts have been made to combine the information, obtained from separate characters, in an objective manner. The method suggested by Penrose (1933b) was to take seven independent traits, such as high cephalic index or fissured tongue, and score each of them equally, presence counting + 1 and absence, zero. Accepted cases of the syndrome scored, on the average, +3.3 points and a control group of retarded patients scored + 0.6. A similar analysis, with ten cardinal signs, was used by Øster (1953) and Gustavson (1964) recommended a list of twenty-one signs.

Such crude methods can only be logically justified if two rules hold good. First, the traits should all be equally characteristic of the condition concerned and, secondly, their occurrences should be mutually independent. The combination of traits with different degrees of specificity can be greatly improved by weighting them accordingly. The correction for intercorrelation is complicated. Theoretically it involves inversion of the covariance matrix in order to obtain the most efficient values for the weightings for discriminative purposes (Fisher 1936). However, very good results are obtained by making the assumption that all intercorrelations

Table 76. Discriminative Efficiency of some Qualitative Traits

Character	Sex	Frequency in Down's syndrome (m)	Frequency in controls (n)	Probability score in favour of Down's syndrome Presence (+) $\log_e m/n$	Absence (−) $\log_e[(1-n)/(1-m)]$	Index of efficiency (I) $(m-n)\log_e \frac{m(1-n)}{n(1-m)}$	Source
Ten ulnar loops on fingers	♂ or ♀	0.320	0.042	+2.0	−0.3	0.67	(a)
Radial loop on digit IV							
Left hand	♂ or ♀	0.524	0.070	+2.0	−0.7	1.23	(b)
Right hand	♂ or ♀	0.454	0.060	+2.0	−0.5	0.99	
Distal loop in 3rd inter-digital area							
Left hand	♂ or ♀	0.540	0.313	+0.5	−0.4	0.22	(c)
Right hand	♂ or ♀	0.854	0.555	+0.4	−1.1	0.45	
Tibial arch on sole							
Left foot	♂ or ♀	0.466	0.003	+5.0	−0.6	2.64	(c)
Right foot	♂ or ♀	0.474	0.003	+5.1	−0.6	2.69	
Four-finger crease							
Left hand	♂ or ♀	0.656	0.013	+3.9	−1.1	3.22	(d)
Right hand	♂ or ♀	0.710	0.008	+4.5	−1.2	4.10	

Sources: (a) Penrose (1964a), (b) Holt (1964a), (c) Ford Walker (1957), (d) Turpin & Lejeune (1953).

between the variables used are equal to one another (Cavalli 1945). For most practical purposes, provided that the number of traits involved is fairly large, it may be assumed that the common intercorrelation is small, even approaching zero, without diminishing the efficiency appreciably (Penrose 1954c).

Discriminative estimates can be expressed usefully in the form of logarithms. The usefulness is enhanced by using the base e, instead of, as in Ford Walker's (1957, 1958) data (see p. 96), base 10 $\log_e$ probabilities, calculated for qualitative characters in a given patient, can be combined by addition with standardized measurements, assuming that the traits are independent of one another. Thus, as an example, a patient with head length 168 mm. and with a tibial arch on the right foot has a score of 3.9 + 5.0 = 8.9. However, with the same head measurement but with a loop pattern on this sole, he would only have scored 3.9 − 0.6 = 3.3. These $\log_e$ scores can be turned back into probabilities at the end of a calculation by using Table 73. Thus, for $\log_e P = 8.9$, the probability ratio P is 7,500/1, whereas, for $\log_e P = 3.3$, P is 27/1. If the initial risk of Down's syndrome, on the basis of maternal age, is known, the combined probability value obtained, such as 7,500/1 or 27/1, can be compared with it. The two characters combined here give a quite strong probability in favour of the diagnosis even if the mother had been aged 20 to 25 years, in the first example but not in the second.

Combination of characters, for purposes of diagnosis of Down's syndrome, has been applied fairly frequently to dermatoglyphic traits and numbers of dermatoglyphic indices have been devised (see p. 95). In some of these procedures, groups of observations of the same kind are combined by using weightings in the form of a discriminant function. An example is Penrose & Loesch's (1971a, b) application of discriminant function to finger, palm and toe patterns. Another instance of such a procedure, involving radiological measurements, is provided by Nicolis & Sacchetti (1963) in their analysis of pelvic angles.

DIAGNOSIS OF PARTIAL OR INCOMPLETE DOWN'S SYNDROME

If the mean values of the scores for Down's syndrome and controls are known for the given set of characters used in the composite group, then the amount of deviation in the direction of the syndrome can be ascertained and expressed as a proportion or percentage.

In general, for any compound measurement or log probability estimate, X, if $\overline{M}$ is the mean for Down's syndrome and $\overline{N}$ the mean for controls, the percentage deviation towards the syndrome is $100(\overline{N} - X)/(\overline{N} - \overline{M})$. Figures of this kind are shown in Table 40 for the sum of the maximal *atd* angles on both hands. This method can be employed for the measurement of degree of Down's syndrome in cases where the diagnosis is in doubt or in which there is mosaicism.

The ordinary rule, which can be demonstrated by observing intelligence or dermatoglyphs, in a group of mosaic cases is that they are, on the average, intermediate between controls and fully affected patients. In respect of one character a mosaic may be typically normal and in respect of another typical of Down's syndrome. Quantitative combination of traits can be very useful in establishing the degree to which a given case is affected, provided that suitable mean values are available as standards for the traits under consideration.

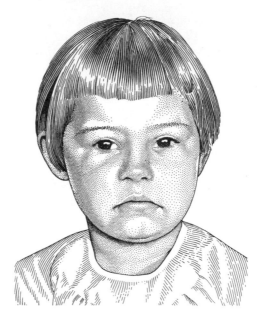

Fig. 47. Mosaic Down's syndrome female aged 10, Binet I.Q. 75. One quarter of the cells in fibroblast culture had normal karyotype and three-quarters had standard trisomy.

Signs of Down's syndrome in a reduced form have often been called microsymptoms (see Fig. 47). These may include facial peculiarities like epicanthic fold, spotting of the iris, protruding lower lip and flattened nose and cheeks. Unless they are carefully scored, they are of little scientific value. However, they can produce a strong enough general impression to make search for mosaicism with respect to trisomy 21 reasonable either in a mentally defective patient or a normal person (Hirsch *et al.* 1967, Kohn *et al.* 1970; also see Fig. 45). The problem is of significance in the study of the genetics of trisomic conditions, especially when mosaicism is suspected in parents or sibs of fully affected cases. Examples of how a variety of traits can be used, by the proposed technique, to indicate the tendency of an individual or a group to deviate

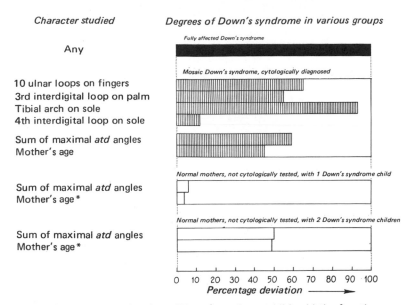

Fig. 48. Degree of deviation of group mean towards Down's syndrome mean.

from the normal in the direction of Down's syndrome are shown in Fig. 48. On the whole, known Down's syndrome mosaics deviate about halfway in that direction.

An example of precise analysis, based upon four uncorrelated discriminative traits, is now given. The family for which these observations are recorded is that described by Blank et al. (1962). Dermatoglyphic patterns and creases are shown in Fig. 49. Scores calculated for the father, the mosaic mother and their affected daughter are shown in Table 77. The combined results, expressed in terms of probabilities, show that on these four tests alone the child's chance of having Down's syndrome outweighs the random risk at birth. The mother is seen to have a higher chance than the father of being diagnosed as a case of the syndrome. She can be said to deviate considerably towards Down's syndrome. This relationship is shown in Fig. 50.

The probability scores of a number of traits combined may give useful information in cases whenever extra chromosomal material of uncertain origin is found by cytological examination, as in the patients described by Dent et al. (1963), Migeon et al. (1962) and Šubrt & Prchliková (1970). A deviation in the direction of Down's syndrome can indicate that chromosome No. 21 is the source of the material rather than No. 22 or some other one. In the absence of cytological tests the diagnosis of incomplete Down's syndrome is very uncertain. However, the ascertainment of the incidence of mosaics or other incomplete types in the

Table 77. Combination of Four Characters for Diagnosis of Down's Syndrome in a Family

Character	Sum of maximal *atd* angles		Ten ulnar loops on fingers		Tibial arch patterns on hallucal pads		Four-finger crease on palms		Total	
	Measurement	$\log_e P$	Presence or absence	$\log_e P$	Presence or absence	$\log_e P$	Presence or absence	$\log_e P$	Combined $\log_e P$	Probability ratio
Father	85°	−3.2	(+)	+2.0	(−)	−0.7	(−)	−1.2	−3.1	1/22
Mother	97°	−1.9	(−)	−0.3	(−) left / (+) right	+2.1	(−)	−1.2	−1.3	1/4
Daughter	138°	+0.9	(−)	−0.3	(+)	+5.0	(+) left / (−) right	+1.4	+7.0	1,096/1
Control average	−3.2 to −2.7			−0.2		−0.6		−1.1	−5.1 to −4.6	−
Down's syndrome average	+2.7 to +3.2			+0.4		+2.5		+2.5	+6.8 to +7.3	−

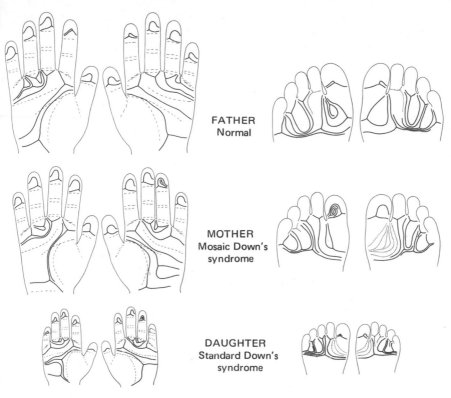

Fig. 49. Dermatoglyphic patterns of normal father, mosaic mother and fully affected trisomic daughter.

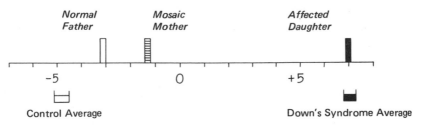

Fig. 50. Combined $\log_e$ probability scores of four traits in members of a family.

population is of importance and there are many different methods which can be used to estimate this.

In a survey of hospital patients, Penrose (1938) diagnosed 63 cases of Down's syndrome without reservation and accepted 9 as incomplete or possible instances wherein only a few signs were present. Cytological surveys, however, have indicated that mosaics are less common than this, mosaicism being found usually in about 2 per cent of cases (Richards

1969). Many partial cases, indeed probably the large majority, are not recognized as abnormal if they occur in the general population.

An estimate of the number of parents of Down's syndrome children who might be mosaic can be obtained from studying dermatoglyphic signs as indicated on p. 96 and in Fig. 48. If known mosaics on the average deviate rather more than halfway towards Down's syndrome, this implies that some 10 per cent of mothers of Down's syndrome children could be mosaics. Similar analysis shows that not more than 1 per cent of fathers would be mosaics.

Another way of estimating the incidence of mosaicism in mothers of Down's syndrome individuals is, using mother's age as a diagnostic sign, by examination of the maternal grandmothers' ages at the births of these mothers. In one survey Penrose (1954b) showed that these grandmothers had ages which were slightly greater than those for control mothers, a 5 per cent deviation towards the mean age for mothers of children with Down's syndrome. Known mosaics have mothers whose ages average considerably higher than control population mothers and may deviate by some 40 per cent towards the mean age for mothers of fully affected cases. Thus, it may be argued again that at least 10 per cent of mothers of Down's syndrome cases are themselves mosaic.

It is possible to infer, from the proportion of partially affected mothers, the approximate population incidence of incomplete Down's syndrome. If it were supposed that only half the mothers who were anomalous in this way actually gave birth to affected offspring, their true incidence might be of the order of 1/4000 in the total population of mothers. Besides this, there are the patients who, though classified as examples of Down's syndrome, are found on examination to be only partially affected. The total incidence of incomplete cases may therefore be as high as 1/3000 in the general population at birth.

10. Cytology

An initial account by Lejeune *et al.* (1959a) described the finding of 47 chromosomes in tissue cultures of three Down's syndrome individuals. Shortly after this, the same authors (1959b) reported nine further examples of the syndrome (5 males and 4 females), all of whom had an additional small acrocentric chromosome (see Fig. 51). It was not certain whether the extra chromosome should be described as supernumerary or homologous with one of the smallest pairs. Ford *et al.* (1959a) examined the chromosomes from bone marrow of a patient with Down's and Klinefelter's syndromes and found 48 chromosomes. Karyotype analysis showed two X chromosomes, one Y and five small acrocentric autosomes. Jacobs *et al.* (1959) examined the somatic chromosomes of six cases of Down's syndrome (3 males and 3 females) and also found a similar extra

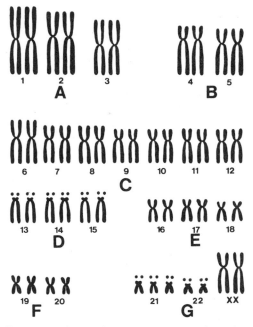

Fig. 51. Karyotype of a standard trisomy 21 Down's syndrome female.

169

acrocentric autosome in each. Böök *et al.* (1959) also studied the somatic chromosomes of three Down's syndrome individuals and concluded that the extra chromosome was morphologically similar to chromosome 21 and, in addition, that three of the five chromosomes in group 21-22 contained satellites. It was thought by most of these investigators that the additional acrocentric chromosome was similar to the larger of the two pairs of small acrocentrics and that it carried satellites, i.e. No. 21 in the Denver classification. Later reports have shown that both chromosomes 21

Table 78. Chromosomal Surveys of Down's Syndrome*

Reference	No. of cases	Country
Benirschke *et al.* (1963)†	67	U.S.A.
Hayashi (1963)	83	U.S.A.
Gustavson (1964)	98	Sweden
Hall (1964)	58	Sweden
Sergovich *et al.* (1964a)	240	Canada
Chitham & MacIver (1965)	105	England
Forteza Bover & Báguena Candela (1965)	50	Spain
Giannelli *et al.* (1965)	96	England
de Grouchy & Roubin (1965)	57	France
Hamerton *et al.* (1965)	157	England
Richards *et al.* (1965b)	225	England
Loftus & Mellman (1965, 1966)	52	U.S.A.
Edgren *et al.* (1966)	73	Finland
Hustinx (1966)	99	The Netherlands
Kleisner *et al.* (1966)	97	Argentina
Pfeiffer (1966)	312	Germany
Tonomura *et al.* (1966)	127	Japan
Zellweger *et al.* (1966a)	171	U.S.A.
Degenhardt & Franz (1967)	52	Germany
Emberger (1967)	78	France
Huang *et al.* (1967)	77	Taiwan
Mikkelsen (1967a)	93	Denmark
Ricci *et al.* (1967)	140	Italy
Wright *et al.* (1967)	180	U.S.A.
von Greyerz-Gloor *et al.* (1969a)	272	Switzerland
Higurashi *et al.* (1969)	321	Japan
Kahn & Abe (1969)	86	England
Engel *et al.* (1970)	365	Germany
Wahrman & Fried (1970)	53	Israel
Morić-Petrović *et al.* (1971)	180	Yugoslavia
Hongell *et al.* (1972)	174	Finland
Lee & Jackson (1972)	120	U.S.A.
Newton *et al.* (1972)	105	Scotland
Sutherland & Wiener (1972)	271	Australia
Aula *et al.* (1973)	425	Finland
Gardner *et al.* (1973)	972	New Zealand

*Studies having 50 or more cases in series
†Quoted by Polani *et al.* (1965)

and 22 have satellites, as do also the D-group acrocentric chromosomes 13, 14 and 15 (Ferguson-Smith & Handmaker 1961). It therefore became questionable whether or not satellites were reliable morphological features for distinguishing between chromosomes 21 and 22.

STANDARD TRISOMY

Chromosomal studies on Down's syndrome series have been extensive since the original work of Lejeune *et al.* (1959a) (see Table 78). All show that the syndrome is always associated with extra chromosomal material which can be identified as chromosome 21 (see below) or part of this chromosome. Two questionable cases of Down's syndrome with normal chromosomes have been reported (Hall 1962, Cowie & Kahn 1965); however, both of these cases are sufficiently unconvincing clinically to be reasonably considered as exceptions to the rule. Previously described patients with an additional G-group-like chromosome, but without the clinical features of Down's syndrome, will have to be restudied using the newer chromosomal staining techniques (G-banding and fluorescence) before any firm conclusions about them can be reached. It is very probable, however, that extra G-group-like chromosomal material found in these cases will be other than a number 21 chromosome, or will consist of only a portion of a number 21 (see also Mosaicism, page 200).

Based upon its size and morphology, chromosome 21 was thought to be trisomic in Down's syndrome. However, initially the precise identification of the extra chromosome was lacking and in certain cases of Down's syndrome the smaller pair, No. 22, had been implicated rather than 21 (Barnicot *et al.* 1963). It was proposed by some that, by definition, the chromosome which was trisomic in Down's syndrome was to be designated as chromosome 21 whether or not it was later found to be a smaller or larger G group chromosome. At the time, it was thought possible that chromosomes 21 and 22 may have some homology and, if so, this could account for irregularity in meiotic behaviour. Ordinary cytological techniques then were inadequate for resolving the problem and it was hoped that autoradiography (Yunis *et al.* 1965), the use of the electron microscope (Barnicot & Huxley 1965), or the finding of a genetic marker on chromosome 21 or 22 would make certain the identification of the extra chromosome. A study of the replication pattern of two kinds of translocated chromosomes, G/D and G/G, in Down's syndrome was carried out by Yunis *et al.* Interestingly enough, it was concluded that the chromosome involved for both translocations was likely to be No. 22.

Autoradiography of chromosomes, after growing cultures in medium containing tritiated thymidine, was used to study the G group (Nos. 21 and 22). Yunis (1965) showed that, in a standard trisomic Down's syndrome individual, three of the chromosomes in the G group were late-replicating over the long arms and they could be differentiated from the remaining two which replicate late over the centromeric region. However, in consequence of the small size of the chromosomes in the G group, identification by use of autoradiography was difficult and imperfect (Back *et al.* 1967, Fraccaro *et al.* 1967).

Quinacrine mustard and quinacrine hydrochloride have proved to be of much greater value in the study of human chromosomal abnormalities. These compounds bind deoxyribonucleic acid (DNA) and form fluorescent regions in the chromosomes resulting in specific fluorescent patterns for each individual chromosome. Of the two chromosome pairs in the G group, bright fluorescence is a property of pair number 21, while weak fluorescence is characteristic of the number 22 pair (see Fig. 52).

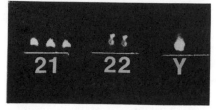

Fig. 52. A comparison of the fluorescence of chromosomes 21, 22 and Y. Chromosomes 21 are trisomic and show an increased fluorescence compared with chromosomes 22.

Caspersson *et al.* (1970b) showed that the extra chromosome in Down's syndrome was a "bright-G" and identical with the number 21 chromosome in fluorescence. Similar results were observed by Alfi *et al.* (1971), O'Riordan *et al.* (1971) and Schwinger *et al.* (1971). Photometrically determined fluorescence patterns, using a quinacrine mustard stain, are seen in Fig. 53.

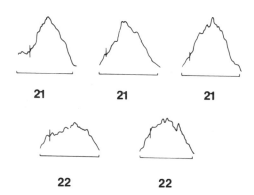

Fig. 53. Fluorescence distribution curves, after labelling with quinacrine mustard, of chromosomes 21 and 22 from a Down's syndrome individual.

Characteristic banding patterns of stained metaphase chromosomes are obtained by using a denaturation technique followed by Giemsa staining (see Fig. 54). By this procedure, chromosomes 21 and 22 can be identified by the difference in the areas of banding on the two chromosomes (see Fig. 55). Ridler (1971), using this technique, showed that the smaller of

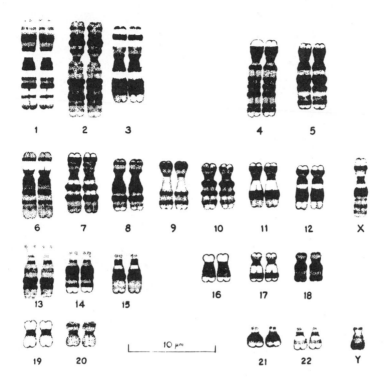

Fig. 54. Drawing of G-banded chromosomes illustrating the different bands associated with the various chromosomes.

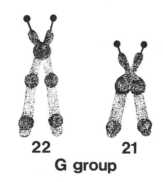

Fig. 55. Metaphase group G chromosomes showing comparative chromosome size and G-band patterns. (After Ridler 1971).

the G group chromosomes was trisomic in Down's syndrome. He noted that the larger G group chromosome pair was lightly stained with a prominent darkly stained centromeric area, together with the occasional occurrence of one or two less dense regions in the long arms. The trisomic group of chromosomes in Down's syndrome was usually smaller and more densely stained, frequently showing a dark band in the proximal part of the long arm. Occasionally, a less intense band was observed in the distal part of the long arm.

Ridler pointed out that the smaller of the G group chromosomes normally would be identified as chromosome number 22, so that Down's syndrome *could* be described as trisomy 22. However, as Baikie (1971) and others have observed, a new chromosomal designation for Down's syndrome would be confusing. The term *trisomy 21* has been used for over a decade in reference to Down's syndrome and the term *trisomy 22* has become associated with a quite different clinical complex (Hsu *et al.* 1971b).

The Fourth International Conference on Standardization in Human Cytogenetics, held in Paris in 1971, accepted the fluorescent patterns, as delineated by Caspersson *et al.* (1971b), for recognition of the chromosome connected with Down's syndrome. This chromosome, though the smaller of the G group, is defined as a number 21, and the larger pair of the G group as number 22. The designation of the smaller G chromosomes as 21, and the larger ones as 22, is a departure from the original 1960 Denver Conference notation (Hamerton 1971a) in which the progressive numbering of the autosomes increases as the size of the autosomes decrease. However, the exception avoids confusion, is relatively convenient and is generally accepted. The cytogenetic equivalent term for Down's syndrome thus remains *trisomy 21*.

It is of interest that Prieto *et al.* (1970), using autoradiography, identified the extra chromosome in Down's syndrome as being one of the later replicating chromosomes of group G, while the Philadelphia (Ph[1]) chromosome appeared to be derived from the early replicating pair. Their work suggested that the extra chromosome in the syndrome was a member of the shorter G group pair, but methodology did not permit unquestionable identification on size alone (Egozcue 1971). Similar findings were obtained by Caspersson *et al.* (1970a, 1970b) and O'Riordan *et al.* (1971) using a fluorescence technique. O'Riordan *et al.* showed that the extra chromosome in Down's syndrome belongs to the shorter pair of the group G chromosomes and that the Ph[1] chromosome is derived from the longer pair.

Hungerford *et al.* (1970) studied pachytene chromomere patterns in Down's syndrome. These studies showed that trivalents in trisomic spermatocytes, and thus the extra chromosome, were compatible in length and chromomere pattern with the shorter of the two G group chromosomes at the pachytene stage.

According to the 1971 Paris Conference classification referred to

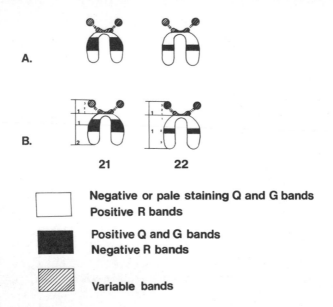

Fig. 56. Illustration A: showing banded areas of chromosomes 21 and 22.
Illustration B: landmarks which divide the chromosomes in defined regions
(After *Paris Conference* 1971).

previously, the G group chromosomes are subdivided into specific regions.
Figure 56 compares the identifiable regions on the numbers 21 and 22
chromosomes.

MECHANISMS PRODUCING STANDARD TRISOMY

Standard trisomy 21, as opposed to translocations and mosaicism, is
found in about 95 per cent of Down's syndrome cases. Asynapsis,
desynapsis, precocious separation and non-disjunction in meiosis are some
of the possible mechanisms underlying the origin of small acrocentric
trisomy. In general terms, asynapsis is the failure of homologous
chromosomes to pair while in desynapsis the chromosomes fall apart after
pairing in zygotene in the absence of chiasma formation. In precocious
separation there is early separation of the chromosomes, probably due to a
reduction of attracting forces within the chiasma after terminalization of
the chiasma has been completed. Non-disjunction strictly implies failure of
homologous chromosomes to separate during the first of the two meiotic
divisions or failure of chromatids to separate during the second meiotic
division (see Fig. 57). The results of non-disjunction were first observed in
plants by Gates (1908), but the cytological process was not demonstrated
until eight years later (Bridges 1916). Since it is not yet possible in man to
distinguish between different types of aberrant chromosomal behaviour by

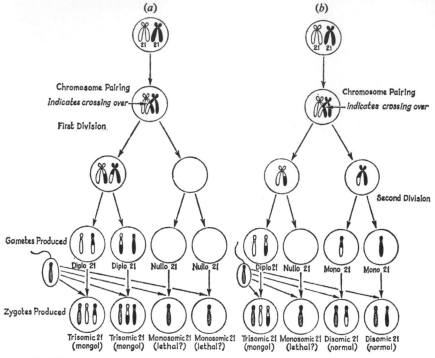

Fig. 57. Schematic representation of non-disjunction occurring during (*a*) the first and (*b*) the second divisions of meiosis. Theoretically the stage of non-disjunction can be identified by observing results of crossing over, but this has not been possible yet in Down's syndrome.

observation of the end product of the meiotic division, they are included, for convenience, under the general term of non-disjunction. In all these types of aberrant chromosomal behaviour the germ cell retains both members of a chromosome pair, so the gametic chromosome number is 24 instead of 23.

It would seem that non-disjunction is related to the increasing age of the mother in respect of both autosomes (Patau 1963) and the sex chromosomes (Court Brown *et al.* 1964). It has been estimated that in approximately 60 per cent of the mothers of Down's syndrome individuals there is an age-dependent factor in the causation (see Chapter 12).

CENTRIC FUSION OF t(Dq21q) TYPE

Although standard trisomy occurs in the majority of Down's syndrome individuals, there is a group in which one of the small acrocentric chromosomes has, by translocation, been fused with either a large, or another small, acrocentric. Fractures are assumed to have taken place at or near the centromeres of the two chromosomes concerned and been followed by translocated rejoining. This process, first observed by Robertson (1916), has been termed centric fusion (White 1954) because the chromosomes rejoin in regions close to the centromeres. Centric fusions have been known to occur in plants and animals (Ford *et al.* 1957). In man, such a translocation was demonstrated in a Down's syndrome child by Polani *et al.* (1960). They reported a typical female with 46 instead of the standard 47 chromosomes. The patient was selected because of the youth (21 years) of her mother at the time of the child's birth. Examination revealed 4 chromosomes in the 21-22 group instead of 5, which would have been expected in a standard Down's syndrome patient, and 5 chromosomes instead of 6 in the 13—15 group. An additional sub-metacentric chromosome was present in group 6—12. The interpretation of these findings was that a reciprocal translocation had taken place between a chromosome 21 and a large acrocentric chromosome of the D group which was designated No. 15.

This translocation is the commonest type of centric fusion found in Down's syndrome. The complementary chromosome formed by fusion of the two short arms of the participating chromosomes seems almost invariably to disappear after a few cell generations. Clinically, the result of having a long arm of chromosome 21 as extra chromatin material is almost the same whether it is attached to another chromosome or isolated, as in the standard trisomic karyotype. Gibson & Pozsonyi (1965) compared physical and mental signs in 10 translocation and 10 standard trisomic patients and found very slight differences in favour of the translocation cases. Dermatoglyphic variation is discussed in Chapter 5.

Table 79. Ages of Parents with Normal Karyotypes who have produced (13—15):21 Translocation Down's Syndrome Children

Source	Age of Father (yr.)	Age of mother (yr.)
Polani *et al.* (1960)	23	21
Ellis & Penrose (1960)	32	31
Makino *et al.* (1960)	–	22
Ellis (1962)	30	26
Priest *et al.* (1963a)	25	28
Ford Walker *et al.* (1963)	–	25
Sergovich *et al.* (1964a)	32	28
Sergovich *et al.* (1964a)	32	29
Sergovich *et al.* (1964a)	35	28
Gustavson (1964)	26	27
Forteza Bover & Báguena Candela (1965)	36	30
Berg (1969)	40	38
Berg (1969)	38	36
Berg (1969)	24	21
von Greyerz-Gloor *et al.* (1969a)	25	23
Mean age	30.6	27.5

Chromosomal studies (using peripheral blood) on the parents of the translocation case, reported by Polani *et al.*, showed normal karyotypes (Carter *et al.* 1960). A similar type of D:21 translocation has been found in other instances of Down's syndrome whose parents had normal chromosome complements (see Table 79). When parents with normal karyotypes produce a translocation Down's syndrome child, the chromosomal mechanism is obscure. It is possible that chromosomal interchange occurs in the germinal tissue of one or other parent and both tend to be young (mean ages, father 30.6 and mother 27.5 years) at the time of birth of the translocation child.

There are three different types of (Dq21q) translocations, since there are three chromosomes in the D group onto which a number 21 chromosome can be translocated. The translocation types are t(13q21q), t(14q21q) (see Fig. 58) and t(15q21q). Autoradiographic studies by Mikkelsen (1967b) and Hecht *et al.* (1968) suggest that the translocation usually involves a number 14 chromosome, rarely number 15 and never number 13. However, by quinacrine mustard fluorescent analysis, Caspersson *et al.* (1971a) subsequently found, in four individuals with a translocation of a number 21 onto a D, that the D chromosome was a number 13 in one instance; it was a number 14 in the other three cases.

PROPORTIONS OF ROBERTSONIAN TRANSLOCATIONS

Depending upon data collection methods and other factors, there are

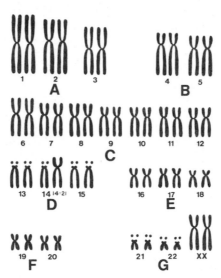

Fig. 58. Karotype of a translocation Down's syndrome female: 46,XX,14-, t(14q21q)+.

Table 80. Proportions of Robertsonian Translocations

Series	Total Number D.S.	Translocations	t(DqGq)	t(GqGq)	t(DqGq)		t(GqGq)	
					Sporadic	Inherited	Sporadic	Inherited
				Percentages				
Hamerton (1971a)	2,594	3.5	44	56	51	49	94.4	5.6
Mikkelsen (1970), Matsunaga & Tonomura (1972)	4,330	5.0	55.3	44.7	55	45	91.3	8.7

D.S. = Down's Syndrome

slight differences in the ratio of translocation cases to standard trisomic cases of the syndrome (see Table 80). Hamerton (1971a) summarized data from 34 separate series comprising a total of 2,594 affected individuals. After making certain adjustments for bias in data collection—and assuming that 35 per cent of all Down's syndrome individuals are born at maternal ages of less than 30 years—the frequency of interchange trisomy is 3.5 per cent. This is slightly lower than the 5 per cent of interchange trisomy found in 4,330 Down's syndrome individuals in the combined series of Mikkelsen (1970) and Matsunaga & Tonomura (1972). In Hamerton's series, t(GqGq) translocation occurred more frequently (56 per cent) than t(DqGq) (44 per cent). In the combined series of Mikkelsen and Matsunaga & Tonomura, the opposite was found, that is, t(GqGq) comprised 44.7 per cent and t(DqGq) 55.3 per cent. The ratios of sporadic to inherited cases for t(DqGq) and t(GqGq) were similar in the two series. In the t(DqGq) group there is nearly an equal number of sporadic and inherited cases. For sporadic t(DqGq) cases the range is 51–55 per cent and for inherited cases it is 45–49 per cent. This is in contrast to t(GqGq) where the range for sporadic cases is 91–94 per cent and for inherited cases between 6–8 per cent. Polani *et al.* (1965) calculated that the new mutation rate of all types of translocations related to Down's syndrome is 2.71×10^{-5} chromosomes 21 per gamete per generation.

Matsunaga & Tonomura (1972) examined the parental ages of 102 translocation Down's syndrome individuals in Japan. They found that the age of the mother, but not of the father, had an effect upon the birth of sporadic cases. With advancing maternal age, the relative risk was apparently increasing for the t(GqGq) while it was decreasing for the t(DqGq) trisomics.

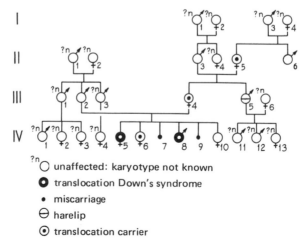

Fig. 59. Pedigree of family with 15:21 translocation carriers and Down's syndrome individuals (after Penrose & Delhanty 1961a).

TRANSMISSION OF t(Dq21q) TYPE OF FUSION

The familial transmission of the (13–15):21 type of translocation was first demonstrated by Penrose *et al.* (1960) and additional information was published by Penrose & Delhanty (1961a). In this family (see Fig. 59) there were 2 Down's syndrome children (IV.5 and 8) in one sibship. Two of the remaining 4 pregnancies resulted in normal children and 2 in miscarriages. The only other abnormality found in this family was one case of harelip in a healthy male (III.5). The two Down's syndrome children (see Fig. 60) exhibited karyotypes similar to that in the case reported by

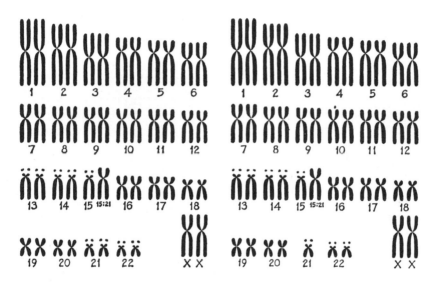

Fig. 60. Chromosomes of Down's syndrome female (Fig. 59–IV.5) with centric fusion: 46,XX,15–,t(15q21q)+.

Fig. 61. Female carrier with normal phenotype (Fig. 59–II.5, III.4, IV.6): 45,XX,15–,21–,t(15q21q)+.

Polani *et al.* (1960) Three phenotypically normal females (II.5, III.4, IV.6) were found to have 45 chromosomes (Fig. 61) Karyotype analysis showed that they each had one extra chromosome in the 6–12 group which was considered to be a fusion between chromosomes 15 and 21. Each lacked one large and one small acrocentric chromosome. Similar families were reported by Carter *et al.* (1960), Makino *et al.* (1960), Buckton *et al.* (1961), Hamerton *et al.* (1961b), Ek *et al.* (1961), Lehmann & Forssman (1962), German *et al.* (1962), Atkins *et al.* (1962), MacIntyre *et al.* (1962), Shaw (1962a) and by Sergovich *et al.* (1964a). Mean maternal age for 16 translocation Down's syndrome cases was 27.3 years.

In an individual who is a heterozygous carrier, the formation of many gametic types is theoretically possible (see Fig. 62). Some would be

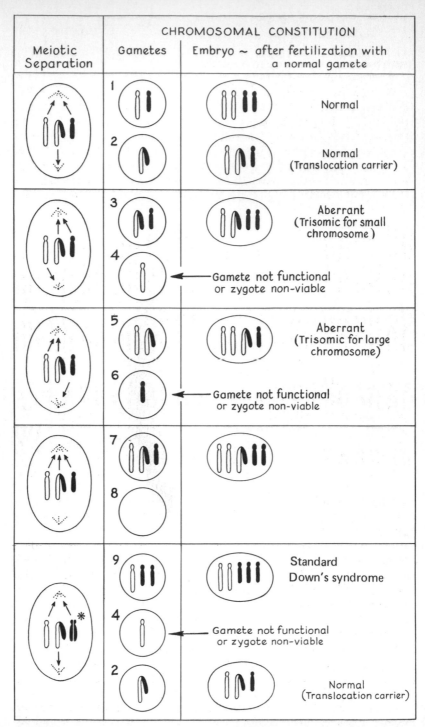

Fig. 62. Representation of meiosis showing the results of translocation on the gametic chromosomes. *indicates precocious separation into chromatids in the first meiotic division followed by non-disjunction in the second.

extremely rare and others would probably be non-viable either as gametes or zygotes. For example, types 7 and 8, which depend on total non-disjunction, would be rare. Gametic type 9, if fertilized by a normal gamete, would form a zygote which would be standard trisomic Down's syndrome. This type of meiotic behaviour could explain the case of a mother with D:21 translocation who has a trisomic child. Gametes of types 4 and 6 would not be rare, but if they were able to form zygotes with normal gametes, the zygotes would be monosomic for a D group chromosome or a 21 chromosome and probably would not be viable. Gametes of type 5, when fertilized, would be effectively trisomic for a D group chromosome, with fusion of a similar D group chromosome and a chromosome 21. This type of zygote has not yet been found. Gametes of types 1, 2 and 3 are known from the zygotes they form when fertilized by normal gametes. Gametic type 1 leads to a normal zygote; gametic type 2 leads to a translocation heterozygous carrier and gametic type 3 to a translocation Down's syndrome individual. Information about pairing during meiosis in a male translocation heterozygous carrier has been obtained from testicular biopsy (Hamerton *et al.* 1961b). Meiotic chromosomes at diakinesis showed 21 bivalents (including the unequal sex bivalent) and one trivalent (Fig. 63).

Three types of viable offspring (normal, carriers and Down's syndrome individuals) of heterozygous translocation carriers, male or female, might be expected in equal numbers, provided that no selective force is operating. The theoretical expected risk of one in three pregnancies resulting in an affected child is not observed (Penrose & Smith 1966, Hamerton 1971a). Estimates of the types and numbers of offspring produced by heterozygous carriers have been obtained by pooling family data (Hamerton & Steinberg 1962, Penrose & Smith). Probably the most accurate estimates of risk of heterozygous carriers producing affected offspring are derived from the data of Hamerton (1971a) (see Table 81). Heterozygous carriers have to be considered separately, according to whether the carrier is female (maternal transmission) or male (paternal transmission). Hamerton has shown that, when the mother is the heterozygous carrier (maternal transmission), for any future pregnancy there is about a 90 per cent chance of a normal child or a balanced heterozygote and about a 10 per cent chance of an infant with Down's syndrome being produced. When the father is the heterozygous carrier (paternal transmission) there is a marked decrease in the risk of producing an affected infant, that is, a 97.6 per cent chance of either a normal infant or a balanced heterozygote and a 2.4 per cent chance of an infant with Down's syndrome. There seems to be an excess of heterozygote carriers produced in families where there is paternal transmission.

The reasons why male and female heterozygotes do not produce as many affected offspring as would be expected or why male heterozygotes have a particularly low risk of producing affected offspring (see Table 81) are not clear. However, from the data of Penrose & Smith, which showed

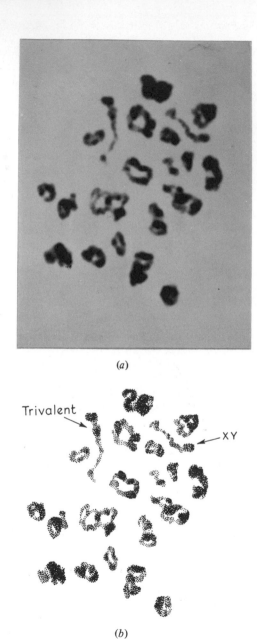

(a)

(b)

Fig. 63. (a) Photograph of diakinesis in a normal male carrier of a D:21 type of translocation. (b) Explanatory drawing (after Hamerton *et al.* 1961b)

Table 81. Karyotypes of Offspring of (Dq21q) Balanced Translocation Carrier Parents (After Hamerton 1971a)

Translocation carrier parents		Phenotypically normal 46,XX or XY	45,XX or XY, D-,21-,t(Dq21q)+	Down's syndrome 46,XX or XY, D-,t(Dq21q)+	Totals	Risk of Down's syndrome
Sex	No.					
Mothers	62	45	37	10	92	1:9
Fathers	32	33	50	2	85	1:42

that there was an increased number of miscarriages and stillbirths among female heterozygotes, it is possible to conclude that many of the affected zygotes are lost during pregnancy. This explanation is not sufficient to account for the low risk of male heterozygotes having affected offspring. In this circumstance, the sperm which would produce an affected child is carrying extra No. 21 chromosomal material which puts it at a physical disadvantage in joining with the normal ovum to form the abnormal zygote. The same type of inheritance has occurred in the mouse. Female mice, heterozygous for the reciprocal translocation t(14;15)6C2, have a high frequency of translocation trisomic offspring. Male mice, heterozygous for the same translocation, have not produced translocation trisomic offspring. Thus, the laboratory mouse may provide a model for studying the causes of this phenomenon (Eicher 1973).

Stene (1970a) has demonstrated how different types of ascertainment influence the segregation ratios in the t(DqGq) translocation. The proportion of translocation Down's syndrome individuals categorized by maternal age is seen in Table 82.

Some of the conclusions derived from pooling family data may not be applicable to all families. For example, the family studied by Hamerton *et al.* (1961b) had phenotypically normal individuals, in three segregating sibships, all of whom were found to carry the translocation (see Fig. 64). In contrast is the family reported by Atkins *et al.* (1962) where the

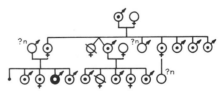

Fig. 64. Pedigree showing transmission of a 15:21 type of translocation (after Hamerton *et al.* 1961b).

O   unaffected

?n   not tested

⊙   translocation carrier

●   translocation Down's syndrome

⊘   stillbirth

Table 82. Proportion of Down's Syndrome Individuals with Translocations, Categorized by Maternal Age*

Maternal age		Total Down's syndrome cases	Translocation Down's syndrome cases						Total translocations
			D/21			G/21			
			de Novo	Familial	?	de Novo	Familial	?	
<30	No.	1792	52	31	10	46	7	5	151
	%		2.9	1.7	0.6	2.5	0.4	0.3	8.4
≥30	No.	1669	5	6	1	9	1	2	24
	%		0.3	0.4	0.1	0.5	0.1	0.1	1.5

*From data of Mikkelsen (1971) and Gardner et al. (1973).

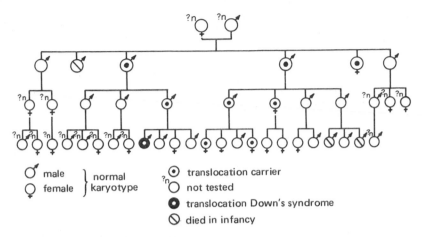

Fig. 65. Pedigree showing transmission of a 15:21 type of translocation (after Sergovich *et al.* 1962).

mother was a translocation carrier and gave birth to 3 Down's syndrome children (2 boys and a girl) all of whom had 46 chromosomes with the 15:21 translocation. A family reported by Shaw (1962a) showed a segregation ratio of one to one for translocation carriers to normal offspring. Transmission of translocation to a Down's syndrome child through a male carrier is seen in the large family studied by Sergovich *et al.* (1962) (see Fig. 65).

A case of (13–15):21 translocation mosaicism has been reported in a phenotypically normal male and his Down's syndrome daughter (Tips *et al.* 1963). In a similar type of case Ferrier (1964) reported that the father's leucocyte chromosomes showed translocation mosaicism. Most of the cells were normal, but 7 out of 34 had 46 chromosomes with a karyotype similar to that found in his translocation Down's syndrome son. Waller & Waller (1973) reported a chromosome (ploidy) mosaic with diploid and tetraploid cells in the ratio of 2:1. There was a t(DqGq) chromosome in all the cell lines. It was concluded that the tetraploid cells originated from explants of lung. Atkins & Bartsocas (1974) reported an unusual chromosomal mosaic with two cell lines in both blood and skin. One cell line carried a balanced translocation, t(15q21q), and the other cell line was trisomic for chromosome 21 with a t(21q21q) translocation.

CENTRIC FUSION OF t(GqGq) TYPE

Another translocation found in Down's syndrome involves two chromosomes of the 21–22 group. Fraccaro *et al.* (1960) described a Down's syndrome boy who had 46 chromosomes which, on karyotype analysis, showed 3 in the 21–22 group and an additional chromosome, morphologically resembling one of the 19–20 group. The patient was born at maternal and paternal ages of 37 and 58 respectively. A fibroblast culture from the phenotypically normal father revealed 47 chromosomes in some cells. Analysis showed that the extra chromosome was morphologically similar to those of the 19–20 group. The data indicated that the additional small metacentric chromosome observed in both the father and the son represented either an isochromosome of the long arm of a No. 21 or a translocation between 21 and 22. The father's peripheral blood showed a normal karyotype, implying a mosaic constitution.

A similar type of case also revealed evidence of mosaicism and transmission through the father (Hamerton *et al.* 1961a). The patient was a male with Down's syndrome whose peripheral blood cultures showed mainly 46 chromosomes, but some cells contained 47. Karyotype analysis of cells with 46 chromosomes showed 5 in the 19–20 group, and the 3 in the 21–22 group. Cells with 47 chromosomes showed 5 in the 19–20 group and 4 in the 21–22 group. Studies on the father showed mainly 46 chromosomes but a few cells with 47 like those found in his Down's syndrome son. The mother's chromosomes were normal. The extra chromosome in the 19–20 group could be an isochromosome for the long arm of No. 21, a 21:21 or a 21:22 centric fusion.

Four types of rearrangements can occur in this chromosomal group. They are: t(21q22q), t(21q21q), 21qi (isochromosome of long arms of No. 21) and tan(21q21q) (tandem of long arms of No. 21). These chromosomal rearrangements must be determined cytologically, since physically and biochemically these individuals cannot be differentiated from standard trisomics. Affected individuals with these rearrangements will have 46 chromosomes and examples of their karyotypes are seen in Fig. 66. The majority of these types of structural change arise *de novo* with only about 6–8 per cent occurring as the result of a familial transmission. Familial transmission occurs almost exclusively as the t(21q22q) type. Differentiation between the t(21q22q) and t(21q21q) was difficult before the advent of fluorescence and chromosomal banding.

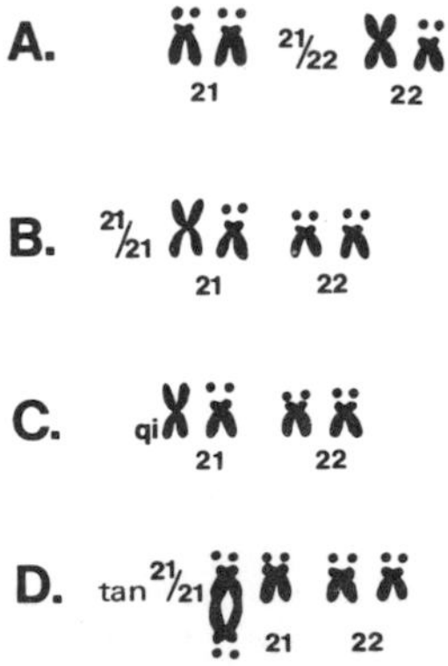

Fig. 66. Four types of G group chromosome rearrangements which result in Down's syndrome.
A: t(21q22q)
B: t(21q21q)
C: 21qi
D: tan (21q21q)

Ten cases of Down's syndrome with sporadic (GqGq) translocations were reported. Nine cases were available for fluorescent study. In all nine cases, two number 21 chromosomes were involved in the translocation (Ying 1973).

TRANSMISSION OF t(GqGq) TYPE OF FUSION

Of the t(GqGq) types of chromosomal rearrangements, the t(21q22q) type may be transmitted through a balanced heterozygous parent. Even in the t(21q22q) type, the majority arise *de novo* and in only about 6 per cent are the structural changes inherited. The t(21q22q) appears to behave like the t(DqGq) Robertsonian translocation and, in the familial form, balanced heterozygous, Down's syndrome and chromosomally normal sibs can be found. The karyotypes of a balanced heterozygous female and a translocation Down's syndrome individual are seen in Figs. 67, 68.

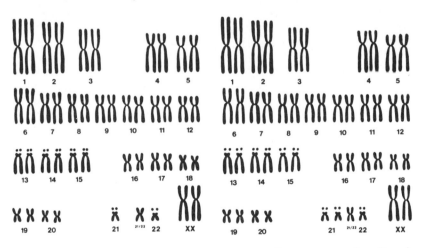

Fig. 67. Female carrier of 21:22 centric fusion with normal phenotype: 45,XX,21-,22-,t(21q22q)+

Fig. 68. Chromosomes of a Down's syndrome female with a 21:22 type of centric fusion: 46,XX,22-,t(21q22q)+.

Penrose *et al.* (1960) reported a Down's syndrome male with 46 chromosomes and t(GqGq) translocation. Some of the cells contained an additional centric particle. A testicular biopsy indicated that spermatogenesis was fairly active. At diakinesis, fewer than the normal number of 23 masses were identified and it was thought that a quadrivalent could be seen in some cells (Miller *et al.* 1960). The quadrivalent during meiosis suggested that the extra metacentric had arisen by a reciprocal translocation between chromosomes 21 and 22. There is some suggestion that the t(21q22q) type of centric fusion is transmitted more frequently through

Table 83. Data on Parental Age in Down's syndrome with a 21:21−22 Fusion

Source	Age of Father (yr.)	Age of Mother (yr.)
	N	N
Hirschhorn *et al.* (1961)	−	36
Penrose & Delhanty (1962)	40	26
Gray *et al.* (1962)	40	36
Benirschke *et al.* (1962)	30	30
Gustavson (1962)	40	30
Sergovich (1962)	38	36
Hamm *et al.* (1963)	23	20
Sergovich (1963)	27	27
Warkany *et al.* (1964)	24	24
Warkany *et al.* (1964)	39	39
Gustavson (1964)	24	24
Gustavson (1964)	50	36
Mean	34.1	30.3
	T	N
Fraccaro *et al.* (1960)	58	37
Forssman & Lehmann (1961)	42	37
Hamerton *et al.* (1961a)	33	21
Shaw (1962b)	35	−
Mean	42.0	31.7
	N	T
Shaw (1962b)	−	28
Pfeiffer (1963)	23	25
	N?	N?
Penrose *et al.* (1960)	41	33
Sergovich (1962)	24	20
Sergovich (1962)	29	24
Bavin *et al.* (1963)	42	39
Gustavson (1964)	−	18

N = Normal karyotype.
T = Translocation carrier.

the father. With such a fusion, Penrose (1962a) noted a significant increase in the paternal age. This trend is seen in Table 83. If the transmission of the aberrant chromosome is through the father, the mean age at birth of the affected child is 42 years but, if both the mother and the father have normal karyotypes, the father's mean age is still increased (34.1 years) though to a lesser degree. The balanced heterozygous carriers of the t(21q22q) produce three types of offspring, though additional gametes and nonviable zygotes are probably formed. In the family containing a t(21q22q) rearrangement reported by Shaw (1962b), there were two Down's syndrome children, 8 translocation carriers and 7 normal offspring (see Fig. 69). Similar types of families were reported by Chapman *et al.* (1973).

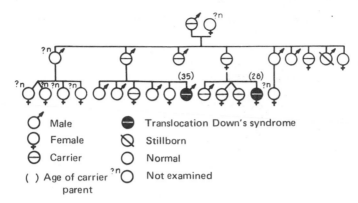

Fig. 69. Pedigree showing transmission of a 21 : 22 type of translocation
(after Shaw 1962b).

The t(21q21q) and 21qi types of chromosomal rearrangements cannot produce balanced heterozygous carriers and all the offspring of carriers would be expected to have Down's syndrome, because every viable gamete would contain the centric fusion or the isochromosome (see Fig. 70). The balanced heterozygous parent must arise from a postfertilization mitotic error of a normal zygote. The gamete produced by the heterozygote must be either disomic or nullisomic–21 (see Fig. 70). Fertilization of these gametes will produce, respectively, a zygote which is trisomic or monosomic–21. The latter zygote is most likely to be non-viable and will be lost as a spontaneous abortion. Families of this type have been reported by Hamerton *et al.* (1961) and Dallaire & Fraser (1964). Dallaire & Fraser reported a sibship with four Down's syndrome individuals, one abortion and one stillbirth. The Down's syndrome cases had 46 chromosomes and a t(GqGq). The father had 45 chromosomes and a similar t(GqGq)

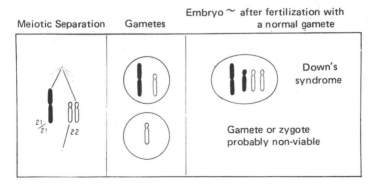

Fig. 70. Representation of gamete formation in the presence of an isochromosome or a 21 : 21 translocation.

chromosome. A t(21q21q) rearrangement would best account for the families in both of these reports.

Hamerton (1971a) has offered an explanation for the origin of the balanced 21qi heterozygote. He postulated that the isochromosome could be formed during gametogenesis in a normal subject. If this were followed by postzygotic non-disjunction, both normal and secondary trisomic cell lines could be produced. Families with a phenotypically normal mixoploid father and an isotrisomic offspring have been reported by Fraccaro *et al.* (1960) and Hamerton *et al.* (1961a).

Family data are still limited in regard to this Robertsonian translocation (Hamerton 1968, 1971a, Chapman *et al.* 1973, Zergollern 1974), but the data suggest an excess of carriers compared with Down's syndrome individuals. Stene (1970c) estimated the risk of Down's syndrome for female carriers to be 8.9 per cent. He was unable to calculate a risk figure for male carriers.

The cases of tandem translocation tan (21q21q) (see Fig. 71) reported

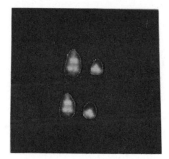

Fig. 71. Quinacrine mustard stained tandem 21 : 21 chromosome compared with a regular chromosome 21 (after Sachdeva *et al.* 1971).

have all been nonfamilial (Warkany & Soukup 1963, Zellweger *et al.* 1963, Lejeune *et al.* 1965, Richards *et al.* 1965a, Vogel *et al.* 1970, Garson *et al.* 1970, Kadotani *et al.* 1970b, Sachdeva *et al.* 1971, Vogel 1972, Bartsch-Sandhoff & Schade 1973, Schuh *et al.* 1974). The case of Cohen & Davidson (1967) was familial, resulting from a balanced G/G translocation in the mother with subsequent trisomy in her children. The unusual family presented by Soudek *et al.* (1968) (see Fig. 72) is best explained as being the result of a pericentric inversion of a familial G/G Robertsonian translocation chromosome (see Fig. 73) Schuh *et al.* thought that the formation of a tandem chromosome with satellites at both ends could best be accounted for as seen in Fig. 74.

OTHER CHROMOSOMAL REARRANGEMENTS

While translocations of the (Dq21q) and (Gq21q) types are the most frequent centric fusions in Down's syndrome, other chromosomal rearrangements also have been noted. Some examples are referred to here and illustrated in Fig. 75.

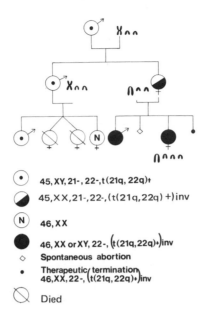

Fig. 72. Modified pedigree of family reported by Soudek *et al.* (1968) in which a t(21q22q) and an inversion of the translocation chromosome are segregating. Diagrammatic configuration of chromosome is demonstrated in pedigree.

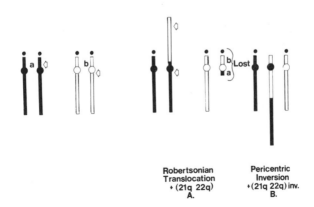

Fig. 73. Drawing of the probable mode of origin of translocated chromosome (A) and the inverted translocated chromosome (B). See Figure 72. (After Hamerton 1971a)

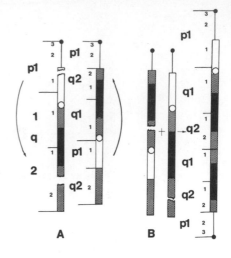

Fig. 74. Schematic representation suggested by Schuh *et al.* (1974) of the formation of a tandem chromosome with satellites at both ends.

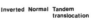

A   **B**

Inverted Normal Tandem
translocation

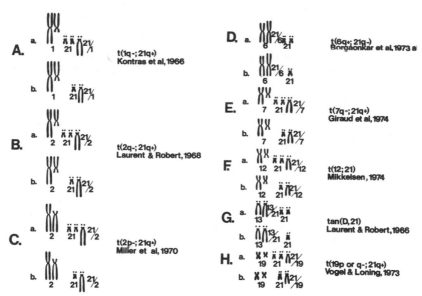

A. a.   t(1q-;21q+)
Kontras et al,1966

b.

B. a.   t(2q-;21q+)
Laurent & Robert,1968

b.

C. a.   t(2p-;21q+)
Miller et al,1970

b.

D. a.   t(6q+;21q-)
Borgaonkar et al,1973 a

b.

E. a.   t(7q-;21q+)
Giraud et al,1974

b.

F. a.   t(12;21)
Mikkelsen,1974

b.

G. a.   tan(D,21)
Laurent & Robert,1966

b.

H. a.   t(19p or q-;21q+)
Vogel & Loning,1973

b.

Fig. 75. Representation of translocations associated with Down's syndrome. (a) is the unbalanced form producing the syndrome and (b) is the balanced form having a normal phenotype.

Kontras *et al.* (1966) studied 19 members of a family in which translocation between chromosomes No. 1 and No. 21 had occurred [t(1q-;21q+)] (see Fig. 75A). Two had Down's syndrome with 47 chromosomes [47,XX,t(1q-;21q+),21+], eleven were balanced translocation carriers with 46 chromosomes [46,XX or XY,G-, t(1q-;21q+)] and six had apparently normal karyotypes.

Laurent & Robert (1968) reported a family in which an uncle and niece each had Down's syndrome and in which a t(2q-;21q+) translocation was present in three generations (see Fig. 75B). The recurrence risk of trisomy was approximately 1 in 5. The same authors (Laurent & Robert 1966) also reported segregation of a D/G translocation, in tandem, in three generations of a family. Of the family members examined, two had trisomy 21 with 46 chromosomes and a tan (D,21), five were balanced translocation carriers and two had apparently normal karyotypes (see Fig. 75G).

Borgaonkar et al. (1973a) described a family with a C/G, probably 6/21, translocation chromosome (see Fig. 75D). Ascertainment was through an individual with Down's syndrome. Genetic linkage analysis suggested the possibility of localization of the Gm locus on chromosome No. 6.

Giraud et al. (1974) investigated a mother with a reciprocal translocation [t(7q-;21q+)]. Out of seven pregnancies, there were no normal children; there were three Down's syndrome children and four spontaneous abortions. Two of the affected children had the identical translocation chromosome as the mother (see Fig 75E).

Miller et al. (1970) described a Down's syndrome boy with the karyotype 47,XY,t(2p-;21q+),21+. His phenotypically normal maternal grandmother, maternal great-aunt, mother and two sisters showed a balanced reciprocal translocation of the type 46,XX,t(2p-;21q+). (See Fig. 75C).

Vogel & Löning (1973) & Chaganti et al. (1975) found familial 19:21 translocation associated with Down's syndrome (see Fig. 75H). Mikkelsen (1974) observed a translocation of the type t(12q21q) in a typical Down's syndrome male. Members of his family carried the balanced form of the translocation (see Fig. 75F). The breakpoints on the chromosomes were 12q14 and 21q22 which were identified by fluorescence studies. A 21 chromosome was translocated to a deleted part of the short arms of a B chromosome in a Down's syndrome child studied by Aarskog (1966).

ASSOCIATED TRANSLOCATIONS

Gardner et al. (1973) reported two Down's syndrome individuals each of whom had a balanced translocation not involving a chromosome 21; in another Down's syndrome individual, there was a translocation between chromosome 3 and a G group chromosome. The karotypes were, respectively, 47,XY,21+,t(1p-;3q+); 47,XY,21+,t(16q-;?+); and 47,XY,G+,t(3?;Gq+). In the latter two cases, the translocations were familial. A 47,XY,G+,t(3?;Gq+) karyotype had been noted earlier by Soukup et al. (1969). They described a balanced translocation (3?-;G?q+)

in two unrelated families. The translocations in both kinships were ascertained through a propositus who had Down's syndrome (standard trisomy 21), in addition to having the balanced translocation.

A t(14q22q) was observed in the mother of a trisomic 47,XY,+21 individual. Interchromosomal interaction was considered as a possible explanation for the occurrence of the trisomy 21 child (Forabosco *et al.* 1973).

Because of the small numbers involved, it is not possible to say if there is an association between a balanced translocation in a parent and the production of a standard trisomic child. The incidence of translocation in the general population could be as high as 1 in 200 (Court Brown 1967); therefore, a small proportion of Down's syndrome cases would be expected to have a balanced translocation in addition to standard trisomy 21. Hamerton (1968) has shown that, despite the fact that many t(DqDq) cases have been ascertained through a propositus with Down's syndrome, there is no evidence of more than a chance relationship in these cases.

OTHER CHROMOSOMAL ABNORMALITIES AND TRISOMY 21

The simultaneous occurrence of Down's syndrome and a structural sex chromosome anomaly was first described by deGrouchy *et al.* (1965b) in a boy with Down's syndrome. The karyotype suggested a pericentric inversion of an X or number 6 chromosome, in addition to trisomy 21. Luthardt & Palmer (1971) reported a female with Down's syndrome who had a deletion of the long arms of one of her X chromosomes. Her karotype was considered to be 47,XXq-,21+.

Bargman *et al.* (1970) described a Down's syndrome child with a small marker chromosome in addition to standard trisomy 21. The mother had the same marker chromosome. The child's karyotype was 48,XY,21+, mar+mat.

Šubrt (1970) noted the transmission of the enlarged short arm of a small acrocentric chromosome through three generations. In the third generation, a child with Down's syndrome was produced. Enlargement of the short arm or the satellites of acrocentric chromosomes has been detected in many individuals, usually without phenotypic effect. The structural change occasionally has been associated with trisomy 21 (see Table 84). Some authors (Cooper & Hirschhorn 1962, deGrouchy *et al.* 1964, Therkelsen 1964) suggested that the enlargement on the short arms of an acrocentric chromosome may be a predisposing factor to meiotic non-disjunction.

Hamerton (1971b) reported a two per cent incidence of short arm enlargement in Down's syndrome individuals and their parents. Edgren *et al.* (1966) noted a much higher incidence (6.8 per cent) and Sands (1969) found an incidence of 3.4 per cent. Court Brown *et al.* (1965) observed 7 (1.6 per cent) out of 438 normal individuals with enlarged short arms on

Table 84. Reported Cases of Enlarged Short Arm of D or G Group Chromosome Associated with Down's Syndrome (After Šubrt 1970)

Author		Short Arm Enlargement D or G	Familial Transmission
Nichols*	1961	G	+
Edwards*	1961	G	?
Hungerford et al.*	1961	G	+
Cooper & Hirschhorn	1962	D	+
Gray et al.	1962	G	+
Therkelsen	1964	G	+
Wolf et al.	1964	D	+
Chaptal et al.	1966	D	+
Vamos–Hurwitz et al.	1967	G	+
Pepler et al.	1968	G	?
Šubrt et al.	1968	D	+
Sands	1969	G	+
Sands	1969	D	+
Šubrt	1970	G	+

*Reference: Šubrt (1970)

acrocentric chromosomes. A comparison of the Hamerton and Court Brown et al. series showed no significant difference between the two studies.

Hamerton et al. (1965) and Edgren et al. (1966) attempted to assess the indirect effects that acrocentric short arm enlargement might produce at meiosis which could lead to non-disjunction. The incidence was investigated in Down's syndrome and normal populations of varying sizes but no conclusive statistical effect was obtained. The comprehensive study by Sands (1969), in which she observed structural abnormalities in the short arms of acrocentric chromosomes, revealed that these abnormalities

Table 85. Standard Trisomy 21 and a Translocation In the Same Individual

Authors		Type of Rearrangement
Hustinx	1963	D/D
Zergollern et al.	1964	D/D
Gripenberg & Airaksinen	1964	D/F
Richards & Stewart	1965	D/D
Brown et al.	1967	D/D
Slavin et al.	1967	D/D
Weiss & Wolf	1968	C/G
Palmer et al.	1969	D/D
Ridler et al.	1969	D/D
Soukup et al.	1969	t(3?;G?q+)
Gardner et al.	1973	t(1p-;3q+);t(16q-;?+); t(3?;Gq+)

occurred in 3.4 per cent of Down's syndrome cases and 2.8 per cent of a control population. These frequencies were not significantly different and lent no support to the hypothesis that the abnormalities in question are correlated directly with non-disjunction of the acrocentric chromosomes.

Table 85 provides a list of published standard trisomy 21 cases in which an associated translocation was present (see also pages 195 and 221). If Down's syndrome in these cases is not coincidental, then an explanation may be sought in the meiotic segregation of the balanced translocation chromosome carrier parent (Soukup *et al.*)

TRISOMY IN FAMILIES WITH t(Dq21q) TRANSLOCATION

Moorhead *et al.* (1961) reported a family in which the mother and her first 4 children each had 45 chromosomes with a karyotype that showed 5 in the 13−15 group, 3 in the 21−22 group and an extra one in the 6−12 group. The mother was phenotypically normal, but the 4 children showed varying degrees of mental retardation and speech defect. A fifth child was chromosomally and phenotypically normal, but the sixth was a standard trisomic Down's syndrome child (see Fig. 76). The authors suggested that the extra chromosome, in the 6−12 group, present in the cells of the mother and the first 4 children, was a translocation between chromosomes 13 and 22. It was postulated that the translocation in the mother's chromosomes was in some way related to the causation of non-disjunction during meiosis which led to the birth of the child with Down's syndrome. Other explanations might be suggested (Hamerton 1962) but the concurrence may have been coincidental.

Another unusual sibship, in which there were two cases of Down's syndrome, was reported by Barnicot *et al.* (1963). One had 45 chromosomes with a (13−15) : (21−22) translocation and the other showed standard trisomy 21 (see Fig. 77). Both the parents had normal

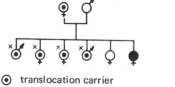

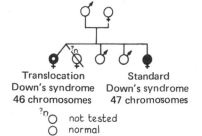

⊙   translocation carrier

○   normal karyotype

●   standard Down's syndrome

x   indicates a speech defect

Translocation Down's syndrome 46 chromosomes

Standard Down's syndrome 47 chromosomes

?n○   not tested

○   normal

Fig. 76. Pedigree showing possible 13:22 translocation and standard trisomic Down's syndrome child (after Moorhead *et al.* 1961).

Fig. 77. Pedigree showing Down's syndrome with a D:21 type of translocation and a standard trisomy 21 in the same sibship (after Barnicot *et al.* 1963).

karyotypes. Another family of the same kind, in which there were two Down's syndrome brothers in the sibship, was described by Ingalls & Henry (1968).

A somewhat similar finding was noted by Priest *et al.* (1963a) in a family in which a 15 : 21 translocation Down's syndrome child was born to parents with normal chromosomal complements. The father had a sister with standard trisomy 21. Another family was reported by Ford Walker *et al.* (1963), in which the father of a 15:21 translocation Down's syndrome female had a brother with standard trisomy 21 (see Fig. 78). Both the

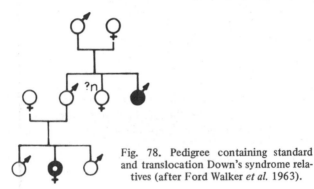

Fig. 78. Pedigree containing standard and translocation Down's syndrome relatives (after Ford Walker *et al.* 1963).

father and the mother of the translocation child had normal karyotypes. It would seem that the transmission of Down's syndrome was through the father of the translocation case. Increased *atd* angles, however, were found on the palms of the mother and of various members of her family, so that it is possible that the translocation was of maternal origin. Hamerton *et al.* (1963) reported a standard trisomic Down's syndrome child whose mother had 45 chromosomes with a translocation affecting two chromosomes in the 13–15 group. The authors suggested that the occurrence of an affected child in this family was either a chance event, or the presence of the translocation in the mother had, in some way, caused a predisposition to non-disjunction. Lele (1964) reported a mosaic 15:21 translocation carrier mother who gave birth to a standard trisomic Down's syndrome male at the age of 30 years. (See also Fig. 62). Ricci *et al.* (1968) described

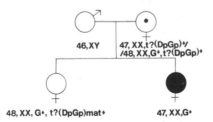

Fig. 79. Partial pedigree of family described by Ricci *et al.* (1968).

the cytogenetic findings in two sisters with trisomy 21 and their phenotypically normal mother. One child had standard trisomy, while the other had, in addition to standard trisomy, a small doubly satellited supernumerary chromosome. The mother had the same abnormal extra chromosome in all cells and a trisomy G in 13 out of 100 metaphases (see Fig. 79).

MOSAICISM

Mosaicism was first definitely reported in Down's syndrome by Clarke *et al.* (1961). Prior to this, mosaicism had been proved in sex chromosomal abnormalities (Ford *et al.* 1959b). For a pictorial example of a mosaic Down's syndrome patient, see Fig. 47. Clarke *et al.* reported a 2-year-old female with some physical findings suggestive of Down's syndrome. Her intelligence seemed to be higher than that of the average child with the syndrome. Both leucocyte and fibroblast cultures showed a mosaic pattern consisting of cells with 46 and 47 chromosomes. The cells with 47 chromosomes were trisomic for chromosome 21. In 13 per cent of the cells from leucocyte cultures and in 34 per cent from fibroblast cultures 47 chromosomes were found (Clarke *et al.* 1963). In other instances of

Table 86. Studies on Mosaicism in Down's Syndrome (Penrose 1967)

Serial number	Sex	Cytology % trisomic†		Parental ages in years		Source
		Leuc.	Fibr.	Father	Mother	
1	♀	20	67	.	19	Nichols *et al.* (1962)
2	♀	13	34	26	26	Clarke *et al.* (1961)
3	♀	63	29	29	38	Lindsten *et al.* (1962)
4	♀	5	75	34	32	Hinden (1961)
5*	♀	15	23	43	40	Blank *et al.* (1962)
6*	♀	27	75	.	39	Smith *et al.* (1962)
7	♀	67	99	29	25	Edwards (1963)
8	♂	.	70	29	24	Gustavson & Ek (1961)
9	♂	50	.	.	17	Hayashi *et al.* (1962)
10	♂	.	40	25	32	Bonham Carter (1962)
11	♂	58	.	.	38	Fitzgerald & Lycette (1961)
12	♂	2	98	45	45	Ridler *et al.* (1965)
13*	♀	10	.	.	38	34	Verresen *et al.* (1964)
14*	♀	20	22	.	39	Weinstein & Warkany (1963)
15	♂	18	.	31	27	Gerald (1963)
16	♀	16	.	39	36	Gerald (1963)
17	♀	17	.	40	31	Gerald (1963)

*Mosaic mothers of Down's syndrome children.
†(No. of cells with 47 chromosomes) x 100 ÷ (No. of cells with 46 or 47)
(See also Table 40)

mosaicism the proportions of cells with 47 chromosomes varied considerably from patient to patient (see Table 86), though usually these proportions were greater in fibroblasts than in leucocytes. Down's syndrome individuals with mosaic chromosome patterns consisting of 46 and 47 chromosomes have also been reported by Aula et al. (1961), Hayashi et al. (1962), Lindsten et al. (1962), Richards & Stewart (1962), Giraud et al. (1963), Zellweger & Abbo (1963), Biscatti (1964), Báguena Candela et al. (1965), Chaudhuri & Chaudhuri (1965), Chitham & MacIver (1965), Hamerton et al. (1965), Richards et al. (1965b), Brøgger & Gundersen (1966), Edgren et al. (1966), Finley et al. (1966) and Reinwein et al. (1966). With an incidence of detected mosaicism in Down's syndrome of about 2 per cent (Richards 1969), many additional examples have since been noted, particularly as large series of karyotyped individuals with the syndrome began to accumulate (see Table 78). In some instances, the blood was found to be almost free of abnormal cells while the skin culture was predominantly trisomic (Hinden 1961, Ridler et al. 1965, Zellweger et al. 1966b, Haberlandt & Wunderlich 1972). In another case (Warkany et al. 1964), no trisomic cells were observed in the blood and the fibroblasts showed only a small proportion (17 per cent) of such cells. An unusual type of 46/47 mosaicism was noted in a Down's syndrome child by Reisman et al. (1966). In leucocyte culture, one cell line showed 47 chromosomes with trisomy 21, whereas the other revealed 46 chromosomes with what was considered to be a probable translocation between a No. 21 and a No. 2 chromosome. Both parents and three sibs had apparently normal karyotypes.

Trisomy 21 mosaicism also has been found, on occasion, in more than one sib. Weiss & Wolf (1968) reported two Down's syndrome brothers with trisomy 21 in some cells and a balanced (Cq-;Gq+) reciprocal translocation in both cell lines. The balanced translocation was transmitted by the phenotypically normal mother. The authors suggested that balanced translocations can result in an increased incidence of mitotic nondisjunction. In a family studied by Hsu et al. (1970a), two children with mosaic trisomy 21 Down's syndrome were born to a young couple with normal chromosomes in their leucocyte cultures.

Gustavson & Ek (1961) reported a triple stem-line mosaic Down's syndrome male. In the skin fibroblasts 30 per cent of the cells contained 46 chromosomes and had a normal male karyotype, 30 per cent had 47 chromosomes with standard trisomy and 40 per cent had 48 chromosomes, i.e. standard trisomy with an extra chromosome in group 19–20. The boy with many clinical features of Down's syndrome reported by Mauer & Noe (1964) had triple stem-line mosaicism, in leucocyte culture, of a 46/47/48 type in the proportions of 1:5:1. The extra chromosomal material in both the 47 and 48 cell lines was considered to belong to the G group. Tonomura & Karita (1964) described another male case in which leucocyte cultures showed cell lines with 47 and 48 chromosomes and also a few normal cells. Edgren et al. (1966) found 45,XO/46,XY/47,XY,G+

mosaicism in both leucocytes and fibroblasts from a Down's syndrome adult male. He was born to a mother aged 32 years and a father aged 26 years. Tsuboi *et al.* (1968) gave an account of a Down's syndrome girl with normal/trisomy 21/trisomy 21 plus telocentric G chromosome mosaicism in leucocyte culture. The mother was 38 years and the father 44 years old at her birth; they had apparently normal karyotypes. Other Down's syndrome cases with mosaic chromosomal patterns and additional stem-lines have been reported by Fitzgerald & Lycette (1961), Blank *et al.* (1963) and by Valencia *et al.* (1963). In the case of mosaicism in Down's syndrome reported by Nichols *et al.* (1962), the mother of the Down's syndrome child had 46 chromosomes with an XX/XY pattern in her leucocytes.

Mosaicism of the 46/47 type has been reported in mothers, who have given birth to standard trisomic Down's syndrome children, by Blank *et al.* (1962), Smith *et al.* (1962), Weinstein & Warkany (1963), Ferrier (1964), Makino (1964), Verresen *et al.* (1964), Turner *et al.* (1966), Taylor (1968), Aarskog (1969), Izakovic & Getlik (1969), Mikkelsen (1970), Krmpotic & Hardin (1971), Timson *et al.* (1971) and Sutherland *et al.* (1972). Smith *et al.* (1962) reported a mother with a mosaic pattern who gave birth to two Down's syndrome children. She was 19 years old at the birth of the first and was herself born when her mother was 39 years of age. An almost identical circumstance was described by Aarskog. In this instance, the mosaic, phenotypically normal mother also gave birth to two Down's syndrome children, the first when she was 22 years old; she too was born to a 39 year old mother. Similarly, in Weinstein & Warkany's case, the mosaic mother gave birth to her affected child at 17 years and was born when her mother was 39 years old. Mosaicism may be missed without extensive investigation. In the phenotypically normal, mosaic mother described by Mikkelsen, mosaicism was not detected in leucocyte culture after she had her first Down's syndrome child at the age of 20 years. When her second affected child was born at the age of 29 years, cytological examination showed trisomy 21 in 3 per cent of leuocytes and 13 per cent of fibroblasts. Sutherland *et al.* reported a mother with some clinical features of Down's syndrome who had three standard trisomic children with the syndrome. Cytological examination of blood and bone marrow samples on three occasions, comprising a total of 59 cells, showed only a normal karotype. Several years later, a further leucocyte culture revealed trisomy 21 in five out of 70 cells.

The tendency for mosaic mothers to be born when their own mothers are relatively old was examined by Richards (1970) who found the mean age of the latter, in 11 cases, to be 33.7 years. This suggested to him that most or all of these mosaic mothers arose from trisomic zygotes. It is probable that mothers with mosaic chromosome patterns have primary oocytes which contain 46 or 47 chromosomes. Reduction division would result in the formation of some gametes with 24 chromosomes (inevitable secondary nondisjunction). Trisomy for chromosome 21 in their children would result from the fertilization by a normal sperm of an ovum with the extra chromosome 21.

A number of fathers with a low degree of trisomy 21 mosaicism, who have had Down's syndrome children, have been documented in recent years (see Table 87). With the exception of the father reported by Walker & Ising (1969), who was said to closely resemble his mosaic Down's syndrome daughter, all the other fathers were phenotypically normal and produced standard trisomic children. None of the mothers showed abnormalities in their karyotypes. The mean age of the fathers and mothers at the birth of their affected children was 24.8 years and 22.8 years, respectively. In the first family described by Hsu *et al.* (1971a), there were two sibs with standard Down's syndrome. A testicular biopsy obtained from the father indicated the presence of a cell line with 47 chromosomes in the germinal tissue. As Hsu *et al.* observed, paternal trisomy 21 mosaicism may be responsible for a significant percentage of standard Down's syndrome infants born to younger mothers.

Table 87. Fathers with Trisomy 21 Mosaicism Who Have Produced Down's Syndrome Children

| Source | % of cells with trisomy 21* | | | | Parental ages at child's birth | |
| | Father | | Child | | | |
	Leuc.	Fibr.	Leuc.	Fibr.	Father	Mother
Massimo *et al.* (1967)	- -	- -	- -†	- -	- -	- -
	- -	- -	- -†	- -	- -	- -
Walker & Ising (1969)	23	- -	15	- -	- -	- -
Hsu *et al.* (1971a) : Family No. 1	0	8	100†	- -	24	20
	0	8	100†	- -	26	22
Hsu *et al.* (1971a) : Family No. 2	6	- -	100	- -	21	22
Hsu *et al.* (1971a) : Family No. 3	5	4	100	- -	30	28
Méhes (1973)	7	- -	100	- -	23	22
Mean Parental ages					24.8	22.8

*(No. of cells with 47 chromosomes) x 100 ÷ (No. of cells with 46 or 47)
†Sibs

Mosaic carriers of translocations have also produced Down's syndrome children with translocations. Reference has been made on p. 187 to two fathers with (Dq21q) translocation mosaicism who have had such children (Tips *et al.* 1963, Ferrier 1964). In another instance, a healthy mother who was a mosaic carrier of a (Dq21q) translocation gave birth to a (Dq21q) translocation Down's syndrome child (Aarskog 1969). Waxman & Arakaki (1966) have reported a mosaic G/G translocation carrier mother who had three Down's syndrome children by two different fathers. One of these children died before chromosomal examination could be undertaken and the other two showed translocation Down's syndrome of the G/G type.

Penrose (1967) gave mean ratios of trisomic cells to normal cells for 17 cases (6 males and 11 females) of cytological mosaicism in Down's syndrome (See Table 88). His criterion for mosaicism was that not less than 9 per cent, or more than 91 per cent, of the cells counted were trisomic for the small acrocentric chromosome. In making his assessment of mosaicism, only cells with 46 or 47 chromosomes were compared. The

Table 88. Mean Ratios of Trisomic Cells to Normal Cells (Penrose 1967)

No of patients	Cells cultured	
	Leucocytes	Fibroblasts
	Trisomic:Normal	Trisomic:normal
9	25.8 : 74.2	58.0 : 42.0
6	28.2 : 71.8	–
2	–	55.0 : 45.0
All	26.7 : 73.3	57.5 : 42.5

results showed that, altogether, the proportion of trisomic cells in the fibroblasts was about twice as great as that of trisomic cells in the leucocytes. There was no appreciable difference between males and females in these proportions. A greater proportion of trisomic cells in fibroblasts, compared to leucocytes, has been noted also with relative frequency in other series of Down's syndrome (Ford 1967, Taylor 1968, 1970, Richards 1969, Taysi et al. 1970). These proportions are not constant at all ages (Taylor, Richards, Taysi et al.); such variations must be taken into account in comparing ratios of trisomic to normal cells in different tissues, and in attempting to correlate phenotypic manifestations with different degrees of mosaicism. Moreover, the apparent absence of trisomic cells in occasional cases were they would be suspected on clinical grounds may be due to the disappearance of such cells with the passage of time. Patients are known in whom leucocyte culture revealed mosaicism at some time and the apparent disappearance of the mosaicism later on (LaMarche et al. 1967, Neu et al. 1969).

Bowen et al. (1974) reported a 14 year old female with mild clinical features of Down's syndrome. Her dermatoglyphic patterns were highly suggestive of the diagnosis. She was functioning in the mildly retarded range with an I.Q. of 70. Lymphocyte and skin cultures were normal (46,XX). One No. 21 chromosome had enlarged short arms (21p+). A paternal uncle had Down's syndrome and 47 chromosomes with trisomy 21. The uncle with Down's syndrome, the patient's father and other normal family members carried the 21p+ marker chromosome. The authors speculated on various explanations of this case. They chose to describe the affected girl as having Down's syndrome with normal chromosomes (DSNC) and as being one of a small but important group of patients. Similar patients were described by Sergovich et al. (1964b) and Day & Miles (1965). Possibly the best explanation for the patient of

Bowen *et al.*, at this time, is that she is an undetected mosaic. However, other explanations may be sought in terms of the previously mentioned *in vivo* instability of mosaic cell populations (Taylor, Richards, Taysi *et al.*) and the disappearance of a trisomic cell line from peripheral blood of mosaic individuals (LaMarche *et al.*, Neu *et al.*)

Mosaicism in Down's syndrome can occur from a normal zygote containing 46 chromosomes or from an abnormal zygote containing 47 chromosomes with trisomy 21 (see Fig. 80). If the zygote is normal and

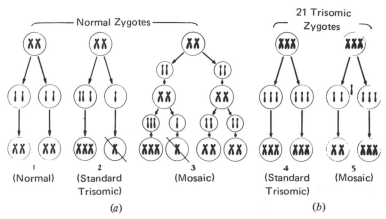

Fig. 80. Representation of origin of standard trisomic and mosaic Down's syndrome by mitotic error in (*a*) normal zygotes and (*b*) trisomic zygotes.

non-disjunction occurs at the first cleavage, two cell lines are formed (45 and 47 chromosomes); however, mosaicism will probably not be found since the monosomic cell-line with 45 chromosomes will probably be inviable. Non-disjunction occurring in a normal zygote after the first cell division would probably result in the production of a Down's syndrome mosaic with both normal and trisomic cell lines. In an abnormal trisomic zygote some cells may become normal by loss of a chromosome at mitotic division.

PARTIAL TRISOMY 21

In an attempt to evaluate which portions of the number 21 chromosome are genetically active in producing the physical and mental characteristics of Down's syndrome, Aula *et al.* (1973) studied five individuals with Down's syndrome and partial trisomy 21. Their study was aided by the use of chromosomal banding. They concluded that trisomy of the band segment and the distal portion of the long arm of chromosome 21 (see Fig. 56) is necessary for the phenotypic features of Down's syndrome. Partial trisomy of the long arm of chromosome 21, without the band segment, was associated with many, but not all, of the typical stigmata of the syndrome. Mental retardation was usually less severe in the affected individuals. Previous reports (Ilþery et al. 1961, Dent et al. 1963, Dekaban & Zelson 1968, Šubrt & Prchliková 1970) on partial trisomy 21 were less informative, since chromosomal banding techniques were not available.

Aula et al. reported the following karyotypes on their five cases: two patients had 47,XX,(21q-)+ and the three remaining had 46,XX/47,XX,(21q-)+; 46,XX,21qi/46,XX,21p-; and 46,XY,15p+, respectively. The 15p+ chromosome, in the last case, was thought to contain part of the long arm of a number 21 chromosome translocated to the short arm of a number 15 chromosome. One of the cases [46,XX/47,XX(21q-)+] previously had been reported by Hongell & Airaksinen (1972). In general, Aula et al. found that their patients with deletions were less retarded and less clinically affected than typical Down's syndrome individuals in their age group.

Niebuhr (1974) suggested that a gradation of clinical features in the syndrome is due to the loss of varying amounts distally from the long arms of a 21 chromosome and, consequently, that trisomy of the most distal segment, 21q22 (Paris Conference Nomenclature), may be pathogenetic in the syndrome.

An unusual family was reported by O'Donnell et al. (1975) in which there were three children with typical Down's syndrome. In this family, the distal half of the long arm of chromosome 21 was inserted on to a chromosome 15. The mother was a balanced translocation carrier. From the chromosomal rearrangements in the family, the authors concluded that trisomy for the distal half of chromosome 21 produces the full phenotypic expression of the syndrome—and that the remainder of chromosome 21 does not cause the syndrome and is compatible with normal mental and physical development. The authors suggested that other cases of the syndrome with karyotypes which were considered to be "normal" actually may have been the result of a small undetected translocation.

Williams et al. (1975), in a study of a family with a reciprocal t(10;21) translocation, provided further evidence that the Down's syndrome phenotype is attributable to trisomy of the distal portion of the long arm of chromosome 21. Three persons in the family with such trisomy had the typical Down's syndrome phenotype; whereas another relative with trisomy of the short arm-centromere-proximal long arm segment of chromosome 21, though mildly retarded, did not show the phenotypic features of Down's syndrome.

COMBINED DOWN'S AND KLINEFELTER'S SYNDROMES

A double chromosomal abnormality, resulting in both Down's and

Klinefelter's syndromes in the same person, was first reported by Ford *et al.* (1959a) (see Fig. 2 and Fig. 81j). The patient's mother and father were 42 and 40 years of age respectively at the time of his birth. Cytological tests on bone marrow, skin and blood all showed 48 chromosomes with 2 X's and 5 small acrocentrics. Monozygotic twin boys with cytological evidence of both conditions were reported by Hustinx *et al.* (1961) and a similar pair of male twins were described by Turpin *et al.* (1964) and Senéze *et al.* (1964). This cytological constitution was noted also in a 10-month-old male infant by Lanman *et al.* (1960). Additional instances of Down's and Klinefelter's syndromes in the same individual (see Table 89) have been reported by Lehmann & Forssman (1960), van Gelderen & Hustinx (1961), Hamerton *et al.* (1962), Milcu & Maicanesco (1963), Court Brown *et al.* (1964), Pfeiffer (1964), de Grouchy *et al.* (1965a), Taylor & Moores (1967), Hecht *et al.* (1969), Gardner *et al.* (1973) and Efinski *et al.* (1974). An unusual patient with D/21 translocation Down's syndrome and XXY/XY mosaicism was described by Punnett & Di George (1967). Two cases of XXY/XY mosaicism were also noted in Gardner *et*

Table 89. Down's Syndrome Individuals with Additional Chromosomal Anomaly

Down's syndrome, plus	Maternal Age	Paternal Age	Authors
XXY	42	40	Ford *et al.* (1959a); Harnden *et al.* (1960)
XXY	20	–	Lanman *et al.* (1960)
XXY	41	–	Lehmann & Forssman (1960)
XXY (twins)	43	–	Hustinx *et al.* (1961)
XXY	19	–	van Gelderen & Hustinx (1961)
XXY	43	43	Hamerton *et al.* (1962)
XXY	35	38	Milcu & Maicanesco (1963)
XXY	40	42	Court Brown *et al.* (1964)
XXY	42	49	Court Brown *et al.* (1964)
XXY	39	59	Pfeiffer (1964)
XXY (twins)	47	57	Turpin *et al.* (1964); Sénéze *et al.* (1964)
XXY	43	27	de Grouchy *et al.* (1965a)
XXY	–	–	Taylor & Moores (1967)
XXY	26	29	Hecht *et al.* (1969)
XXY (2 cases)	⩾30	–	Gardner *et al.* (1973)
XXY	–	–	Efinski *et al.* (1974)
Mosaic XXY/XY	34	40	Punnett & Di George (1967)
Mosaic XXY/XY (2 cases)	⩾30	–	Gardner *et al.* (1973)
XXX	20	19	Day *et al.* (1963)
XXX	46	47	Pfeiffer (1964)
XXX	47	45	Yunis *et al.* (1964)
Mosaic XXX/XX	23	27	Duillo & Serra (1969)
Mosaic XXX/XX (2 cases)	⩾30	–	Gardner *et al.* (1973)
XYY	35	44	Verresen & van den Berghe (1965)

Table 89 continued on next page

Table 89. (Contd.)

Down's syndrome, plus	Maternal Age	Paternal Age	Authors
XYY	22	33	Uchida et al. (1966)
XYY	28	27	Al-Aish et al. (1971)
XYY	24	27	Laxova et al. (1971)
XYY	20	24	Neu et al. (1971)
Mosaic XO/XX	–	–	Medenis et al. (1962)
Mosaic XO/XX	42	44	Root et al. (1964)
Mosaic XO/XX	26	28	van Wijck et al. (1964)
Mosaic XO/XX	–	–	Báguena Candela et al. (1966)
Mosaic XO/XX	–	–	Taylor (1970)
Mosaic XO/XX	–	–	Grosse et al. (1971)
Mosaic XO/XX	–	–	Cohen & Davidson (1972)
Mosaic XO/XX/XXX	26	26	Zergollern & Hoefnagel (1964)
Trisomy 18	20	21	Gagnon et al. (1961)
Mosaic trisomy 18	44	48	Hsu et al. (1965)
Mosaic trisomy 18	23	–	Marks et al. (1967)
Mosaic trisomy 18	20	22	Zellweger & Abbo (1967); Bodensteiner & Zellweger (1971a)
Mosaic trisomy 18	37	46	Glogowska (1969)
Trisomy 13-15	39	46	Becker et al. (1963)
Mosaic trisomy 13-15	39	38	Smith et al. (1965)
Mosaic trisomy 13-15	34	37	Porter et al. (1969)
Mosaic trisomy 8	18	21	Wilson et al. (1974)
t(DqDq)	24	27	Hustinx (1963)
t(DqDq)	30	29	Zergollern et al. (1964); Corcoran et al. (1964)
t(DqDq)	36	38	Richards & Stewart (1965)
t(DqDq)	29	–	Zellweger & Abbo (1965)
t(DqDq)	27	28	Marsden et al. (1966)
t(DqDq)	31	–	Brown et al. (1967)
t(DqDq)	26	29	Orye & Delire (1967)
t(DqDq)	–	–	Slavin et al. (1967)
t(DqDq)	37	44	Palmer et al. (1969)
t(DqDq)	31	32	Ridler et al. (1969)
t(DqFq)	38	–	Gripenberg & Airaksinen (1964)
Pericentric inversion of X or 6	–	–	de Grouchy et al. (1965b)
Inv(Yp+q-)	24	33	Sparkes et al. (1970)
Mosaic XX/X,iso(Xq)	–	–	Mikkelsen (1970)
Xq-	29	30	Luthardt & Palmer (1971)
Dq+	38	–	Chaptal et al. (1966)
Marker chromosome	21	24	Bargman et al. (1970)

al.'s (1973) extensive survey. The age of the mothers in most of the patients was above the average population level of about 28 years.

A boy with an extra G group chromosome, as well as an extra X, was described by Erdtmann et al. (1971). However, he did not show characteristic Down's syndrome features and the authors speculated that he might be an instance of 48,XXY,22+ double aneuploidy. Another clinically atypical patient with an extra X and an extra G chromosome was reported by Nankin *et al.* (1974). The boy with trisomy 21 and sex chromosome mosaicism reported by Prieur *et al.* (1972) was unusual in showing a 45,X/47,XY,21+ karyotype.

Chromatin-positive live-born males have been found with a frequency of 1/510 (Harnden *et al.* 1964). Using an incidence for Down's syndrome of 1 in 700 births (and not taking into consideration maternal age at the time of the child's birth), the chance association of both Down's and Klinefelter's syndromes in an individual could be expected to be 1 in about 360,000. However, double aneuploidy of the 48,XXY,21+ type seems to occur with greater than chance frequency (1 in about 11,600) in newly born males (Taylor & Moores), although the prospects of survival appear to be reduced (Hecht *et al.*).

Estimated incidences at birth of Down's syndrome individuals with a second chromosomal abnormality are given in Table 90.

Table 90. Estimated Incidence at Birth of Down's Syndrome Individuals with Double Aneuploidy

Second condition	Incidence second condition	Incidence of Down's syndrome*	Incidence of combined conditions considering each event to be independent
1. Klinefelter's syndrome	1 : 510†	1 : 700	1 : 360,000
2. Triple X syndrome	1 : 833†	1 : 700	1 : 580,000
3. XYY syndrome	1 : 489*	1 : 700	1 : '340,000
4. Turner's syndrome	1 : 2,500†	1 : 700	1 : 1,750,000
5. Trisomy 13–15 syndrome	1 : 2,200‡	1 : 700	1 : 1,540,000
6. Trisomy 18 syndrome	1 : 4,300‡	1 : 700	1 : 3,010,000

*Combined estimate covering all maternal age groups.
†Harnden et al. (1964).
*Berg & Smith (1971)
‡Marden *et al.* (1964).

COMBINED DOWN'S AND TRIPLE X SYNDROMES

A Down's syndrome female with triple X chromosomes was initially described by Day *et al.* (1963). Peripheral blood cultures showed 48 chromosomes with trisomy for both 21 and X (see Fig. 81k) and a buccal smear revealed two chromatin bodies in some cells (see Fig. 82). Yunis *et al.* (1964) reported a similar female infant with trisomy 21 and X, autoradiographic studies in this instance showing two late replicating X chromosomes. Two sex chromatin bodies were found in 14 per cent of the buccal cells and 60 per cent contained one sex chromatin body. Another instance of this form of double aneuploidy was mentioned by Pfeiffer (1964). A girl with trisomy 21 and X chromosome mosaicism of the type XXX/XX was described by Duillo & Serra (1969). Two such cases were

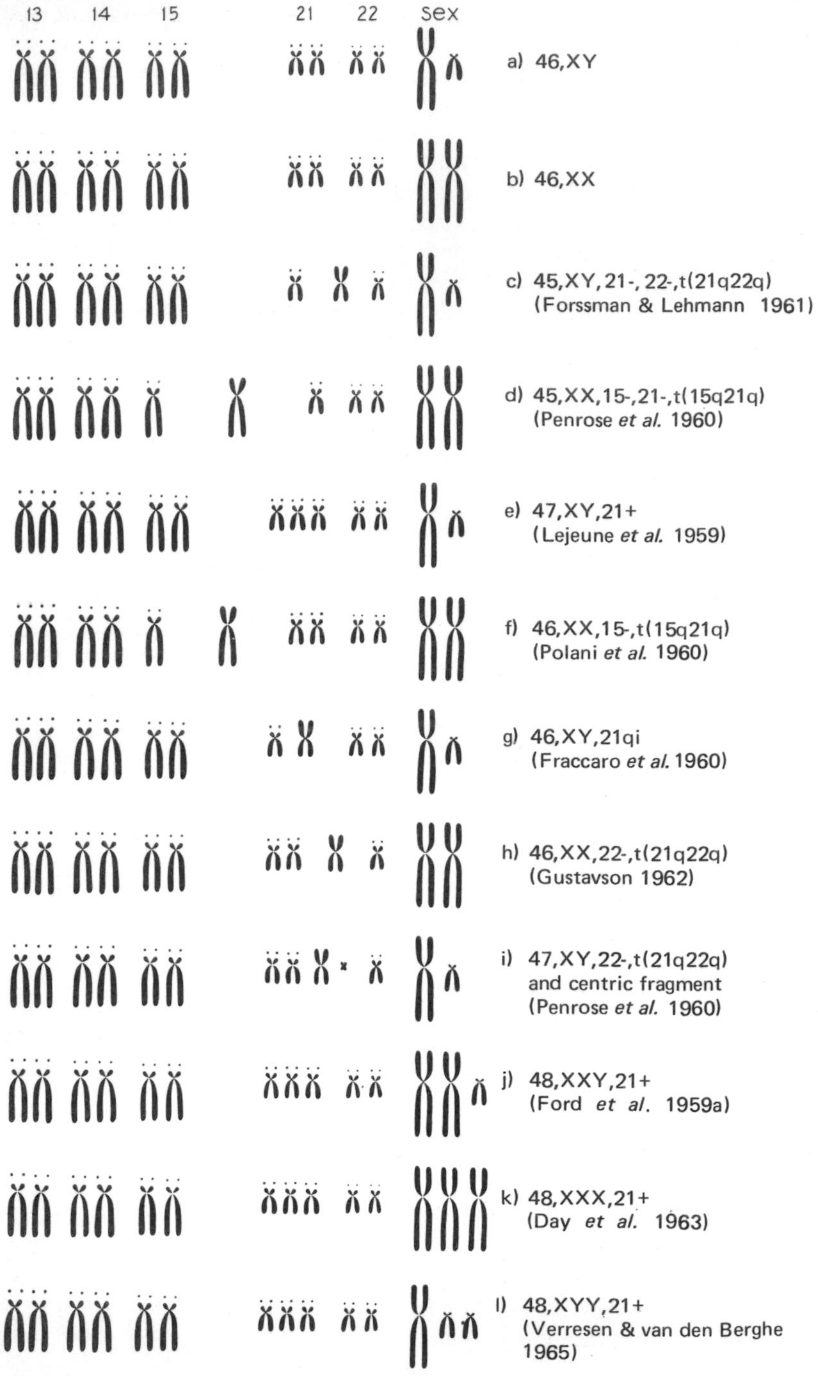

13	14	15		21	22	sex	

a) 46,XY

b) 46,XX

c) 45,XY,21-, 22-,t(21q22q)
(Forssman & Lehmann 1961)

d) 45,XX,15-,21-,t(15q21q)
(Penrose *et al.* 1960)

e) 47,XY,21+
(Lejeune *et al.* 1959)

f) 46,XX,15-,t(15q21q)
(Polani *et al.* 1960)

g) 46,XY,21qi
(Fraccaro *et al.* 1960)

h) 46,XX,22-,t(21q22q)
(Gustavson 1962)

i) 47,XY,22-,t(21q22q)
and centric fragment
(Penrose *et al.* 1960)

j) 48,XXY,21+
(Ford *et al.* 1959a)

k) 48,XXX,21+
(Day *et al.* 1963)

l) 48,XYY,21+
(Verresen & van den Berghe
1965)

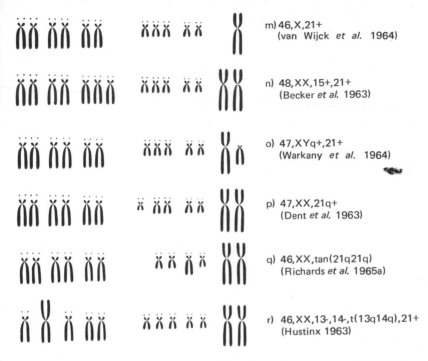

m) 46,X,21+
(van Wijck *et al.* 1964)

n) 48,XX,15+,21+
(Becker *et al.* 1963)

o) 47,XYq+,21+
(Warkany *et al.* 1964)

p) 47,XX,21q+
(Dent *et al.* 1963)

q) 46,XX,tan(21q21q)
(Richards *et al.* 1965a)

r) 46,XX,13-,14-,t(13q14q),21+
(Hustinx 1963)

Fig. 81. Representation of acrocentric and sex chromosomes: (*a*) to (*d*), normal phenotypes; (*e*) to (*r*), Down's syndrome phenotypes.

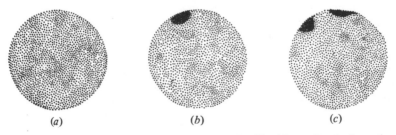

(a) (b) (c)

Fig. 82. Diagram of cells: (*a*) with no Barr body; (*b*) with one Barr body; and (*c*) with two Barr bodies.

found by Gardner *et al.* (1973) among 972 individuals with Down's syndrome, both born to mothers over 30 years of age.

COMBINED DOWN'S AND XYY SYNDROMES

A 9-year-old Down's syndrome boy was noted by Verresen & van den

Berghe (1965) to have an XYY sex chromosome complement as well as standard trisomy 21. Further examples of this form of double aneuploidy in infants were recorded by Uchida *et al.* (1966), Al-Aish *et al.* (1971), Laxova *et al.* (1971) and by Neu *et al.* (1971). The clinical characteristics of Down's syndrome predominated in these cases and no distinctive modifications of the phenotype, consequent on the extra Y chromosome, were apparent. An extra Y appears to be about as frequent in live-born males as an extra X, so that an estimated incidence of each of these conditions combined with Down's syndrome is similar (see Table 90).

COMBINED DOWN'S AND TURNER'S SYNDROMES

A 9-year-old girl with clinical features of Down's and Turner's syndromes was found by Medenis *et al.* (1962) to have standard trisomy 21 and XO/XX mosaicism. Similar cases were reported by Root *et al.* (1964) and by van Wijck *et al.* (1964) (See Fig. 81m). Another infant, with trisomy 21 and a 45,XO cell line was described by Báguena Candela *et al.* (1966). Grosse *et al.*'s (1971) patient, a 7-year-old girl with some features of Down's syndrome and less of Turner's syndrome, showed 45,XO/46, XX/47,XX,21+ mosaicism. Additional patients, with clinical evidence of both Down's and Turner's syndromes, have been found to have 45,X/47,XX,G+ mosaicism (Taylor 1970, Cohen & Davidson 1972). Another type of chromosomal variant was reported by Zergollern & Hoefnagel (1964) in a 12-year-old Down's syndrome female whose sex chromosomes were interpreted as showing XO/XX/XXX mosaicism.

COMBINED DOWN'S AND TRISOMY 18 SYNDROMES

A premature male infant with multiple congenital anomalies was found, on skin culture (see Fig. 83), to be trisomic for both chromosomes No. 18 and No. 21 (Gagnon *et al.* 1961). The infant died shortly after birth and, on post-mortem examination, the following abnormalities were found: hypertelorism, low-set malformed ears, depressed sternum, interventricular septal defect, cystic malformations of the renal cortex, imperforate anus, pronation of forearms and pes valgus. The mother's and father's ages at the time of the child's birth were 20 and 21 years respectively.

Substantially older parents (mother 44; father 48 years) also have produced an infant with trisomy of chromosomes 18 and 21 (Hsu *et al.* 1965). The predominant clinical features were those of trisomy 18 and the child died at the age of 3 months. In this instance, mosaicism was noted in blood culture, about half the baby's cells examined showing the double trisomy and a similar proportion revealing no apparent chromosomal abnormality. Another form of mosaicism was found by Marks *et al.* (1967) in a 6-year-old boy with clinically recognizable Down's syndrome. Of 40

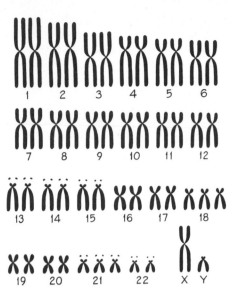

Fig. 83. Representation of karyotype of standard Down's syndrome male with trisomy 18 (after Gagnon *et al.* 1961).

cells studied from leucocyte culture, trisomy 21 was observed in 33 and trisomy 18 in the remaining seven. Mosaicism of such a kind was reported also in a younger boy by Zellweger & Abbo (1967). They detected, in addition, a small proportion of cells with a normal chromosomal complement. Bodensteiner & Zellweger (1971a) subsequently reported additional details about this child who showed phenotypic characteristics of both Down's and trisomy 18 syndromes. They also documented a further case of trisomy G/trisomy E mosaicism in a child whose clinical features were not typical of either Down's or trisomy 18 syndromes. The latter case is somewhat reminiscent of the trisomy 18/trisomy G mosaic infant reported by Toldsdorf *et al.* (1965). That infant, who died at the age of three days, showed the phenotypic peculiarities of trisomy 18 but no convincing clinical evidence of Down's syndrome. A further variant was described by Glogowska (1969) in a 3-year-old Down's syndrome boy. He had standard trisomy 21 and, in some cells, an extra chromosome 18 as well.

COMBINED DOWN'S AND TRISOMY (13–15) SYNDROMES

Karyotype analysis in a 4-year-old girl, with clinical and dermatoglyphic features typical of Down's syndrome, showed 48 chromosomes with apparent trisomy for a No. 21 and for a chromosome in the 13–15 group (see Fig. 81n) (Becker *et al.* 1963). The child's I.Q. was 62 on the Stanford-Binet test. Her mother and father were aged 39 years and 46 years respectively at the time of her birth and both had normal karyotypes.

Another Down's syndrome female, who was severely retarded and died at the age of 19 years, was found to have trisomy 21 in all of 134 cells studied, 16 per cent of these cells also showing trisomy of a 13–15 group chromosome (Smith *et al.* 1965). An unusual finding in this patient was a complete absence of dermal ridge patterns on the hands. Mosaicism of a different variety was reported by Porter *et al.* (1969). They described a male infant, 41 of whose cells were examined in a blood culture. Ten of these cells had 47 chromosomes with trisomy 21, another 31 also revealed 47 chromosomes but with trisomy in the 13–15 group, and two cells had 48 chromosomes with both these trisomies. The baby displayed many of the clinical features of Down's syndrome although he was hypertonic.

DOWN'S SYNDROME WITH ASSOCIATED TRISOMY 8

A child with standard trisomy 21 and mosaic trisomy 8, in both blood and skin cells, was reported by Wilson *et al.* (1974). The extra No. 21 and No. 8 chromosomes were identified by quinacrine fluorescence and Giemsa banding patterns. The combination had not previously been noted in a live-born child. The clinical features were characteristic of Down's syndrome and no phenotypic effects related to the extra No. 8 chromosome were apparent. The young parents showed normal karyotypes.

DOWN'S SYNDROME WITH ASSOCIATED (DqDq) TRANSLOCATION

Translocation of the (DqDq) type has been observed quite frequently in phenotypically normal persons as well as in others with a variety of clinical abnormalities. Until the recent advent of chromosomal banding techniques (see p. 172), it was difficult to establish which of the 13–15 chromosomes were involved in such a translocation in a given instance, although autoradiography was of some help in this regard.

A (DqDq) type of translocation has been found in a number of persons who were also trisomic for chromosome No. 21 (see Table 89). In some instances, the Down's syndrome individual had standard trisomy 21 (see Fig. 81r), as in the cases reported by Hustinx (1963), Zergollern *et al.* (1964), Richards & Stewart (1965), Brown *et al.* (1967), Slavin *et al.* (1967), Palmer *et al.* (1969) and Ridler *et al.* (1969). In other instances, translocation Down's syndrome was present of either the D/G (Zellweger & Abbo 1965, Orye & Delire 1967) or G/G (Marsden *et al.* 1966) type.

Ridler *et al.* undertook a survey of the incidence of (DqDq) translocation in a combined British sample of 2,209 karyotyped cases of Down's syndrome. Four of these (1 in 552) had associated (DqDq) translocation, compared with an estimated general population incidence (Jacobs 1968) of 1 in 800. The result suggested that the association of such a translocation with Down's syndrome is fortuitous.

OTHER ADDITIONAL CHROMOSOMAL ANOMALIES IN DOWN'S SYNDROME

A number of other examples of additional chromosomal anomalies in persons with Down's syndrome are listed in Table 89.

An unusual translocation between a D and F chromosome was described by Gripenberg & Airaksinen (1964). de Grouchy et al. (1965b) found a probable pericentric inversion of an X or No. 6 chromosome in a boy with trisomy 21. Another Down's syndrome boy showed what was interpreted as a pericentric inversion of the Y chromosome (Sparkes et al. 1970). This chromosome was present in several male relatives, including the father, and was without apparent phenotypic effect. Mikkelsen (1970) found a 33-year-old Down's syndrome female with standard trisomy who also had XX/X, iso X mosaicism. Luthardt & Palmer (1971) reported a Down's syndrome girl with a deletion of the long arm of one of her X chromosomes. Her karyotype was 47,XXq-,21+. Chaptal et al. (1966) noted a structural anomaly, in the form of elongation of the short arm of a D group chromosome, in a child with trisomy 21. The phenotypically normal mother had a similar D chromosome. Bargman et al. (1970) described a Down's syndrome infant who had a small marker chromosome in addition to trisomy 21. The same marker chromosome was present in the mother. The infant's karyotype was 48,XY,21+,mar+mat.

RARE ABNORMALITIES OF CHROMOSOME NO. 21

The presence of specially large satellites on one chromosome No. 21 has frequently been observed in normal people. An enlargement of the shorter arm has been considered to be a normal variation; Jacobs (1965) reported it to be present in some 5 per cent of the population. A striking chromosome of this type, however, was present in grandfather, mother and Down's syndrome child in the case recorded by Therkelsen (1964).

Deletion of some part of the chromosome might, however, be expected to be accompanied by abnormal symptoms. German & Bearn (1962) described a female patient in whose cells a member of the pair believed to be No. 21 was very small and was probably a ring chromosome formed after deletion. The patient showed signs which were in some respects the opposite of those found in Down's syndrome (Figs. 84, 85). She had a narrow face and a very long head, a prominent nose, downward outward slope of palpebral fissures and receding chin. There were no transverse creases across the palms and the axial triradii were normally placed. All the digital patterns were arches. The fingers and toes were long. She could be described as partially monosomic.

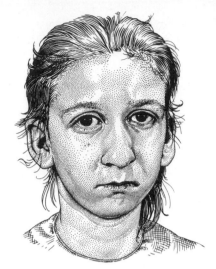

Fig. 84. Female patient with supposed partial monosomy for number 21 chromosome: age 11 years, I.Q. 65.

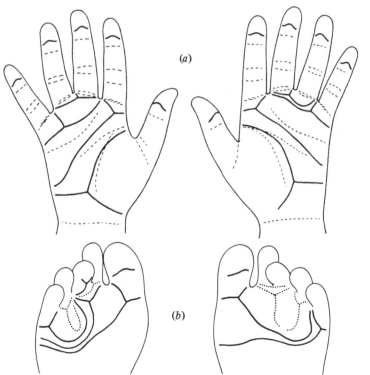

(a)

(b)

Fig. 85. Dermatoglyphic patterns on hands and feet of female in Fig. 84. Contrast with patterns on hands and feet of standard Down's syndrome individual in Fig. 49.

A more striking example of a similar condition was found by Lejeune *et al.* (1964) in a male infant. Again, one of the small acrocentrics was represented by a ring chromosome but in a considerable proportion of the cells this was absent. The child was considered to be a mosaic (as well as a partial) monosomic for No. 21 and many physical signs were present which could be interpreted as being the converse of those found in Down's syndrome. Complete monosomy of No. 21, comparable with Turner's syndrome in the sex chromosomes, would seem likely to be a lethal condition. On the other hand, in *Drosophila melanogaster* (Bridges 1923) the monosomic insect, haplo-IV, is viable and has differences from the normal which are the opposite of those found in the trisomic condition (see Fig. 3).

Crandall *et al.* (1972) reported three individuals with a G ring chromosome. One of them had a 21 ring chromosome and some features of "antimongolism" while the other two, each with a 22 ring chromosome, had minimal and nonspecific physical findings. Kelch *et al.* (1971) reported two cases of deletions of group G chromosomes. One of the infants had a characteristic "antimongoloid" facies suggesting a possible deletion of a No. 21 chromosome. Gripenberg *et al.* (1972) and Halloran *et al.* (1974) reported cases of monosomy 21 and Halloran *et al.* described a (45,XX,G-) female with marked mental and physical retardation, "antimongoloid" slant, low set ears, syndactyly of toes and a cardiac defect.

ANEUPLOIDY IN RELATIVES OF DOWN'S SYNDROME INDIVIDUALS

An aspect of genetical interest in the study of Down's syndrome is the finding of different chromosomal anomalies in close relatives of persons with the syndrome. Some examples are given in Table 91.

Turner's syndrome has been reported in sibs by Zellweger & Mikamo (1961), Johnston & Petrakis (1963) and Casteels-Van Daele *et al.* (1970). In the family described by Zellweger & Mikamo, the third child was a typical case of Turner's syndrome and the youngest had Down's syndrome, the diagnoses being confirmed on chromosomal examination. The parents and three other sibs had normal karyotypes. Johnston & Petrakis surveyed 37 families each of which contained one child with Down's syndrome. One sister was found to be chromatin negative and clinical and chromosomal investigation substantiated the diagnosis of Turner's syndrome. The parents showed normal karyotypes (see Fig. 86). In the sibship reported by Casteels-Van Daele *et al.*, the child diagnosed as Turner's syndrome, born two years after her standard trisomic Down's syndrome brother, was considered to have an isochromosome for the long arm of one of the X chromosomes (46,XXqi).

Miller *et al.* (1961) reported a eunuchoid man with multiple anomalies and 49 chromosomes with an XXXXY pattern. His father, who died of

Table 91. Examples of Chromosomal Anomalies found in Close Relatives of
Down's Syndrome Individuals

Anomaly in relative	Relationship of Down's syndrome individual to relative	Source
Turner's syndrome	Sister	Zellweger & Mikamo (1961)
Turner's syndrome	Brother	Johnston & Petrakis (1963)
Turner's syndrome	Brother	Casteels-Van Daele et al. (1970)
XXXXY male	Paternal aunt and female first cousin	Miller et al. (1961)
Klinefelter's syndrome	Half sister	Benirschke et al. (1962)
Klinefelter's syndrome	Brother	Wright et al. (1963)
Klinefelter's syndrome (fetus)	Brother	Iinuma et al. (1973)
Mosaic Klinefelter's syndrome	Half brother	Wright et al. (1963)
XYY male	Daughter	Hauschka et al. (1962)
XXX female	Brother	Breg et al. (1962)
XXX female	Female first cousin	Breg et al. (1962)
XXX female	Sister	Huang et al. (1967)
XXX female	Offspring	Kadotani et al. (1970a)
XXX female	Offspring	Morić-Petrović et al. (1971)
XXX female	Offspring	Singer et al. (1972)
XXXX female	Daughter	Bergemann (1961)
Mosaic XXX females (4 cases)	Granddaughter, daughter, niece or sister	Bergemann (1961)
Trisomy 17-18	Sister	Hecht et al. (1963)
Trisomy 17-18	Sister	Hecht et al. (1964)
Trisomy 17-18	Sister	Hecht et al. (1964)
Trisomy 17-18	Brother	Turner et al. (1964)
Trisomy 17-18	Brother	Holmgren & Ánséhm (1971)
Trisomy 17-18	Sister	Crandall & Ebbin (1973)
Trisomy 13-15	Maternal uncle	Hecht et al. (1964)
Extra metacentric in a male	Sister	Gustavson et al. (1964)
Extra metacentric in a male	Daughter	Sergovich et al. (1967)
Extra mediocentric chromosome	Daughter and granddaughter	Townes (1968)
(DqDq) translocation	Mother and maternal aunt	Hamerton et al. (1963)
(DqDq) translocation	Son	Chaptal et al. (1965)
(DqDq) translocation	Daughter and granddaughter	Zellweger & Abbo (1965)
(DqDq) translocation	Daughter and sister	Marsden et al. (1966)
(DqDq) translocation	Son	Orye & Delire (1967)
(DqDq) translocation	8 relatives	Palmer et al. (1969)
(DqDq) translocation	8 relatives (see text)	Ridler et al. (1969)
69,XXY triploid fetus	Maternal aunt and 2 distant relatives	Penrose & Delhanty (1961b)
46,XX/47,XX,C+ mosaicism	Son	Bishun (1968)

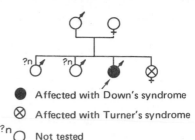

Fig. 86. Sibship with Down's and Turner's syndromes (after Johnston & Petrakis 1963).

● Affected with Down's syndrome

⊗ Affected with Turner's syndrome

?n ◯ Not tested

chronic lymphatic leukaemia, had a sister and niece who were both affected with standard Down's syndrome. The evidence for a common genetical mechanism in this case is weak because the most satisfactory explanation for the XXXXY zygote is fertilization by a Y sperm of an abnormal ovum, but here the Down's syndrome individuals were paternally related. A patient with (21qGq) translocation Down's syndrome was found to have a half brother with Klinefelter's syndrome (Benirschke *et al.* 1962). A third half sib in the family was normal. All three had different fathers. Wright *et al.* (1963) described two sibships in each of which a standard trisomy 21 Down's syndrome child had a brother or half-brother with Klinefelter's syndrome. In the first of these sibships the child with Down's syndrome was one of dizygotic twins, the other twin being normal (see Fig. 87). In the second sibship the boy with Klinefelter's syndrome showed XY/XXY mosaicism. A diagnostic amniocentesis undertaken at 17 weeks gestation on a 42 year old woman, who had previously had a son

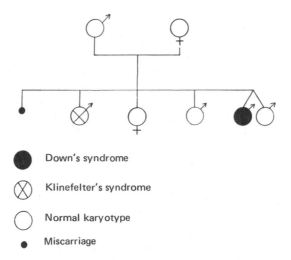

● Down's syndrome

⊗ Klinefelter's syndrome

◯ Normal karyotype

• Miscarriage

Fig. 87. Sibship with Down's and Klinefelter's syndromes (after Wright *et al.* 1963)

with Down's syndrome, revealed a fetus with 47,XXY Klinefelter's syndrome (Iinuma *et al.* 1973). The parents elected to have the pregnancy terminated and the diagnosis was confirmed on cord blood.

Hauschka *et al.* (1962) reported a Down's syndrome girl whose father had 47 chromosomes. Karyotype analysis showed that he had six small acrocentrics, two of which were considered to be Y chromosomes. He had average intelligence and, in two marriages, there had been nine pregnancies. One daughter had Down's syndrome and one was amenorrhoeic with failure of sexual development. She had 46 chromosomes with an XX pattern in blood and bone marrow; however, the possibility that she was mosaic (XX/XO) was not excluded. Mothers with extra sex chromosomes who have produced Down's syndrome children are also known. Such mothers have had three (Kadotani *et al.* 1970a, Morić-Petrović *et al.* 1971, Singer *et al.* 1972) or four (Bergemann 1961) X chromosomes.

A similar chromosomal abnormality in a family, which included a person with Down's syndrome was reported by Breg *et al.* (1962). They examined the buccal mucosa cells of 148 mentally retarded females in institutions and found three with double sex chromatin. All three had a somatic chromosome number of 47 with an extra X and no evidence of mosaicism. Two of them had relatives with Down's syndrome. The first triple-X female had a Down's syndrome brother. The other had a paternal uncle whose daughter was affected with the syndrome. Mosaic triple X females with Down's syndrome relatives also have been reported (Bergemann 1961). An additional variant was the occurrence in a sibship of a triple X child whose sister had Down's syndrome of the t(GqGq) type (Huang *et al.* 1967); three other sibs (two boys and a girl) and the parents showed normal karyotypes.

During their study of trisomy 17–18, Hecht *et al.* (1963) found a trisomic 17–18 female infant with a Down's syndrome sister. The mother was 42 years old when the trisomic 17–18 child was born and a year younger when the child with Down's syndrome was born: the father was 46 and 45 years old respectively. Hecht *et al.* further noted that the mean maternal age for trisomic 17–18 children is increased just as it is in Down's syndrome. Hecht *et al.* (1964) subsequently reported two more such sibships and commented on the likelihood of the noted association not being a random one. Similar types of sibship were reported by Turner *et al.* (1964), Holmgren & Ånséhm (1971) and Crandall & Ebbin (1973). In Holmgren & Ånséhm's sibship, a standard trisomic boy with Down's syndrome had dizygotic twin sisters one of whom showed trisomy 17–18 (see Fig. 88). Trisomy 13–15 has been noted less frequently among relatives of Down's syndrome individuals. In one such family (Hecht *et al.* 1964), a maternal uncle of a child with 13–15 trisomy was found to have standard Down's syndrome. This uncle was the thirteenth child of parents each aged about 42 years at the time of his birth.

A severely retarded, epileptic male, whose younger sister had standard Down's syndrome, was found by Gustavson *et al.* (1964) to have an extra,

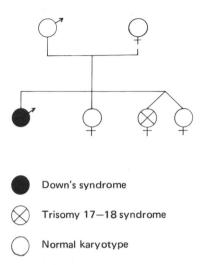

● Down's syndrome

⊗ Trisomy 17—18 syndrome

○ Normal karyotype

Fig. 88. Sibship with Down's and trisomy 17—18 syndromes (After Holmgren & Ånséhm 1971)

small metacentric chromosome of uncertain origin. A standard Down's syndrome daughter was born also to a father who was mosaic for three extra metacentric fragments, each appearing to have satellites on both ends (Sergovich *et al.* 1967). He was a clinically normal man aged 30 years at the time and his wife was two years older. Two previous pregnancies had ended, respectively, in a stillbirth and a spontaneous abortion. An unusual family with an extra mediocentric chromosome was reported by Townes (1968). This extra chromosome was found in a Down's syndrome child, with 48 chromosomes (including trisomy 21), as well as in her phenotypically normal father and grandfather.

Translocations of the (DqDq) type have been noted, from time to time, in relatives of Down's syndrome individuals (Hamerton *et al.* 1963, Chaptal *et al.* 1965, Zellweger & Abbo 1965, Marsden *et al.* 1966, Orye & Delire 1967, Palmer *et al.* 1969, Ridler *et al.* 1969), as well as in the Down's syndrome cases themselves. In the family reported by Ridler *et al.* eight healthy, phenotypically normal relatives of a Down's syndrome child were known to carry such a balanced translocation, i.e. all four sibs, the father, paternal grandmother, a paternal aunt and cousin. The family reported by Palmer *et al.* was very similar.

Examples of other unusual chromosomal anomalies found in close relatives of Down's syndrome cases are given in Table 91. The source of cultures of triploid cells (Penrose & Delhanty 1961b) was a missed abortion from a normal female whose sister had Down's syndrome of the t(21q22q) type (see Fig. 89). An extra C group chromosome in some blood and skin cells was found by Bishun (1968) in a 27 year old phenotypically normal mother of a standard Down's syndrome boy.

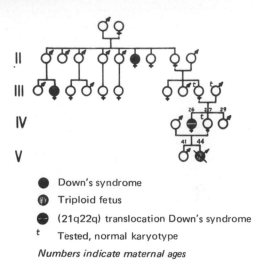

- ● Down's syndrome
- ◉ Triploid fetus
- ⊖ (21q22q) translocation Down's syndrome
- *t* Tested, normal karyotype

Numbers indicate maternal ages

Fig. 89. Pedigree of Down's syndrome and fetal triploidy.

TWINS

When twins are dizygotic and one has Down's syndrome the other is usually unaffected (Allen & Baroff 1955, Zellweger (1968b). There are a few exceptions to this where dizygotic twins have been both affected (Russell 1933, MacKaye 1936, Nicholson & Keay 1957, McDonald 1964, Fielding & Walker 1972, Hirsch *et al.* 1974). An unusual pair of dizygotic twins was reported by Rohmer *et al.* (1970). One, with the clinical characteristics of Down's syndrome, had a 47,XX,21+ karyotype; the other, without clinical features of the syndrome, had 46,XX/47,XX,21+ mosaicism.

Table 92. Distribution of Twins in Down's Syndrome (After de Wolff *et al.* 1962)

| | Monozygotic | Dizygotic | | Same sex but uncertainty about zygotic type | Total |
		Both same sex	Different sex		
One affected (discordant)	1*	46	79	43	169
Both affected (concordant)	18	1†	1‡	12	32
Total	19	47	80	55	201

*de Wolff *et al.* (1962)
†MacKaye (1936)
‡Nicholson & Keay (1957).

Monozygotic twins have been found to be equally affected except on rare occasions (see Table 92). de Wolff *et al.* (1962) reported male monozygotic twins one of which had standard Down's syndrome whereas the other was chromosomally and phenotypically normal. A few similar twin pairs were subsequently reported (Nielsen 1967). They can be thought of as a form of mosaicism expressed as two separate people. These pairs could have arisen from either a normal or an abnormal zygote. de Wolff *et al.* favoured the theory that there was an anomaly in the division of the chromosomes during the first stage of blastogenesis after the fusion of normal gametes.

An unequally affected monozygotic pair of twins has also been described by Dekaban (1965): one twin had a normal karyotype and the other showed 48 chromosomes with trisomy 21 and an additional small "abnormal" metacentric. Another variant in a pair of female twins, considered probably to be monozygotic, was reported by Shapiro & Farnsworth (1972): one twin had a normal karyotype and phenotype, while the other had 46,XX/47,XX,21+ mosaicism without clinical appearances of Down's syndrome.

The incidence of monozygotic Down's syndrome twins is lower than would be expected from the population frequency. It is thought (Keay 1958) that there may be frequent intrauterine death of one or both members of the pair.

OFFSPRING OF FULLY AFFECTED DOWN'S SYNDROME FEMALES

So far, 22 examples of fully affected Down's syndrome females have been reported. Nine of the offspring had Down's syndrome, two were mentally retarded, ten were normal and three were stillborn (see Table 93). The mean maternal age at the birth of these affected mothers of children with the syndrome is about 36 years. The age of the Down's syndrome mothers at the births of their own affected children is much younger, averaging about 22 years.

Cytological studies have been carried out on some of the Down's syndrome mothers and their offspring (see Table 93). Hanhart *et al.* (1961) cultured fibroblasts from such a mother and her affected daughter. They showed that both had standard trisomy. This demonstrated secondary (inevitable) non-disjunction in man. The same phenomenon has been observed since in a number of instances. A Down's syndrome female produces two types of gamete in her germ cells. One type will have 24 chromosomes and, when fertilized by a normal sperm, will become a standard case of Down's syndrome. The other type of gamete will contain the haploid number of 23 and, when fertilized by a normal sperm, will become a normal zygote (see Fig. 90).

The occurrence of inevitable non-disjunction is not related to advancing maternal age. The mean age of a Down's syndrome mother at the time of

Table 93. Offspring of Fully Affected Down's Syndrome Females

Description of child	Age of D.S. mother at birth of her child	Maternal age at birth of D.S. mother	Karyotype		Authors
			D.S. Mother	Child	
Normal female	25	—	—	—	Sawyer (1949); Sawyer & Shafter (1957)
D.S. male	30	42	—	—	Lelong et al. (1949)
D.S. female	19	19	Trisomy 21	Trisomy 21	Rehn & Thomas (1957); Stiles (1958); Stiles & Goodman (1961); Johnston & Jaslow (1963)
Retarded male	30	42	Trisomy 21	Normal	Forssman & Thysell (1957); Forssman et al. (1961)
Retarded female	29	39	—	—	Schlaug (1958)
Normal male	—	—	Trisomy 21	Normal	Levan & Hsu (1959, 1960)
Normal male	22	22	—	—	Mullins et al. (1960)
D.S. male	23	44	Trisomy 21	—	Hanhart (1960b)
D.S. female	21	44	Trisomy 21	Trisomy 21	Hanhart et al. (1961)
Stillborn male twins	14	34	Trisomy 21	Normal (both twins)	Thuline & Priest (1961); Priest et al. (1963b)
Normal male	21	40	—	—	Thompson (1961)
Stillborn female	20	22	Trisomy 21	—	Thompson (1961, 1962)
D.S. male	22	22	Trisomy 21	—	Thompson (1961, 1962)
Normal female	18	46	Trisomy 21	Normal	Foxton et al. (1965)
Normal female	27	35	Trisomy 21	Normal	Tagher & Reisman (1966)
D.S. female	18	—	Trisomy 21	Trisomy 21	Finley et al. (1968)
D.S. male	17	43	Trisomy 21	Trisomy 21	Friedman et al. (1970)
Normal female	19	37	Trisomy 21	Normal	Masterson et al. (1970)
Normal female	30	39	Trisomy 21	Normal	Masterson et al. (1970)
Normal male	16	42	Trisomy 21	Normal	Morić-Petrović & Garzicic (1970)
D.S. female	23	—	Trisomy 21	Trisomy 21	Rethoré et al. (1970)
Normal female	25	40	Trisomy 21	Normal	Reiss et al. (1971)
D.S. male	20	40	Trisomy 21	Trisomy 21	Fuchs-Mecke & Passarge (1972)

D.S. = Down's syndrome

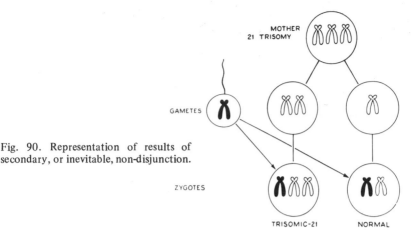

MOTHER
21 TRISOMY

GAMETES

ZYGOTES

TRISOMIC-21   NORMAL

Fig. 90. Representation of results of secondary, or inevitable, non-disjunction.

the birth of her similarly affected child, in the nine recorded cases, is 21.4 years. A similar result is obtained from examining the ages of mosaic mothers at the births of their Down's syndrome children. For Case No. 5, in Table 86, this age was 31 years. For Case No. 6, the corresponding ages were 17, 19 and 21 years; for No. 13 the age was 29 years and for No. 14, 17 years. The mean maternal age at the births of these six children is, thus, 22.3 years.

NON-DISJUNCTION DURING MEIOSIS

de Grouchy *et al.* (1970) reported a 21 marker chromosome (21p-) in duplicate in a Down's syndrome individual and in single state in the mother. They used this family to demonstrate that non-disjunction of chromosome 21 occurred, in this case, in the mother during the second meiotic division of oogenesis (see Fig. 91). A similar family was reported by Juberg & Jones (1970).

Licznerski & Lindsten (1972) and Robinson (1973), using the fact that chromosome 21 demonstrated a heteromorphic quinacrine fluorescence pattern, came to conclusion that non-disjunction occurred during the first meiotic division. The basis for this conclusion was that the Down's syndrome individual seemed to have both the mother's No. 21 chromosomes. The possibility of non-disjunction occurring in the second meiotic division could not be excluded, since a similar type of fluorescence pattern of the 21 chromosomes could be obtained if crossing over occurred between the fluorescent satellite region and the centromere. It is not yet known how often, if at all, crossing-over occurs in this region in female meiosis. However, a chiasma has occasionally been observed in the short arm of chromosome 21 in human male meiosis (Hultén & Lindsten 1970).

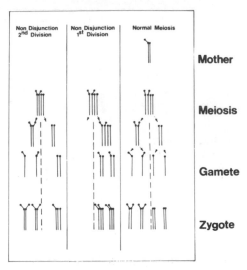

Fig. 91. Schematic representation of a marker 21 chromosome in mother and types of zygotes produced if non-disjunction occurs at first or second meiotic division. (After deGrouchy *et al.* 1970).

In studies similar to Robinson's, Mutton (1973) and Smith & Sachdeva (1973) found evidence from fluorescent chromosome studies that non-disjunction occurred at the second meiotic division in the mother. In the Down's syndrome individual, similar appearing marker chromosomes were identified.

Sasaki & Hara (1973) and Uchida (1973), using the fluorescence technique, showed that in separate families the extra chromosome was of paternal origin and that non-disjunction occurred during the second meiotic division. Uchida raised the consideration that, since the fathers in her study tended to be young, paternal non-disjunction should not be overlooked as a cause of trisomy in the maternal-age-independent group. Another interpretation was suggested by Smith (1973).

MEIOSIS AND SPERMATOGENESIS

The results of investigations on meiosis and spermatogenesis in Down's syndrome males have varied considerably (see Table 94). Lack of good cytological techniques, in the early studies, made morphological inter-pretation and chromosome counting difficult in both spermatogonia and spermatocytes. As demonstrated by Hultén & Lindsten (1970), Kjessler & de la Chapelle (1971) and Schröder *et al.* (1971), the extra chromosome may be part of either a trivalent or a univalent. A pachytene trivalent G chromosome previously had been observed by Hungerford *et al.* (1970). Schröder *et al.* found that, at diakinesis-metaphase I, 41 per cent of cells were normal, containing 2 G-bivalents. The authors argued in favour of the view that an elimination of the supernumerary G chromosome may occur at one of the spermatogonial mitoses or earlier. Such a conclusion was tentative, since it was derived from investigation of small numbers of spermatogonial mitoses. The model for the conclusion is based upon studies of the elimination of supernumerary chromosomes in XYY males (Thompson *et al.* 1967, Melnyk *et al.* 1969, Hultén 1970, Evans *et al.* 1970, Hsu *et al.* 1970b, Tettenborn *et al.* 1970).

Table 94. Meiotic Chromosome Studies

Authors	Number of Patients Studied	Type of Down's Syndrome	Results	Spermatogenic Arrest
Mittwoch 1952*	1	Trisomy 21	Bivalents	-
Miller *et al.* 1960	4	Trisomy 21	Univalents, trivalents, multivalents	Present
Hamerton *et al.* 1961b	1	D/G†	Bivalents, trivalent	-
Sasaki 1965	1	Trisomy 21	G,Bivalents and trivalents	Present
Finch *et al.* 1966	1	Trisomy 21	Bivalents and univalent	Present ‡
Hultén & Lindsten 1970	1	Trisomy 21	Extra chromosome part of trivalent or univalent	-
Hungerford *et al.* 1970	1	Trisomy 21	Pachytene trivalent G chromosome	-
Kjessler & de la Chapelle 1971	2	Trisomy 21	Extra chromosome part of trivalent or univalent	Absent
Schröder *et al.* 1971	3	Trisomy 21		Absent
Hecht *et al.* 1970,1973	2	G/G	21;21 translocation	-

*See Chapter 1.
†Heterozygote carrier (see Fig. 63).
‡Received oestrogen therapy.

Meiotic studies on two sibs with Down's syndrome were suggestive of a 21/21 chromosome rearrangement. Banding of somatic chromosomes of the mother and one of the Down's syndrome individuals established that the chromosomal rearrangement was a 21/21 translocation and not an isochromosome (Hecht *et al.* 1973).

While spermatogenic arrest has been reported (see Table 94), Kjessler & de la Chapelle and Schröder *et al.* were unable to confirm this finding. They observed normal spermatogenesis although a decrease in quantity was noted. On the basis of testicular histology, however, the patients could not be considered sterile.

CELL CYCLE

Mittwoch (1972) presented evidence that different chromosome constitutions may affect mitotic cycle times and hence the rates of cell proliferation. The presence of an additional chromosome in Down's syndrome is likely to slow down mitotic cycle times. In XY cells there is a slight overall increase of cell growth compared with XX cells.

TRISOMIC FIBROBLAST CELLS IN CULTURE

Kaback & Bernstein (1970), using fibroblast cultures derived from individuals with Down's syndrome, observed a decrease in the rate of DNA synthesis in these trisomic cells. They could not determine which of the cell phases were prolonged. Similar findings were observed by Mittwoch (1967), using a different procedure for determining DNA synthesis. These investigators noted an increase in cellular RNA in Down's syndrome cell lines. The effect was evident only during conditions of exponential growth and could indicate that major development effects of the extra 21 chromosome would occur during periods of active cellular division.

Fialkow *et al.* (1973) reported on the replicative life span of cultured skin fibroblasts in mothers of Down's syndrome individuals. No significant differences were observed between Down's syndrome and control mothers or between those women who had offspring with Down's syndrome at younger versus old ages. Preliminary data suggested that fibroblasts from women with thyroid antibodies have greater longevity than those from antibody negative women.

TRANSFORMATION OF FIBROBLASTS AND LYMPHOCYTES

Todaro & Martin (1967) demonstrated that fibroblast cultures from individuals with trisomy 18 or 21 are more susceptible than diploid fibroblasts to *in vitro* transformation by SV40. Lymphoblastoid cell lines also have been established from peripheral blood of persons with Down's syndrome (using the Epstein-Barr Virus (EBV)).

Miyoshi *et al.* (1974) and Smith *et al.* (1975) showed that, although EBV capsid antibody levels were generally higher in Down's syndrome, the frequency of and the period of time to cell line establishment were similar for Down's syndrome and normal persons. Lymphoblastoid cell lines derived from Down's syndrome individuals have been characterized by Fujiwara (1973, 1974), and Woods *et al.* (1973).

CHROMOSOME LOSSES IN CULTURE

Bloom *et al.* (1967) and Neurath *et al.* (1970), working with cells from normal individuals (euploid cell lines), found a linear relationship between chromosome size and the probability of loss for chromosomes of groups A to F. The very small G chromosomes were missing more often than could be predicted on the basis of regression curves. Mikkelsen (1967a) studied the loss of a single chromosome from cells from individuals with Down's syndrome. In these cell lines, she found a significant deficit of cells lacking a large A or B group chromosome; there was also a greater than expected loss of chromosomes in groups G and Y in parents but not in Down's syndrome children. Gall *et al.* (1970) found that, for single chromosome losses from Down's syndrome cell lines, the results were similar to those on normal cell lines reported by Bloom *et al.* and Neurath *et al.* Gall *et al.* found that the loss of the G chromosome in cultured cells from Down's syndrome individuals was no different from the loss of the G chromosome from euploid cell lines. They concluded that there was no significant degree of mosaicism in Down's syndrome cells in culture.

RADIATION EFFECTS ON TRISOMY 21 CELLS

The radiation studies of Dekaban *et al.* (1966) and Chudina *et al.* (1966) suggest that lymphocytes from individuals with Down's syndrome (trisomic cells) are more sensitive than lymphocytes from normal individuals (diploid-21 cells) to radiation. It appears that a change in chromosome number (trisomy 21) will influence the production of aberrations caused by radiation. Chudina *et al.* induced chromatid type of changes by x-ray. Additional studies by Kućerova (1967), Sasaki & Tonomura (1969), and Evans & Adams (1973) extended the observations. Lymphocytes irradiated in G_1, x-ray or γ-irradiated trisomic-21 lymphocytes, had a 50-100 per cent increased incidence of chromosomal aberrations (dicentric and ring aberrations) over normal lymphocytes (diploid-21) from mosaics. The frequency of deletions was the same between the two cell types. It was shown that the increase in aberrations in the trisomic cells was not due to an increased involvement of all the chromosomes in the aberration formations.

Sasaki *et al.* (1970) exposed blood samples of individuals with chromosomal abnormalities, including Down's syndrome, to x-rays. They studied the relationship between chromosome constitution and chromosomal radiosensitivity of lymphocytes. Their results showed that the chromosomal radiosensitivity was consistently higher in cells which were trisomic for the whole or a part of a chromosome than the cells with a normal karyotype. They suggested that the increased chromosomal radiosensitivity of trisomic cells was the effect of altered enzyme activity.

CHROMOSOMAL DAMAGE DUE TO CARCINOGENS

O'Brien *et al.* (1971) demonstrated the susceptibility of chromosomes from Down's syndrome individuals to 7,12-dimethylbenz (a) anthracene (DMBA), in *in vitro* studies. The chromosomal aberrations, chromatid gaps or breaks occurred in both the Down's syndrome and normal cells; however, they were found much more frequently in the former. Isochromatid exchanges and dicentric chromosomes were observed but less frequently. Lymphocytes from Down's syndrome patients were able to repair DNA damage induced by ultraviolet light or 4-nitroquinoline-N-oxide. At the doses used to produce chromosomal aberrations, DMBA did not significantly inhibit either replicative DNA synthesis or the repair of damage induced by ultraviolet light or 4-nitroquinoline-N-oxide in lymphocytes from normal or Down's syndrome individuals. DMBA did not stimulate unscheduled DNA synthesis in the lymphocytes from either group.

LINKAGE OF GENES TO CHROMOSOME 21

Tan et al. (1973) showed that antiviral protein (AVP) and the human dimeric form of indophenol oxidase (IPO-B) are on the No. 21 chromosome. By using mouse-human somatic cell hybrid clones they were able to demonstrate that only those clones protected by human interferon (which stimulated AVP) also contained IPO-B. Chromosomal analysis of the clones indicated that chromosome G-21 was the only human chromosome common to those clones possessing both these character-istics. The loss of chromosome G-21 from a clone shows the loss of both these phenotypes. They concluded from their findings that the gene(s) for indophenol oxidase (IPO-B) and the gene(s) for the antiviral protein are syntenic (present on the same chromosome) and that they are linked to human chromosome G-21. In a later paper, Tan et al. (1974) showed that human primary skin fibroblasts trisomic for chromosome 21 were three to seven times more sensitive to protection by human interferon than normal diploid or trisomic 18 or 13 fibroblasts. The response in trisomic 21 fibroblasts was consistent with the known assignment of the human antiviral gene (AVP) to chromosome 21. So far there has been no substantiation of these observations. If the findings are substantiated, the meaning in terms of pathophysiology in Down's syndrome will remain to be determined. Sichitiu et al. (1974) tested 11 Down's syndrome patients and compared them with a similar number of controls for the red blood cell enzyme levels of IPO-B. The enzymatic studies were performed on starch gel electrophoresis of haemolysates of identical haemoglobin content. The results showed a significant increase in the dimeric form of IPO in Down's syndrome patients. The levels suggested that there is a trisomic gene effect.

Sinet et al. (1974) demonstrated that superoxide-dismutase activity (S.O.D.A.) is increased in erythrocytes of Down's syndrome children. Since the S.O.D.A. was found to be 1.4 times higher in the syndrome compared with normal children, they argued that this is a gene dosage effect (Sinet et al. 1975).

AMNIOCENTESIS STUDIES

Amniocentesis is best performed by the transabdominal route, since the transvaginal approach appears to increase the risk of abortion (Gerbie *et al.* 1971). Many physicians prefer to locate the placenta by ultrasound scanning, before inserting the needle. Even when the placenta is anterior, accurate placental localization may show an area where the needle can be safely inserted. The procedure is performed under local anaesthesia and is usually done on an out-patient basis at 14-16 weeks of pregnancy.

The potential risks of transabdominal amniocentesis include spontaneous abortion which seems to be small, and infection which should be minimal if proper sterile techniques are used. Total risks to both the mother and the fetus are not precisely known but probably amount to less than one per cent (Turnbull *et al.* 1973).

At the present time, exact recurrence risk figures for Down's syndrome based upon amniocentesis studies are difficult to evaluate, since many of the reported studies fail to record the maternal age at the time of the amniocentesis or the maternal age at which a previous child with Down's syndrome was born (also see page 272). These limitations apply to individual amniocentesis series or the pooling of data. Acknowledging these limitations, amniocentesis studies provide the following results. In family studies in Manitoba, Uchida (1970) observed a recurrence rate of 1:57 in standard trisomy 21. Littlefield *et al.* (1971), using the accumulated data on 182 cases of mothers who had previously borne a child with trisomy 21 and later had amniocentesis, found a recurrence risk factor of about 1:60. Milunsky (1973), using data from a national survey, estimated a risk factor of 1:97. The author correctly pointed out that this figure is only an approximation, since it was derived from 485 patients who had previously borne children with Down's syndrome but whose ages were not available for analysis (see Table 95).

Table 95. Amniocentesis Done Because of Advanced Maternal Age

Author	Over 35 Years		Under 35 Years	
	Total	D.S.*	Total	D.S.*
Turnbull *et al.*, 1973	21	1	6	0
Hsu *et al.*, 1973	54	0	–	–

*Down's Syndrome

Because of the increased incidence of Down's syndrome with increasing maternal age, a substantial number of women aged forty and over have had amniocentesis performed. In some clinics, amniocentesis is performed on women thirty-five and over. The reasons for doing amniocentesis on the older maternal age group is that not only is the incidence of Down's syndrome increased but so are some of the other chromosomal anomalies, namely, trisomy 13-15, trisomy 18, and sex chromosome aneuploids 47,XXY, 47,XXX and 47,XYY. It has been calculated (Penrose & Smith

1966) that women over thirty-five constitute only 13.5 per cent of all pregnancies but these women produce over 50 per cent of all infants with Down's syndrome. Bodensteiner & Zellweger (1971b) estimated, from their studies. that there is about 1:66 risk to a mother forty to forty-five years of age and a 1:21 risk to those over the age of forty-five years of bearing a child with Down's syndrome (see also Tables 95 and 96). Similar results have been found in the amniocentesis studies of Milunsky et al. (1970). Gertner et al. (1970), Ferguson-Smith et al. (1971) and Nadler (1972).

Table 96 Results of Amniocentesis on Mothers Who Previously Had Down's Syndrome Children. (After Hsu et al. 1973)

Previous Child with Down's Syndrome	No. of Cases	Normal	D.S.*	Abnormal Other
Maternal Age <35 years	50	49	0	1
Maternal Age 35-40 years	9	8	1	0
Maternal Age >40 years	3	3	0	0

*Down's syndrome

On the other hand, Zellweger & Simpson (1973) found that very young mothers, between 15 and 19 years of age, did not have a significantly greater incidence of offspring with Down's syndrome than mothers between 20 and 30 years of age. They concluded that there was no justification for considering prenatal chromosomal analysis a necessary examination in this age group, except in cases of parental translocation and parental mosaicism. Whether or not mothers below the age of 15 years have a higher risk of having aneuploid infants is not yet known.

While the frequency of maternal mosaicism is uncertain, estimates of as high as 10 per cent have been made (see page 98); this type of estimate is not based upon cytological studies. It is to be expected that mosaic mothers are at an increased risk of having additional children with Down's syndrome. The risk to subsequent children varies from mother to mother and it will be dependent upon the degree of mosaicism in the germ cells. Timson et al. (1971) observed the following, based upon eight mosaic mothers (Aarskog 1969, Timson et al.). Eight 46,XX/47,XX,21+ mothers had eleven children with Down's syndrome and two normal children. After excluding the propositi, the empirical risk was 3 in 5. The average age of the mothers was 23.6 years (range 17-32) and the average percentage of 47,XX,21+ cells was 16.4 per cent (range 5-29) in the peripheral blood lymphocyte cultures. It is of interest that the mothers were relatively young and that the range of percentage of abnormal cells overlaps with the range found in other cases of Down's syndrome mosaics who are physically and mentally affected. Since these mothers were ascertained as the result of having had a child with Down's syndrome, the data are biased. Timson et al. emphasized that in cases where this kind of mosaicism has been detected in a pregnant woman, antenatal diagnosis is indicated.

SPONTANEOUS ABORTIONS

Now that large series of spontaneous abortions have been studied cytogenetically, it is evident that most of the chromosome abnormalities found in live births are present in aborted fetuses. This is particularly true of trisomy 21; this autosomal abnormality is well represented in all studies on abortion material. Group G trisomies were found in 12.4 per cent of the cases reported by the Geneva Conference, (1966) and in 9 per cent of the abnormal abortions reported by Carr (1965). In contrast, Arakaki & Waxman (1970) found only one Down's syndrome fetus in 31 cases of autosomal abnormalities. This case was mosaic 46,XY/47,XY,G+. It has been estimated that, for every infant born alive with Down's syndrome, 2-3 were lost as abortions due to the fact that their physical abnormalities were not compatible with survival.

11. Vital Statistics

INCIDENCE AT BIRTH

At birth the incidence of Down's syndrome in populations of European origin is of the order of 1 in 700. In general, the results of various investigators are in good agreement (see Table 97). Most estimates have been obtained from maternity hospital records. A more complete survey is that reported by Collmann & Stoller (1962a,b) from Victoria, Australia. From 1942 to 1957, 1,134 Down's syndrome children were born in Victoria out of a total of 780,168 registered live births, representing an incidence of 0.145 per cent or 1 in 688 live births. A considerable number of surveys have since been published.

Lilienfeld (1969) summarized the reports of 34 incidence studies. He found that the reported rates range from 0.32 to 3.4 per 1000 births (1:3000 to 1:300). The frequency distribution in these reports is seen in Table 98. There were great differences in the types of populations studied and the methods of ascertainment which undoubtedly account for some of the variation in the different studies.

In Black populations the incidence was considered to be much lower than that in Caucasians; by inference from the figures of Thompson (1939), it may be only 1 or 2 per 10,000 births. However, Parker (1950) and Kashgarian & Rendtorff (1969) noted incidence figures closer to those of European populations. Although Down's syndrome has been reported in nearly all non-European·populations, e.g. Africans, Indians, Chinese, Egyptians, Esquimaux and American Indians, reliable incidence figures usually are not available. Matsunaga (1967a) observed that Down's syndrome now is in Japan, as in Europe and North America, one of the best known abnormalities both to physicians and to other case workers concerned with mental retardation. He thought that the diagnosis of Down's syndrome in the Japanese newborn is probably somewhat more difficult than in Europeans and that accurate data on its incidence at birth are still insufficient. Presumably, the incidence is not less than 1 per 1000 live births.

Marmol et al. (1969), in the Collaborative Project in the U.S.A., also reported that the incidence of Down's syndrome in the white and black populations was nearly equal. Hashem & Sakr (1963) and Thores & Philion (1973) noted a similar incidence in Egyptian and British Columbia Indians respectively. Morris (1971) did a survey of Down's syndrome in the European and Maori populations in New Zealand. The Europeans showed

Table 97. Incidence at Birth of Down's Syndrome.

Number with Down's syndrome	Total number of births in sample	Inci- dence	Source	Type of material	Region
6	3,818	1/636	Jenkins (1933)	H	Chicago
18	13,964	1/776	Malpas (1937)	H	Liverpool
7	4,374	1/629	Penrose (1938b)	S	England
32	27,931	1/873	Parker (1950)	N	Washington D.C.
130	67,645	1/520	Hug (1951)	H	Zürich
107	71,521	1/666	Carter & MacCarthy (1951)	H	London
52	39,788	1/765	Øster (1953)	H	Copenhagen
1,134	780,168	1/688	Collmann & Stoller (1962a)	P	Victoria
91	54,482	1/588	Beolchini et al. (1962)	–	Milan
92	61,821	1/675	Buchan (1962)	H	Newcastle-Upon-Tyne
4	3,000	1/751	Wedberg et al. (1963)	H	Gothenburg
38*	25,038	1/657	Hall (1964)	H	Southern Sweden
134	131,634	1/980	Davidenkova et al. (1964)	–	Leningrad
513	316,954	1/617	Leck (1966)	P	Birmingham
27	15,517	1/588	Spellman (1966)	H	Cork City
37	23,720	1/746**	Stevenson et al. (1966)	–	Santiago
27	20,074	1/495**	Stevenson et al. (1966)	–	Czechoslovakia
22	14,083	1/581**	Stevenson et al. (1966)	–	Mexico City
17	15,852	1/694**	Stevenson et al. (1966)	–	Panama City
39	19,714	1/571**	Stevenson et al. (1966)	–	Madrid
10	8,528	1/853	Brewis et al. (1966)	P	Carlisle, U.K.
13*	11,646	1/892	Robinson & Puck (1967)	H	Denver
97	90,792	1/934	Halevi (1967)	H	Israel
2,432	2,722,774	1/1123	Stark & Mantel (1967)	H	Lower Michigan
1,810	1,287,446	1/709	Fabia (1969)	H	Massachusetts
63	54,761	1/869	Sever et al. (1970)	H	Collaborative Project, U.S.A.
53*	24,245	1/457	Wahrman & Fried (1970)	H	Jerusalem
24	16,605	1/691	Coriat et al. (1971)	H	Buenos Aires
2,398	1,290,244	1/537	McDonald (1972a)	H	Quebec
17	10,493*	1/617	Ingalls (1972)	–	Boston
4*	5,049	1/1262	Friedrich & Nielsen (1973)	H	Århus
34*	31,334	1/921	Robinson (1973)	H	Denver
103	42,340	1/411	Harlap (1974)	–	Jerusalem
42	30,314	1/722	Haynes et al. (1974)	P	Rochester, Minnesota

*All cases investigated cytologically.
**Standardized for maternal age.
H = Hospital data.
S = Sibs of retarded persons without Down's syndrome
N = Hospital data which includes a black population of 25,026 births in which 29 Down's syndrome children were born. Incidence of 1/863.
P = General population.

Table 98. Thirty-four Down's Syndrome Incidence Studies Showing Frequency Distributions (After Lilienfeld 1969)

Incidence	Number of Reports
<1:1000	5
1:1000–1:700	18
1:650–1:500	10
>1:500	1

an incidence of 1:806, but the incidence in the relatively small Maori population was markedly lower (1:8181). Morris noted a maternal age variation for the Europeans but not for the Maoris.

The incidence varies greatly with the age of the mother. At about the maternal age of 20 years the incidence is 1 in 2,300, and at 45 years and over the incidence increases markedly to about 1 in 54 (Cohen & Warland

1960). The distribution of maternal age at births resulting in Down's syndrome, compared with births in the general population, is seen in Fig. 92. Up to the age of 30 the distribution curve rises not appreciably more rapidly than the distribution curve of all births in the population. After this point the numbers of all births diminish steadily, though those for Down's

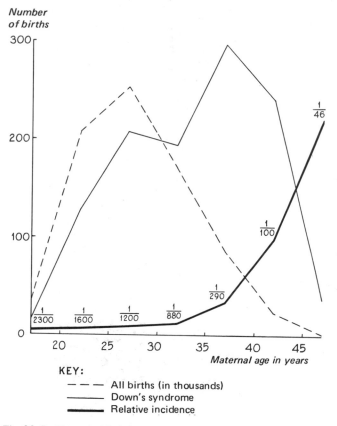

Fig. 92. Incidence at birth from survey by Collmann & Stoller (1962a).

syndrome individuals, after a slight halt, continue to rise until about the maternal age of 40 years. The relative incidence of Down's syndrome continues to rise after the peak of absolute incidence has been passed. Whether or not the incidence would continue to increase if the menopause did not stop the reproductive period in the female is not absolutely clear. The shape of the distribution curve suggests that the relative incidence would continue to advance but at a diminishing rate.

In the Victoria study it was noted that the annual birth incidence was not constant but varied periodically in a five to six year cycle of maxima and minima (Collmann & Stoller 1962a). In addition it was found that there were geographical concentrations of births occurring within any year. The difference between high concentration areas (urban) and low concentration areas (rural) could not be accounted for by the age distributions of the mothers in these two areas (Collmann & Stoller 1963c). The fluctuations were considered to be indicative of environmental influence, such as acute infectious disease, in the causation as suggested by Pleydell (1957). Robinson (1973) showed that for women over 35 years of age there was no difference in the incidence between May to October and November to April, but for women under 35 years of age there was a marked increase in the incidence in the May to October period (see Table 99).

Table 99. Incidence Figures by Season (After Robinson 1973)

Period	Mothers Under 35 Years	Mothers Over 35 Years
May to October	(19/14,123) 1:743	(6/1431) 1:238
November to April	(3/12,805) 1:4268	(8/1299) 1:162

In a perinatal study in Jerusalem comprising the years 1964 to 1970, Harlap (1974) reported an incidence rate of 2.4 per 1000 births. She noted that there was a highly significant short term cycle of 6 months with incidence peaks among Spring and Autumn births in six of the seven years studied. The changes in incidence were independent of maternal age or standard of living. There was also a long-term decrease in Down's syndrome incidence which was considered to be part of a cycle of approximately 10 years. The author felt that the data supported the hypothesis that environmental factors play a major role in the aetiology of the syndrome. The conclusions in the study are based upon a small number of Down's syndrome infants which makes acceptance difficult. This criticism applies also to the data of Robinson (1973). Lander et al. (1964) also reported a decreased frequency of September births of Swedish Down's syndrome babies compared with general population births but, since this was a prevalence study from institutional data, there could have been a differential death rate of Down's syndrome babies born in different seasons.

Leck (1966) and Edwards (1970) showed trends for a lower incidence of Down's syndrome during the early autumn. The cause of this, however, was attributed to a seasonal under-ascertainment. Haynes et al. (1974) found no discernible pattern, for a 37 year period in Rochester, Minnesota, in the incidence rates of Down's syndrome by month of delivery.

McDonald (1972a) did a yearly and seasonal incidence study of Down's syndrome in Quebec and found a yearly rate of 1.86/1000 live births (1:537). This was somewhat higher than the rate in Britain of 1.6 (1:625) and of 1.5 (1:666) in Australia. There was no evidence of seasonal variation in incidence nor of any increase following epidemics of infectious hepatitis. The findings are similar to those of other surveys by Stark & Fraumeni (1966), Leck (1966), Ceccarelli & Torbidoni (1967), Kogon et al. (1968) and Baird & Miller (1968). Thus there is little support for the position that there is a causal association of infectious hepatitis in mothers and an increased risk of having a child with Down's syndrome (Stoller & Collmann 1965a and b, 1966, Doxiadis et al. 1970, Kučera 1971).

A high incidence of chromosomal abnormalities in spontaneous abortions has been reported by Carr (1963, 1965), 44 in 200 specimens. Five had chromosome patterns diagnostic of Down's syndrome. If these findings are confirmed, the incidence of Down's syndrome in spontaneous abortions must be about 1:40. By implication, the incidence of Down's syndrome at conception could be 1/200, three times the incidence at birth. It is estimated that from 65 per cent (Creasy & Crolla 1974) to 80 per cent (Kajii et al. 1973) of Down's syndrome conceptions are lost as spontaneous abortions. If these figures are accurate, and such abortions did not occur, the absolute incidence of Down's syndrome live-births would increase about three-to five-fold.

POPULATION INCIDENCE

Prevalence of Down's syndrome in the general population at a given time is of importance to administrators who have to plan training and care. Penrose (1932b, 1949c) gave prevalence figures and estimated that there were 3.24 living Down's syndrome individuals at all ages per 10,000 population (1 in 3,000). Other prevalence studies have been reported from Denmark (Øster 1956), London (Carter 1958) and Victoria, Australia (Collmann & Stoller 1963a) (see Table 100). A major survey which gave a markedly different value was described by Doxiades & Portius (1938). They found only 58 surviving Down's syndrome individuals in a total general population of 415,413 of all ages in Germany, implying a prevalence of 1 in 7,000.

In the Victoria study the prevalence of Down's syndrome was 10.2 per

Table 100. Population Incidence

Location	Prevalence	Source
Eastern Counties, England	1/10,000	Penrose (1932b)
Germany	1/ 7,000	Doxiades & Portius (1938)
London, England	1/ 3,000	Penrose (1949c)
Copenhagen, Denmark	1/ 4,000	Øster (1956)
London, England	1/ 1,000*	Carter (1958)
Victoria, Australia	1/ 2,200	Collmann & Stoller (1963a)

*Among 10-year-old children

10,000 for the first year of life, but decreased to about 7 for children of school age and to almost zero by 50–54 years of age. The prevalence figures reported by Penrose (1949c) for the age group 10–14 years was 4.6 per 10,000, slightly lower than, but in good agreement with, those reported in the Victoria study. Collmann & Stoller (1963a) noted that 25 per cent of all living affected persons were under 7 years of age, 50 per cent were under 16 years of age and 75 per cent were under 27 years of age. An increase in expectation of life occurred from 1929 to 1949 (Carter 1958). With improved medical care in the future an additional increase in the population incidence is to be expected.

Zeuthen & Nielsen (1973) reported the prevalence of chromosome abnormalities in a Danish male population (19 years of age) of 3,840 conscripts. Only males with small testes and short stature (≦181 cm), and mentally retarded males were examined chromosomally. Total prevalence of chromosome abnormalities in this special group was 4.69 per 1000. It is of interest that the prevalence of males with Down's syndrome and double Y males was equal, 1.30 per 1000 (1:769), and that of Klinefelter males 0.78 per 1000 (1:1282).

LIFE TABLES (SURVIVAL RATES)

Penrose (1932b, 1949c) estimated that the life expectancy of Down's syndrome individuals in 1929 was 9 years (9.5 for males and 8.5 for females) and, by 1947, it had increased to 12 years. Brothers & Jago (1954) found that the average age of death of institutional Down's syndrome patients in Victoria, Australia, was slightly over 10 years. Collmann & Stoller (1963b) reported that the mean age of all living affected persons in Victoria, Australia, was 18.3 years (see Table 101). They calculated survival rates for 729 Down's syndrome babies born from 1948 to 1957.

Table 101. Life Expectation in Down's Syndrome.

Place	Mean survival age in years	Source
London, England	9	Penrose (1932b)
London, England	12	Penrose (1949c)
Victoria, Australia	10	Brothers & Jago (1954)
Victoria, Australia	18	Collmann & Stoller (1963b)
*Surrey, England	35.3	Richards & Sylvester (1969)
*Texas, U.S.A.	30.5	Deaton (1973)

*Institution populations.

Life tables were also published by Record & Smith (1955) based on the histories of 252 cases born in Birmingham, England, from 1942 to 1952, and by Carter (1958) from the data of 725 patients who attended the Hospital for Sick Children in London between 1944 and 1955. Of live born Down's syndrome children, 30 per cent were dead at 1 month of age, 50 per cent were dead at 1 year of age, and 60 per cent were dead at 10 years of age. In the Victoria study the infant mortality rate (deaths under 1 year per 1,000) was 311 for Down's syndrome persons as

Table 102. Mortality Rates and Life Table for Live Born Down's Syndrome Children 1948—52, from Birth up to 3 Years of Age (After Collmann & Stoller 1963b)

Age Period	No. at risk at start of period	No. dying during period	Mortality rate per cent per annum	Life Table % alive at start of each period
Months				
0–	729	174	47.8	100.0
6–	555	53	19.2	76.1
Years				
1–	502	80	15.9	68.9
2–	422	28	6.6	57.9
3–	394	19	4.8	54.0

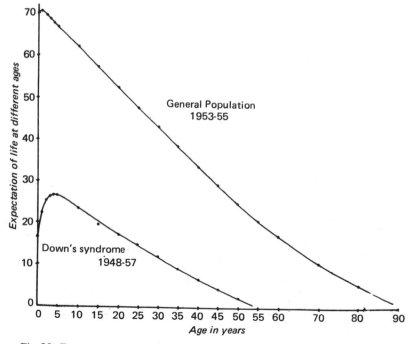

Fig. 93. Expectation of life at different ages for Down's syndrome individuals compared with a normal population. (After Collmann & Stoller 1963b)

compared with 20.8 for the related general population of births. Mortality rates for live born Down's syndrome individuals from birth to 3 years of age are seen in Table 102. As in earlier surveys there was a high mortality rate but here it was reduced to 3 per cent in the first 6 months of life. The expectation of life of Down's syndrome individuals at birth is 16.2 years and at 1 year of age it is 22.4 years. It increases to 26.7 years at 5–9 years of age until at 50–54 years of age it is 2.5 years (see Fig. 93). Secular changes in mortality have been found. Carter (1958) compared the mortality rates for 1944–48 with 1949–55 and noted that the mortality rate had decreased by approximately 40 per cent in the later period. Collmann & Stoller (1963b) divided their data into two periods. 1948–52 and 1953–57, and noted that the main secular difference was a 33 per cent decrease in mortality in the later group for the first 6 months of life.

A decrease in mortality continues, particularly below the age of three years. Continuing improvements in medical care, especially the use of antibiotics and cardiac medical and surgical treatment, have had the greatest effect on reducing the mortality in the syndrome. Improved living conditions are also a factor.

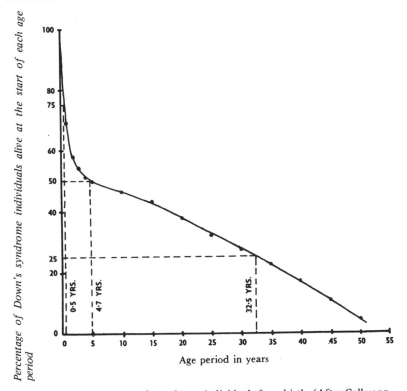

Fig. 94. Survival of Down's syndrome individuals from birth. (After Collmann & Stoller 1963b)

Survival rates as seen in Fig. 94 were given by Collmann & Stoller (1963b). They are low in the first years of life but improve thereafter. Almost 25 per cent of the Down's syndrome infants born alive were dead by the end of the first six months of life, 31 per cent died before they were one year of age and 50 per cent by the age of four to five years. After this age, survival rates did not show such a marked fall with age and 25 per cent reached the early thirties—with 4 per cent surviving to the age of 50 to 54 years. Later studies by Fabia & Drolette (1970a) gave survival rates for infants with and without congenital heart disease which is probably a more useful way of evaluating survival in the early years of life. Fabia & Drolette collected data on 2,421 Down's syndrome individuals born alive, from 1950 through 1966, to residents of Massachusetts. The authors produced sex specific life tables for Down's syndrome children up to 10 years of age. In addition, they constructed life tables for patients with and without congenital heart disease. In their series, 353 of 1,180 (29.9 per cent) of girls and 338 of 1,241 (27.2 per cent) of boys had congenital heart disease.

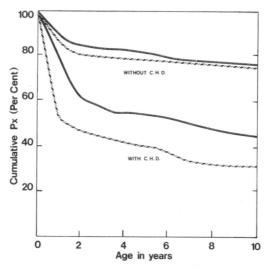

Fig. 95. Survival rates for first 10 years of life for Down's syndrome children with and without congenital heart disease. Solid lines represent males and hatched lines females. (After Fabia & Drolette 1970a)

The study showed that, regardless of congenital heart disease, approximately two-thirds (67.2 per cent of boys and 61.9 per cent of girls) of Down's syndrome children were still alive at 10 years of age. The cumulative survival rate for females with the syndrome became significantly lower at one year of age and remained so throughout the rest of the first ten years of life. Of those Down's syndrome individuals with congenital heart disease, only 44.9 per cent of boys and 32.0 per cent of girls survived the first ten years of life. On the other hand, nearly three-quarters of the Down's syndrome children without congenital heart disease were still alive at age 10—76.4 per cent of boys and 76.6 per cent of girls (see Fig. 95).

For the Down's syndrome children with congenital heart disease, survival of the females was significantly lower from age two onward. Except for the first week of life, the conditional probabilities of death were higher for females at all ages. However, the differences were statistically significant only in the age group 6—11 months (see Fig. 96). This finding was similar to that of Allen (1968) who showed a higher proportion of deaths among Down's syndrome girls with congenital heart disease (53.5 per cent) than among non-Down's syndrome girls with congenital heart disease (43.1 per cent). Because of the difference in mortality rates, the possibility was raised that girls with Down's syndrome have different and more severe cardiac defects. However, Cullum & Liebman (1969) found no evidence to support this view (see also Chapter 2).

Life expectancy studies on institutionalized Down's syndrome patients have been made by Richards & Sylvester (1969) and Deaton (1973). The mean age at death of institutionalized Down's syndrome individuals was 35.3 years in Surrey, England and 30.5 years in Texas, U.S.A. (see Table 101). Mean survival ages on institutionalized affected persons are not comparable with those reported by Collmann & Stoller and Fabia & Drolette, since the selection favours institutionalized Down's syndrome individuals, because high death rates in the early age groups have precluded these individuals from being institutionalized.

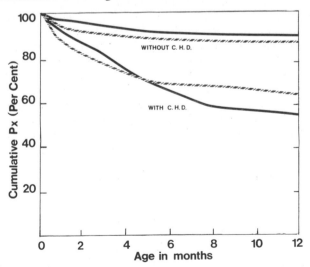

Fig. 96. Survival rates for first year of life for Down's syndrome infants with and without congenital heart disease. Solid lines represent males and hatched lines females. (After Fabia & Drolette 1970a)

Table 103. Causes of Death in Institutionalized Down's Syndrome Patients (Deaton 1973)

Cause	No. of Deaths	%
Heart disease	32	35.1
Pneumonia	21	23.1
Stroke	8	8.8
Infection (other than pneumonia)	6	6.6
Cancer and leukaemia	5	5.5
Asphyxiation from choking on food	4	4.4
Gastrointestinal diseases	4	4.4
Kidney failure	3	3.3
Pulmonary embolus	2	2.2
Endocrine diseases	2	2.2
Unspecified	4	4.4
Total	91	100.0

Deaton studied a total of 1,018 Down's syndrome patients in institutions during the ten year period 1960 to 1969. Of these, 927 were alive at the end of the study and 91 had died (see Table 103 for causes of death). The study indicated that the survival rate of Down's syndrome persons had been increasing during the past two decades and was in agreement with the findings of Forssman & Åkesson (1965a), Jackson et al. (1968) and Richards & Sylvester.

A sex difference in the mortality rate was noted by Record & Smith, who in agreement with Penrose (1932b) found that the rates in infancy and in early childhood were higher for females than for males. It was found that the percentage of male survivors increased with age. Collmann & Stoller (1963b) had slightly different findings, in that the mortality rate for the first 6 months of life was higher in females (275.8) than in males (202.7); however, at later age periods, the rate for males tended to be higher than for females, though the difference was not statistically significant. The percentage of males at birth was 50.8 and increased to 53.2 at 6 months of age, but by 5 years of age it had dropped to 51.9.

A careful survey of the mortality rate in a group of 1,263 patients with Down's syndrome was carried out by Forssman & Åkesson (1965a). The group had a mortality 6 per cent higher than that for the general population (less than 1 per cent). There was no appreciable difference between males and females. In the early years from 1 to 5, the excess mortality was 11 per cent but thereafter until the age of 40 the excess ranged from 3 to 7 per cent in different groups. Above the age of 40 years the rate increased again and after 50 years it exceeded the population standard by 30 per cent. These investigators emphasized the improved health and increased longevity of such patients in recent years. Forssman & Åkesson's (1967) further analysis of Swedish mortality data agrees well with that of 1964 Danish data of Øster et al., for deaths of males, but for females the latter study shows deaths in the early age group (1–4 years) as much higher and those in the later age groups lower than in the Swedish data.

CAUSES OF DEATH

Infections of the respiratory tract have been the commonest causes of death. In the 1954 report of Brothers & Jago bacillary dysentery was the second most common cause; however, in later reports (Record & Smith 1955, Carter 1958) cardiac malformations were second. The cause of death varies with age of the Down's syndrome individual and, from the data of Record & Smith, in the neonatal period cardiac malformation was most significant.

In a 10-year follow-up study of 524 affected persons who were living in 1949, Øster et al. (1964) found that 73 of them died during the period whereas only 7 deaths would have been expected on the basis of general population statistics. In the age group 0–4 years the mortality rate was 52 times the expected figure, in the age group 5–9 years it was 37 times greater but, for Down's syndrome individuals over 10 years of age, it was only 7 times greater than that in the general population (see Table 104). There was a slightly higher number of deaths of female

Table 104. Number of Deaths Compared with the General Population Corrected for Age. (After Øster et al. 1964)

Age of Down's syndrome individual	Observed number	Expected number	Proportional increase (Obs./Exp.)
0–4	17	0.33	52
5–9	13	0.35	37
10–14	3	0.31	10
15–44	20	3.03	7
45–	20	2.66	8
All	73	6.68	10.9

over male affected persons which was especially noticeable below 10 years of age. In addition the death rate of institutional Down's syndrome persons was slightly higher than that of Down's syndrome individuals living at home. The main cause of death was pneumonia and none died of tuberculosis (see Table 105), in contrast to the frequent mortality from tuberculous infection in the early part of the century (Pearce et al. 1910).

Causes of death for institutionalized Down's syndrome patients in Deaton's study, as seen in Table 103, differ somewhat from those listed in Table 105. Some of the differences between the two studies can be accounted for by the way the primary cause of death was determined. For

Table 105. Causes of Death in Down's Syndrome Compared with the General Population. (After Øster *et al.* 1964)

Causes of death	Observed number	Expected number	Proportional increase (Obs./Exp.)
Respiratory disease	37	0.3	123
Infectious disease (excluding tuberculosis)	5	0.1	50
Cardiac anomalies	13	1.2	9
Apoplexy and senile diseases	3	0.4	8
Other causes	9	2.6	3
Malignancies	4	1.2	3
Accidents	2	1.1	2
Tuberculosis	0	1.3	0
Suicide	0	0.7	0

example, in Deaton's study, if pneumonia was accompanied by heart disease and cardiac congestion, the death was attributed to heart disease rather than pneumonia. In Deaton's data, there were two deaths due to acute leukaemia and three to cancer. One patient died of cancer of the testicle which has also been reported in the studies of Holland *et al.* (1962) and Jackson *et al.* (1968). Deaton suggested that there may be a propensity for cancer of the testicle in Down's syndrome. The association with leukaemia is well known and is discussed in detail in Chapter 6.

MATERNAL AGE

The incidence of Down's syndrome varies considerably with maternal age. The maternal age distributions from eleven different countries can be seen in Table 106 and Fig. 97. Selection of data was influenced by reliability of the control populations. Some of the groups are small, but of intrinsic interest. The relative incidence figures show consistency of pattern, though there is variation in the steepness of rise with increasing age. The steepness is associated with the proportion of age-dependent cases in different samples. Moreover, small samples are very variable at the extremes of maternal age. Inconsistencies in selection of cases from hospitals or through public health ascertainment make it difficult to compare the distributions from different countries satisfactorily. Fluctuations in the control population statistics also have to be considered. To some extent the relative incidence ratios will be greater in countries where the mean control maternal age is low, as in Germany (27.1 years) and less in Sweden, where the mean control maternal age is high (28.7 years). Altogether there is much more variation in the ratio figures from different sources than could be attributed to chance sampling; but some of the circumstances affecting selection of data may counterbalance one another in the total for all countries. The ratios for the different age groups in the

Table 106. Distribution of Down's Syndrome by Mother's Age in 11 Countries.

In each sample the control distribution is reduced in numbers so that the total agrees with that of the observed total number of cases. The central maternal ages of the groups, which are used for the calculation of means, are adjusted at the extremes to 18 instead of 17 and 46 instead of 47.

	Mother's age	Australia	Canada	Denmark	England	Finland	Formosa	Germany	Japan	Sweden	U.S.A.	U.S.S.R.	All countries
Group	Centre												
Down (M)													
-19	18	15	12	11	32	21	0	6	3	22	61	1	184
20-24	22	128	24	56	220	99	1	24	44	118	225	49	988
25-29	27	208	42	68	360	119	2	36	59	138	278	54	1,364
30-34	32	194	49	79	422	148	4	35	60	193	326	59	1,569
35-39	37	297	80	142	731	235	5	54	89	324	490	100	2,547
40-44	42	240	85	145	708	266	6	63	54	383	357	76	2,383
45-	46	37	20	17	132	58	2	7	12	64	51	6	406
Total		1,119	312	518	2,605	946	20	225	321	1,242	1,788	345	9,441
Mean		33·7	34·9	34·6	35·1	34·9	36·6	34·2	33·2	35·4	33·3	33·7	34·43
Control (N)													
-19	18	50·8	24·5	29·0	105·9	47·0	0·3	12·8	6·6	67·5	112·0	6·0	462·4
20-24	22	298·3	84·4	131·1	663·6	258·3	4·3	70·0	83·6	293·6	477·1	101·4	2,465·1
25-29	27	363·6	89·3	157·5	821·7	270·1	8·1	75·4	113·8	353·2	550·0	118·0	2,920·7
30-34	32	245·2	64·5	111·9	584·0	198·7	5·1	42·1	70·3	280·0	407·6	73·5	2,082·9
35-39	37	123·4	36·5	64·2	323·5	114·0	1·8	19·6	35·9	175·3	196·7	37·6	1,128·5
40-44	42	35·2	11·7	22·8	98·4	52·8	0·4	4·9	10·2	66·8	42·6	7·9	353·7
45-	46	2·5	1·1	1·5	7·9	5·1	0·0	0·2	0·6	6·2	2·0	0·6	27·7
Total		1,119·0	312·0	518·0	2,605·0	946·0	20·0	225·0	321·0	1,242·0	1,788·0	345·0	9,441·0
Mean		28·0	27·8	28·3	28·4	28·2	28·3	27·1	28·2	28·7	27·7	27·9	28·17
Ratio (M/N)													
-19	18	0·30	0·49	0·38	0·30	0·45	0·00	0·47	0·45	0·33	0·54	0·17	0·398
20-24	22	0·43	0·28	0·43	0·33	0·38	0·23	0·34	0·53	0·40	0·47	0·48	0·401
25-29	27	0·57	0·47	0·43	0·44	0·44	0·25	0·48	0·52	0·39	0·51	0·46	0·467
30-34	32	0·80	0·76	0·71	0·72	0·73	0·78	0·83	0·85	0·69	0·80	0·80	0·753
35-39	37	2·40	2·19	2·21	2·26	2·06	2·78	2·76	2·48	1·85	2·49	2·66	2·257
40-44	42	6·82	7·26	6·36	7·20	5·04	13·64	12·86	5·29	5·73	8·38	9·62	6·737
45-	46	14·80	19·05	11·33	16·71	11·37	58·82	35·00	20·00	10·32	25·50	10·00	14·657
Ratio for totals (M/N)		1·00	1·00	1·00	1·00	1·00	1·00	1·00	1·00	1·00	1·00	1·00	1·000

Sources:

Australia	:	Collmann & Stoller (1962a)
Canada	:	{Beall & Stanton (1945), Newcombe & Tavendale (1964)
Denmark	:	Øster (1953)
England	:	Penrose (1965c)
Finland	:	Renkonen & Donner (1964)
Formosa	:	Tsuang & Lin (1964)
Germany	:	Lenz et al. (1959)
Japan	:	Matsunaga (1964)
Sweden	:	{Forssman & Åkesson (1965b), Milham & Gittelsohn (1965)
U.S.A.	:	Malzberg (1950)
U.S.S.R.	:	Davidenkova et al. (1964)

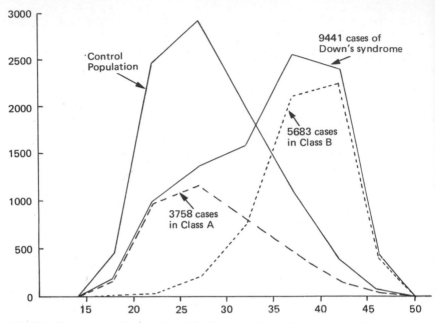

Fig. 97. Maternal age distribution of 9,441 cases of Down's syndrome with control population (see Tables 106 and 109).

Australian sample, the only one attempting to cover a large population exactly, agree well in every five-yearly maternal age group with the ratios of the totals for all countries. Åkesson & Forssman (1966) studied a large Swedish population of Down's syndrome individuals (1242) and concluded that one-third of them belonged to the age-independent class and the remaining two-thirds were in the age-dependent class. James (1970) pointed out some possible limitations of interpreting probabilities of Down's syndrome births based upon the available curves until age-specific fertility and spontaneous abortion rates are critically determined.

Variables associated with maternal age, like age of the father and order of birth, when taken by themselves, are also significantly related to the incidence of Down's syndrome. The increase in paternal age, however, was shown to be probably a secondary effect of the increase in maternal age (Jenkins 1933). Penrose (1933a), using a covariance analysis, concluded that paternal age had no detectable influence in a pooled sample of cases. Partial correlations gave the same result. In 150 sibships each containing at least one Down's syndrome child, the correlation for maternal age and incidence of Down's syndrome among the children (r_{mi}) was +0.36, and that for paternal age and Down's syndrome (r_{fi}) was +0.29. Since the correlation between paternal age and Down's syndrome for a constant maternal age (r_{fim}) was −0.01 ± 0.04, no paternal age effect could be inferred. Matsunaga (1967), using data obtained from 834 cases of Down's syndrome in institutions in Japan, showed a similar pattern to that for Caucasians in the increase in relative incidence of the syndrome with maternal age. He noted that the pattern did not vary with the socioeconomic status of the mothers. When the influence of maternal age was eliminated, paternal age had no effect. Similar results were found by Sigler *et al.* (1965a). However, some data seem to indicate that there may be an exception to this finding. The increase in paternal age found in cases with the 21:(21–22) or G/G type of translocation (Penrose 1962a) would be hidden, if data from every type were pooled, since this group of Down's syndrome individuals only represents about 1 per cent of the total.

The fluorescent chromosome studies of Sasaki & Hara (1973) and Uchida (1973) show that, for some standard trisomic Down's syndrome cases, the extra chromosome came from the father and not the mother. The number of these cases is likely to be small. Since only a few have been reported, it is too early to know if they are more likely to occur in the younger or older paternal age group. (See Non-Disjunction During Meiosis, Chapter 10).

BIRTH ORDER

The incidence of Down's syndrome increases with maternal age but also

Table 107. Incidence of Down's Syndrome in Relation to Birth Order and the Effect of Correcting for Maternal Age (After Penrose 1933b)

Birth order	(a)	(b)	(c)
1	21	29.9	14.7
2	17	32.5	21.7
3	16	22.0	17.6
4	16	16.1	16.4
5	9	12.4	13.9
6	17	10.1	13.7
7	15	9.7	14.1
8	12	7.2	12.2
9	10	4.6	8.7
10	8	3.7	7.4
11	4	1.3	3.2
12	2	1.6	3.2
13	4	1.6	3.7
14	2	0.7	1.7
15 and above	1	0.4	1.6
Totals	154	153.8	153.8
Means	5.51	4.04	5.50

(a) Observed number affected
(b) Expected number affected: first estimate
(c) Expected number with effect of maternal age eliminated

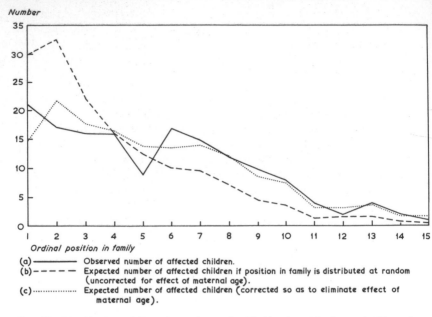

Fig. 98. Distribution of Down's syndrome by birth order: (a) observed; (b) crude expectation; (c) expectation corrected for maternal age.

with birth order which is correlated with the mother's age. It was shown statistically (Penrose 1933b, 1934a and b) that when the influence of maternal age was eliminated the birth order was not in itself a contributing cause (see Table 107 and Fig. 98). Exceptions have been found by Smith & Record (1955) who considered that primogeniture was significant in mothers under 40 years of age

Jenkins (1933) observed that sibships containing Down's syndrome children had fewer members than average; however, it was later shown that sibships, selected by the presence of a Down's syndrome child, were larger than those selected by the presence of a child with another type of mental retardation (Penrose 1938a). The observation has been often made that the interval between the Down's syndrome and the preceding child is longer than is usual between sibs. Penrose (1934a) showed that the lengthened interval might be merely an expression of the fact that the age and not the parity was of causal significance. Matsunaga noted a significant decrease in the relative incidence according to birth rank, irrespective of the socioeconomic conditions. This, he felt, was not an effect of birth order, as such, but probably due to some selection practiced by parents having a retarded child, since the same tendency was found in the families of other varieties of mentally retarded individuals. There was no indication that either too short or too long an interval free from pregnancies, before birth of infants with Down's syndrome, was of aetiological significance.

12. Aetiology

Down's syndrome has presented many problems, but none of these problems has been more difficult than that of understanding the aetiology of the syndrome. In spite of this, there now are some known conditions that will lead to the birth of a Down's syndrome infant. Outstanding among these conditions is the inevitable trisomy which occurs in half the children when a mother is herself trisomic. Balanced translocation carrier and mosaic parents also belong in this group. There are a multiplicity of cytological types, many of which represent specific causal mechanisms and these are demonstrated in Chapter 10. The association of maternal ageing with non-disjunction, however, defies suitable explanation. What makes an understanding of this association of the utmost importance is the fact that maternal ageing is of aetiological significance in practically all of the trisomic conditions and certain of the sex chromosome abnormalities.

The distinction between the pathology and the aetiology of Down's syndrome is not always made clear. The existence of an extra acrocentric chromosome, or its equivalent, in the somatic cells is an essential pathological feature but the primary aetiological factors are those which cause the aberrant chromosome to be present. A careful appraisal of environmental and genetical factors, such as parental age and familial interrelationship, can be used as accurate guides to the differentiation of specific causes of the syndrome.

FAMILIAL INCIDENCE

Before anything definite was known about the chromosomal anomalies responsible for Down's syndrome much had been learned from family investigation. First, there was the indication that, in a proportion of familial cases, transmission was of the irregularly dominant or collateral kind (Hanhart 1944); that is to say, a patient's sibs, cousins, uncles, aunts, nephews and nieces were occasionally affected. Direct transmission from parent to child was also known, and first described by Lelong et al. (1949). The collateral pattern in certain heavily affected pedigrees (Fig. 99) (Fantham 1925, Penrose 1938a) strongly suggested chromosomal anomaly, an inversion or a translocation with balanced carriers (Penrose 1939), rather than a heterozygous gene as the cause. However, the low familial incidence, especially in sibships, made it seem likely to many

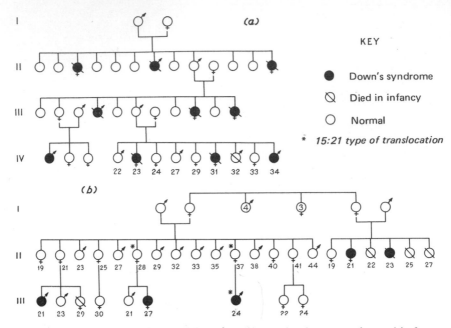

Fig 99. Two pedigrees of familial Down's syndrome showing maternal ages: (*a*) after Fantham (1925); (*b*) after Penrose (1938b)

observers that coincidence of two or more cases in a family was merely the result of the random distribution of a relatively common disease in the general population (Øster 1953). Indeed, even if some familial cases were conceded to be evidence of a genetic process, others had still to be attributed to coincidence.

At this point a second salient fact comes into consideration, namely, that in familial cases there is, on the average, a weakened influence of maternal age. The effect is particularly noticeable in first cousin pairs whose mothers are sisters (Table 108). The tendency for lowering of mother's age is much less marked when relationship is through the father than when it is through the mother. This suggests that most examples of apparent paternal line inheritance are coincidental.

The distributions of mothers' ages for control births and in unselected samples of Down's syndrome individuals, when expressed as percentages, form two curves which cut at a point between 33 and 34 years (Fig. 97, Chapter 11). The distributions of mothers' ages for selected groups of patients (those with affected sibs, and those with a maternal or paternal affected relative), treated in the same way, form a set of curves all of which pass through approximately the same point. Such a set of distribution curves is shown in Fig. 100 (Penrose 1964b). From this it can be reasonably concluded that all the distributions are composed of the same two basic distributions combined in different proportions.

Table 108. Distribution of Maternal Age in 41 Pairs of First Cousin Down's Syndrome Individuals Classified by Type of Relationship (Penrose 1961b)

Type of relationship between relevant parents	Maternal age group						Totals	
	15 to 34 years			35 to 49 years				
	Obs.	Exp.	x^2	Obs.	Exp.	x^2	Obs.	Exp.
Brothers	3	6.5	1.9	11	14.0	0.6	14	20.5
Brother and sister	12	13.0	0.1	28	28.0	0.0	40	41.0
Sisters	15	6.5	11.1	13	14.0	0.1	28	20.5
All types*	30	26.0	–	52	56.0	–	82	82.0

* The expectations are based on 1,038 cases; 332 were born to mothers less than 35 years of age. There is significant excess of affected children of young sisters.

ANALYSIS OF MATERNAL AGE DISTRIBUTIONS

When he compared the distributions of mothers' ages in samples of affected individuals and controls, Jenkins (1933) observed that, after the age of 30, the incidence behaved almost as a "logarithmic" function, i.e. the rise in risk with age was exponential or of the compound interest type. He explained this by the hypothesis of diminishing viability of ova and he thought that the modified pattern in the younger maternal age groups was caused by different factors also causing diminished viability with age.

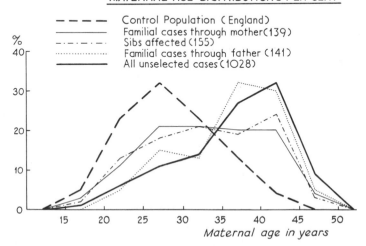

Fig. 100. Maternal age percentage distributions of different Down's syndrome samples and of a control population (Penrose 1964b).

the distribution curve of mothers' ages in Down's syndrome is
ome samples, this is unusual and the general pattern can best
d as bitangential (Haldane 1952). It has a characteristic
Bleyer 1938) resembling the outline of a crouching animal or

In view of the indications, based upon the set of curves shown in Fig.
100, it is natural to suppose that one of the two main distributions which
contributes to the final result is likely to agree with the control
distribution and to include all cases in which maternal age is not a
significant factor. The remainder will then represent the distribution of
cases in which maternal age is a fundamental causal influence.

The question immediately arises as to how the relative proportions of
the two classes, which have been termed A and B, can be correctly
ascertained. It is clear that the control population sample, by definition,
must be almost 100 per cent class A and zero per cent class B. One can then
ask what is the maximal proportion of Down's syndrome individuals
who, by virtue of their maternal age distribution in any given sample,
could be assigned to class A. This can be done by assuming that in the
youngest age group there are no age-dependent cases. In a small sample it
may be necessary to pool the first two five-yearly groups to obtain a
satisfactory estimate. In the sample of 9,441 cases (Table 106, Chapter
11), the age group 15−19 has the lowest incidence, 0.398. This implies
that, on the average, nearly two-fifths of all patients could belong to class
A, in which the cause is independent of age. This class would include all
the hereditary cases and some hypothetical instances of environmental
origin. The remaining three-fifths would be caused by some process closely
related to ageing of the ovum (see Fig. 97).

Judging by the relative incidence figures, for different countries, in the
combined maternal age groups 15−24, the proportion of patients who
could be allocated to class A may approach 50 per cent in Japan, the
United States and the U.S.S.R., but it is less than 33 per cent in England,
Canada and Formosa.

Another way of making a similar comparison is to subtract the control
mean maternal age from the corresponding mean in a sample of Down's
syndrome cases. This difference is an indication of the proportion of older
mothers in the sample. It varies from 4.2 years in Japan and 5.2 years in
the United States to 7.5 years in England and 8.3 years in Formosa.

CAUSES INDEPENDENT OF THE MOTHER'S AGE (CLASS A)

(i) *Secondary non-disjunction*

The most definitely identified cause of Down's syndrome is trisomy in
the mother (see Table 93, Chapter 10). The classical situation in which the
mother is fully affected is very uncommon. However, a parent may be
mosaic for trisomy and, in so far as the gonads are affected in this way, the

same type of inevitable non-disjunction would occur during oogenesis. If one-quarter of the oogonia were trisomic, for example, one-eighth of the offspring would be affected provided that there was no selection against aneuploid cells. Instances of standard trisomic mosaic mothers with affected children continue to be identified but the identification of correspondingly mosaic fathers is exceedingly rare (see Table 87). There are also rare known examples of translocation mosaic Down's syndrome fathers of affected children (Fraccaro et al. 1960, Ferrier 1964). Possibly there is more selection against aneuploid sperms than against aneuploid ova.

The average maternal age in the nine instances of Down's syndrome with fully affected mothers is approximately 22 years. In the seven affected children of five mosaic mothers, the corresponding average is approximately 23 years. Thus there is no indication of increased maternal age here; indeed, the reverse is the case and it might be reasonably supposed that, in secondary non-disjunction, the maternal age is usually below the normal. Such an effect could be produced if trisomy in the mother tended to reduce fertility by shortening the reproductive period.

The incidence of Down's syndrome caused by mosaic trisomy in the mother has been estimated, on the basis of frequency of dermatoglyphic microsymptoms in parents of patients, to be 10 per cent of all cases (Penrose 1965a). For fathers the estimate is 1 per cent.

There are likely to be several different origins of mosaicism. When the zygote starts normal and becomes trisomic by somatic non-disjunction the effect would not be dependent upon maternal age. Conversely, if the zygote started trisomic and reverted in some cell lines to the normal karyotype, the same aetiological considerations would apply as for fully affected cases.

(ii) *Translocation or other anomaly of the critical chromosome in a parent*

As shown in Chapter 10 (Table 79), there is no indication of any maternal age effect for Down's syndrome individuals with the (Dq21q) type of translocation. As these cases are found much more frequently to have a carrier mother than a carrier father, they help to account for the phenomena described in relation to familial incidence. The origin of the translocation, like that of a gene mutation, must be sought in the ancestral germ line. It may occur in the parental germ cells. If so, the case appears sporadically. In spite of the selective disadvantage for the children of female carriers, the anomaly can persist for many generations. Under closely inbred conditions, it might, in theory, occasionally become homozygous and it is not necessarily disadvantageous (Penrose 1962b). However, the high proportion of sporadic instances, approximately one-half of all those recorded, suggests that selection against heterozygotes is strong.

The incidence of the (Dq21q) translocation type among all cases of Down's syndrome is probably about between 2 and 3 per cent (Turpin & Lejeune 1965) and this is equivalent to a population frequency at birth of

2½/100 X 1/660 or 1/26,000. The fertility of zygotes with unbalanced translocations is effectively zero. Thus, the total loss of abnormal chromosomes in each generation is proportional to the number of translocation Down's syndrome individuals plus possible stillbirths with other unbalanced karyotypes caused by the same fusion. In a steady-state population this loss must be compensated by equivalent mutation rate per haploid set of chromosomes per generation which will be more than half the incidence of translocation Down's syndrome individuals. This question has been discussed by Brøgger et al. (1964).

Similar considerations apply to the (21qGq) type of translocation though, here, there are complicating factors. There is uncertainty as to whether an isochromosome is sometimes formed and the father's age may be a factor in causation. The incidence of Down's syndrome associated with this kind of fusion is about 1 per cent of all cases; 1.2 per cent is given by Turpin & Lejeune (1965).

Closely allied to the abnormalities in gametogenesis, which can follow from a heterozygous translocation, is non-disjunction caused by failure of pairing because of heterogeneity. A heterozygous inversion may interfere with pairing in a small chromosome and so also might a duplication or other anomaly (Therkelsen 1964). The point has been emphasized by Patau (1963). Some pedigrees even suggest that abnormalities associated with large acrocentrics may interfere with normal pairing of the small acrocentrics at meiosis and consequently lead to their non-disjunction. That is, balanced translocation of the (Dq21q) type (Moorhead et al. 1961) or of the (DqDq) type (Hamerton et al. 1963) in a parent could lead to standard G-trisomy in the offspring. Many variations in chromosome morphology are being found in normal members of the population, particularly in relation to Nos. 9 and 16, Y and acrocentric satellite structures (Court Brown et al. 1964). In respect of No. 21, undetected structural polymorphism could predispose to the formation of abnormal gametes (see p. 196). When this produces Down's syndrome it would have an incidence independent of the age of the mother. The number of cases caused in this way might be as many as those caused by visible translocations.

(iii) *Genes which tend to produce non-disjunction*

Another hypothetical cause of Down's syndrome, which would act independently of the mother's age, is a specific gene which disturbs the process of cell division. Genes which can cause non-disjunction during oogenesis in homozygous females have been described by Sturtevant (1929) and by Lewis & Gencarella (1952) in *Drosophila*. The error could affect any chromosome and multiple non-disjunction occurred.

In man, the presence of such a gene would be manifested by familial incidence of one or more kinds of non-disjunction, multiple trisomy and increased frequency of these conditions in the children of sisters. Moreover, there would be, if the gene were rare, a detectable increase in consanguinity among maternal grandparents of trisomics as compared with paternal grandparents. In a series of many hundreds of Down's syndrome individuals whose family histories were investigated by Penrose (1962b, 1964a), there were five instances of parental consanguinity (mean age of mother 39.0 years) and five of paternal grandparental consanguinity (mean age of mother 35.6 years). Maternal grandparents were consanguineous in 12 cases (mean age of mother 33.5 years) but the excess here above 5 expected is not statistically very remarkable. Furthermore, studies by Forssmann & Åkesson (1966) have not disclosed any excess of consanguinity in the parents of mothers in a large series of cases. Studies by Juberg & Davis (1970) of all the Down's syndrome individuals in an inbred Amish community revealed no evidence of greater inbreeding among families with Down's syndrome children than was found in the community in general. These results indicate that, if maternal homozygous genes cause Down's syndrome, they must be of common occurrence.

Evidence pointing to genes, which predispose to non-disjunction when carried by heterozygous father or mother, has been found (Miller et al. 1961) but it is difficult to know how far such familial concentrations should be attributed to chance coincidence. The likelihood, that they are manifestations of genes which favour non-disjunction, is increased if the mothers of the patients concerned are relatively young. The same consideration applies to instances of double trisomy in the same patient.

The gene studied by Beadle (1932) in maize, called "sticky", was not only responsible for non-disjunction and other types of chromosomal error in oogenesis but it was also associated with aberrations in somatic mitoses. This means that mosaicism itself can have the properties of an inherited trait. The assumption that such genes occur in man could explain the origin of many known types of mosaicism, in particular, those instances of mosaicism which start as zygotes with normal karyotypes and become trisomic at an early stage in development. Familial mosaics would be expected to exist but no autosomal instances of this have yet been fully described.

It is very difficult to estimate what proportion of Down's syndrome individuals owe their origin to genes of the types discussed here but it might altogether amount to as large a proportion as from 5 to 10 per cent.

(iv) *Environmental influences*

Many suggestions have been made concerning external influences which might cause non-disjunction or equivalent errors in the absence of any genetical predisposition (Davidenkova et al. 1964). Illness in the mother during pregnancy, however, was practically excluded by Øster's (1953) extensive enquiries. Among more recent theories, those involving infection (Robinson & Puck 1965) or exposure to radiation (Uchida & Curtis 1961, Sigler et al. 1965b) are the most favoured. However, evidence for the significance of maternal radiation, either before or during pregnancy, is equivocal. Carter et al. (1961) found no significant relationship between the two events, and Stevenson *et al.* (1970) reported there was no evidence that maternal diagnostic irradiation before conception had any influence on the subsequent birth of a Down's syndrome infant. Emotional stress in the mother has been blamed by Drillien & Wilkinson (1964b). Androgenic hormone increase has been reported by Rundle *et al.* (1961) in mothers of patients. Similarly, attempts have been made to relate maternal urinary oestriol excretion and fetal chromosome abnormalities (Jørgensen & Trolle 1972, Blumenthal & Variend 1972). Aetiological significance has been attributed to high fluoride content of water supplies by Rapaport (1963) and to atmospheric pollution by Greenberg (1964). Aetiological factors related to thyroid autoimmunity in mothers have been proposed by Fialków (1964, 1970), as well as to an increased incidence of thyroid disease in these women (McDonald 1972b). A faulty immune mechanism has also been postulated in the mothers of Down's syndrome individuals (Zsako & Kaplan 1969, Pollard *et al.* 1970, Kerkay *et al.* 1971).

It has been observed that aneuploidy can be generated in cell cultures by exposure to a great variety of poisons which disturb mitosis, to radiation with X-rays or ultraviolet light and to virus infection (Russell 1964). It is natural to transfer such ideas to the aetiology of Down's syndrome but so far there is no direct evidence pointing to any of these factors (Schull & Neel 1962). Nevertheless, in view of the inherent liklihood from experimental evidence that environment can cause genetical changes of the types responsible for Down's syndrome, it must be conceded that a substantial number might originate in this manner.

El-Alfi *et al.* (1964) showed that an agent in the plasma of patients with viral hepatitis could cause chromosomal breaks in human leucocyte cultures. Though disputed (see p. 238), indirect evidence of the causal significance of infectious hepatitis in Down's syndrome has been produced by Stoller & Collmann (1965, 1966) in Australia. It was observed that the fluctuations in the incidence of this virus disease and Down's syndrome were closely correlated over a 12-year period. In view of all these considerations, probably at least 10 per cent of all Down's syndrome cases might be supposed to fall into the environmentally determined sub-group of Class A. It is not, however, generally accepted that environmental effects are all age-independent. Some influences might be supposed to act especially on older mothers. Thyroid antibodies, which could have arisen in consequence of infectious disease, were found by Fialkow *et al.* (1965) to occur, however, with unusual frequency in young mothers of Down's syndrome children.

INFLUENCE OF THE MOTHER'S AGE (CLASS B)

(i) *Oocyte deterioration*

After removing as large as possible a number of patients from a sample whose maternal age distribution agrees with that of the control popula-

Table 109. Distribution of Mothers' Ages in Down's Syndrome.

Partition of classes A (age-independent) and B (age-dependent) with expected values for class B based upon three different hypotheses.

	Mother's age in years (t) Central value	Control distribution (N)	Down's syndrome (M)	Age-independent (A)	Age-dependent (B)	Expected values for distribution (B)		
						Chance occurrence of 17 or more events	Increase with power of age: t^{10}	Exponential rise with age: 4^t
Absolute numbers	18	462·4	184	184	0	0	4	4
	22	2,465·1	988	981	7	10	23	61
	27	2,920·7	1,364	1,163	201	149	218	286
	32	2,082·9	1,569	829	740	784	850	817
	37	1,128·5	2,547	449	2,098	2,055	1,968	1,769
	42	353·7	2,383	141	2,242	2,275	2,192	2,219
	46	27·7	406	11	395	410	428	527
	All Total	9,441·0	9,441	3,758	5,683	5,683	5,683	5,683
	error + or −	...	...	...	...	190	360	704
	Mean age	28·17	34·43	28·17	38·57	38·59	38·40	38·39
Relative incidence	18	1·000	0·398	0·398	0·000	0·000	0·001	0·008
	22	1·000	0·401	0·398	0·003	0·004	0·009	0·025
	27	1·000	0·467	0·398	0·069	0·051	0·075	0·098
	32	1·000	0·753	0·398	0·355	0·377	0·408	0·392
	37	1·000	2·257	0·398	1·859	1·821	1·744	1·568
	42	1·000	6·737	0·398	6·339	6·432	6·199	6·274
	46	1·000	14·657	0·398	14·259	14·791	15·417	19·022
	All	1·000	1·000	0·398	0·602	0·602	0·602	0·602

Note: Class (A) contains 0·398 of the cases in sample (M), distributed by mother's age as in sample (N). Observed numbers in class (B) are obtained by subtraction of class (A) from (M) in each age group. Expected total of (B) in each of the three examples are made to agree with the observed total number, 5,683. Good agreement with observed values in all age groups is obtained when expectation empirically is based on the hypothesis that non-disjunction is the result of 17 or more chance events occurring at either one of two sites (paired centromeres). It is assumed here that the true incidence of Down's syndrome at the maternal age of 46 is 0·0222. The relative incidence values are proportional to the sums of terms of Poisson distributions from $i = 17$ to $i = \infty$, where $m = 0·19565$.

tion, a residual class (B) is obtained. The analysis of this distribution is of special interest because, in it, a clue may be found leading to the explanation of the process. The mean is usually about 38 years, that is 10 years more than that for the control group. In the combined distribution of Down's syndrome cases from 11 countries (Table 109), 5,683 patients out of 9,441 or 60.2 per cent would belong to class B after a section of 3,758, supposedly belonging to class A, and 39.8 per cent of the total, had been removed. The mean maternal age, $\bar{B}$, in this class B is 38.57 years as compared with $\bar{A}$, the corresponding mean, 28.17 years in class A. It follows formally that the mean, $\bar{M}$, for the whole group of cases, given by the equation $\bar{M} = 0.398\bar{A} + 0.602\bar{B}$, is 34.43. Moreover, in any group of patients the proportions in class B can be quickly estimated by finding the difference between the two means $\bar{M}$ and $\bar{A}$ and dividing by $\bar{B}-\bar{A}$, which is usually almost exactly 10 years, and, here, 10.40 years.

It is generally accepted that, since the father's age has no appreciable independent significance, non-disjunction in class B must necessarily always come through the mother. The view is strengthened by the knowledge that, in mammals, oogonia only proliferate until some time late in the intrauterine period; meiosis begins shortly before birth or in early postnatal life (Franchi et al. 1962). After leptotene, zygotene, pachytene and diplotene phases have been passed, the resting stage of dictytene is reached. The oocyte remains in this condition until its final maturation at the time of formation of the Graffian follicle. The first meiotic division is then completed with extrusion of the first polar body. The human female reproductive capacity lasts from roughly 15 to 50 years and the oocytes are in the dictytene stage from birth and during the whole length of this period. The chances of damage or of age-deterioration of the nucleus during dictytene do not apply to the sperms, which proceed rapidly through the meiotic cycle (Ford 1960b).

The distribution of mother's age in the three-fifths or so of Down's syndrome individuals in class B, when directly compared with the general population distribution, gives a relative incidence curve which rises very rapidly with increasing years. Since most patients born after the maternal age of 34 belong to this class, the incidence curve at late ages is similar to that found for all Down's syndrome individuals and which was shown by Jenkins to rise almost exponentially. The class B cases from a sample of 1,038 (Penrose 1961a) showed that an exponential or compound interest rise over the whole range gave a fairly good approximation to the incidence observed; the rate of increase of risk rose about four-fold every five years. Data from some other sources agree better with the assumption that the rate of increase of risk is, on the average, about 3.5-fold every five years. The observed rise is not quite in agreement with any exponential or compound interest rate for it tends to slow down after the age of 40 years.

A more satisfactory agreement with observation is obtained on the assumption that the incidence rises with the tenth power of the mother's age (see Table 109).

Theoretical considerations follow if it is known which type of curve the rise of incidence with age in class B really represents. An exponential rise suggests some slowly growing infective factor gradually disturbing more and more cells. Alternatively there could be failure of nucleolus breakdown in the meiotic prophase, caused by some chemical or physical process connected with age, affecting especially the acrocentric chromosomes because they carry nucleolar organizers (Ford 1960b). A rise of incidence with a power of the age suggests that the error in the ovum, which leads to non-disjunction, depends upon a succession of independent accidents. A sufficient number in a given cell causes the meiotic divisions to become inaccurate, on account of degeneration of the spindle mechanism which relies upon the integrity of an exact number of separate parts or strands (Penrose 1965b).

Very good agreement with the observed relative incidence figures for different maternal age groups is provided on the basis of the assumption that 17 or more breaks (deleterious events of chance occurence which affect one or other centromere of the critical pair of chromosomes) cause non-disjunction (see Table 109). If the number of strands, at metaphase, attached to a centromere is not less than 20 (Barnicot & Huxley 1965), this number of breaks might be mechanically significant.

Such a theory of progressive deterioration by accidental occurrences would be equivalent to postulating a natural ageing of the nucleus of the ovum. After a certain number of breaks the spindle mechanism would be unable in the first meiotic division to overcome the resistance required to separate the paired chromosomes, especially those supplied with nucleolus organizers like the acrocentrics in man. A maternal age effect similar to

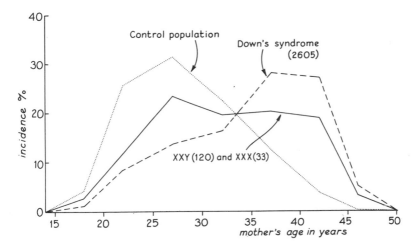

Fig. 101. Maternal age percentage distributions of sex trisomy (Court Brown *et al.* 1964) and Down's syndrome compared with that of a control population.

that found in Down's syndrome has been observed in other autosomal trisomies (Smith *et al.* 1961) and also in some sex chromosome aberrations, XXY males and XXX females (Court Brown *et al.* 1964). An indication that the same causal process, which operates in Down's syndrome, may be responsible is shown by the tendency for the distribution curves for controls, Down's syndrome and X-trisomic types to intersect at approximately the same point (Penrose 1964c) (see Fig. 101).

The hypothesis of uterine selection receives little or no support at the present time (Matsunaga 1967). The assumption is made, in this hypothesis, that non-disjunction occurs at an equal rate in all maternal age groups but that rejection of trisomic fetilized ova decreases with maternal ageing.

German (1968) postulated that delayed fertilization of an ovum may permit non-disjunction to occur at second meiotic metaphase. It was assumed that the maternal age effect was a reflection of decreasing frequency of coitus with increasing duration of marriage, thereby delaying the time of fertilization of the ovum in older women. German's statistical data gave support to his hypothesis; however, a subsequent study by Penrose & Berg (1968) did not (see Table 110). Cannings & Cannings

Table 110. Duration of Marriage in Years by Age of Mother at Birth of Child
(Penrose & Berg 1968)

Age of Mother	Down's syndrome			Controls			Differ- ence of Means	Standard Error Difference
	Number of Cases	Mean Duration	δ	Number of Cases	Mean Duration	δ		
15–24	96	2.13	1.18	282	2.06	1.13	+0.07	±0.1
25–29	152	4.32	2.58	364	4.35	2.59	−0.03	± 0.2
30–34	147	6.84	3.82	271	7.11	3.78	−0.27	± 0.3
35–39	281	11.04	5.30	166	10.52	5.08	+0.52	± 0.4
40–49	312	14.28	6.25	63	13.15	6.03	+1.13	± 0.5
All	988	9.54	6.45	1,146	5.82	4.66	+3.72	± 0

(1968) found that the age dependency for the frequency of coitus was not closely enough related to the incidence of Down's syndrome to support German's theory. In addition, data collected from a Baltimore study (Sigler *et al.* 1965a) also failed to support the hypothesis (Lilienfeld 1969). Ingalls (1972) proposed that delayed fertilization of the oocyte in older women could be the consequence of erratic endocrine function or infections. Henderson & Edwards (1968) suggested that the number of chiasmata per cell at diakinesis and metaphase-I decline with increasing maternal age, leading to a localization of chiasmata to the ends of bivalents and the presence of univalents. A high frequency of non-diploid embryos may arise from older oocytes from such a mechanism. As yet, in human oocytes, it has not been possible to relate chiasma frequency and maternal age, though such a relationship appears to occur in mouse oocytes.

Emanuel *et al.* (1972) suggested that mothers who give birth to children with Down's syndrome at a chronologically early age may, in some way, be characterized by an acceleration of the biological ageing process. In support of their hypothesis, the authors suggested that there is an increased prevalence of gray hair in young mothers of children with Down's syndrome. They also offered other examples to support their position.

(ii) *The risks for very young mothers*

It is found empirically that, when simple rules are applied to explain the distribution of mothers' ages in class B, some slight discrepancy often occurs in the groups of young mothers aged 15 to 29. This is consistent with the fact that, in some individual surveys, a slight relative excess of Down's syndrome cases seems to occur in the very youngest maternal age groups; that is to say, they show a slightly greater risk than for those aged, say, about 25 years. This is specially noticeable in Øster's (1953) sample of first born Down's syndrome children. The same type of effect is found in German and North American unselected samples and it also appeared in the incidence curve calculated from 224 English families (Penrose 1934b). The suggestions made by Smith & Record (1955) and Renkonen & Donner (1964) concerning the first born in the family should be considered in this connection.

One of the difficulties in assessing the significance of data involving order of birth comparisons is that official statistics usually fail to give an accurate picture. Not only are illegitimate births usually excluded but stillbirths are also left out. Thus the control data bias results in favour of finding excess of observed first born abnormal children.

(iii) *Partition of causes*

It is convenient to classify the definitely known and theoretically probable causes of Down's syndrome in relation to the maternal age factor. Table 111 shows how this can be attempted. Some very rough estimates of proportions of patients in each aetiological category are also given.

PATERNAL CAUSES

Paternal causes of Down's syndrome are few compared with maternal causes. In fact, the maternal ageing effect is so great that it would completely mask any small paternal effect. It is now possible to identify and, in some cases, predict the paternal origin of a Down's syndrome infant. The following considerations apply.

(a) Balanced translocation carriers of the (13-15):21 type and translocation mosaic fathers of the 21:22 type are known. A few fathers with 46,XY/47,XY,21+ mosaicism, who have had Down's syndrome children, are also known (see Table 87).

(b) A significant increase in the paternal age has been noted in the 21:22 type of centric fusion when the abnormality is transmitted through

Table 111. Partition of Causes of Down's Syndrome

Class		Cause	Possible proportion in an unselected group
(A)	Independent of mother's age	(i) Inevitable non-disjunction (parent partly or wholly trisomic)	10%
		(ii) Abnormality in chromosome pairing (inherited translocation, inversion or other anomaly of the critical G-chromosome)	10%
		(iii) Abnormal meiosis or mitosis (specific genes which cause non-disjunction)	10%
		(iv) Environmental disturbance of cell division (infection, poison, radiation)	10%
(B)	Dependent upon mother's age	Non-disjunction during oogenesis (deterioration of meiotic cell-division mechanism)	60%

the father (see Table 83). If the transmission of the aberrant chromosome is through the father the mean age at the birth of the Down's syndrome infant is 42.0 years, but if both the mother and the father have normal karyotypes, the father's mean age is still increased (35.6 years), though less so (Penrose 1962a). However, in Japan, an examination of the parental age of 102 translocation trisomics by type and origin of the translocation showed that in sporadic translocation cases the age of the mother, and not of the father, was significant (Matsunaga & Tonomura 1972).

(c) In a few families it has been demonstrated that the extra chromosome in the Down's syndrome infant was of paternal origin (Sasaki & Hara 1973, Uchida 1973). It is too early to know if these fathers are mosaic individuals or if some other mechanisms are responsible for the transmission of the chromosome. Priest (1969), in her dermatoglyphic study of parents of Down's syndrome individuals, observed that the fathers of affected individuals had significantly higher dermal indices than the fathers of her control group. She suggested as a possible explanation that mosaicism may be present in this group of fathers of Down's syndrome children.

(d) A paternal chromosomal abnormality may give rise to the birth of a Down's syndrome infant. Sergovich et al. (1967) reported a chromosomal abnormality in a father of such an infant. The father was a mosaic. In one of his cell lines, he had 49 chromosomes with three metacentric fragments and the other cell line was normal.

(e) An epidemiological study of parents of Down's syndrome individuals and matched controls suggested a relationship for Down's syndrome and paternal exposure to radar (Cohen & Lilienfield 1970).

(f) While inevitable or secondary non-disjunction has been demonstrated in fully affected Down's syndrome mothers (see p. 223), fully affected males have not been known to father affected or even chromosomally normal children.

13. Prevention and Treatment

Since the advent of antenatal diagnosis, it has been possible to determine the chromosomal status of the fetus and, in certain circumstances, prevent the birth of a Down's syndrome infant. At the present time, the preventative aspects of the syndrome are limited in scope to well defined high risk situations. In general, this form of prevention applies to potential parents who have a chromosome translocation or are themselves mosaic, and to older women or females with the syndrome who become pregnant. Presently, antenatal diagnosis is being recommended for women 35-40 years of age and older to prevent Down's syndrome and other chromosomal abnormalities. Prevention of the syndrome, in the more classical sense, could only be accomplished once we have understood those factors which are producing non-disjunction in association with ageing in the female.

Most therapies used in treating Down's syndrome have not lived up to their initial claims when put to the test of scientific investigation. Others, about which beneficial claims have been made, have not yet been subjected to satisfactorily controlled investigation so that unbiased evaluation is not possible. Indeed, correct evaluation of drug therapy presents many problems and pitfalls for the investigator. Mental improvement is a frequently used standard for measuring a Down's syndrome individual's response, which may be done either by looking for changes in I.Q. or S.Q. Down's syndrome individuals are highly responsive to their environments so that small changes in test scores could be accounted for by added stimulation or merely new developmental changes associated with maturation. In addition, it is not certain that I.Q. and S.Q. tests are the best means of evaluating responses to therapy. There is no form of medical treatment which has yet been proved to have significant merit. In the broadest sense, treatment comprises the application of medical, social and educational measures to improve the welfare of the patient (Smith 1975). Social and educational aspects are considered in Chapter 14, whereas the implications of medical treatment are discussed in the present chapter.

INDIVIDUAL TREATMENT

(a) Medicinal
The earliest form of therapy to be widely used was administration of dried thyroid gland. This evolved naturally because Down's syndrome

265

individuals were classified as cretins until their condition was recognized as a separate clinical entity. The efficacy of thyroid therapy has not been substantiated by clinical research except in a small number of patients who have intercurrent hypothyroidism (Benda 1960). Pituitary extract has been claimed to have a beneficial effect (Benda 1946, 1960); however, these claims were not supported in the results of studies conducted by Berg et al. (1961). Allied to this therapeutic attempt is that suggested by Jaensch (1930) who reported, without giving details, that cases of mental deficiency, with supposed endocrine disorder, were improved by taking large quantities of organically combined iodine. Other drugs, such as thymus extract and glutamic acid, have been fashionable in the treatment of the mentally retarded and they were tried without success in the syndrome. It was suggested (de Moragas 1958) that, by using dehydro-epiandrosterone, the facies and the neuromuscular performance of Down's syndrome individuals could be improved. Controlled studies testing this claim did not validate it (Diamond & Moon 1961). Many unusual combinations of drugs and vitamins (Turkel 1963) have been used without success (Bumbalo et al. 1964). A form of treatment which employs cellular extracts (Siccacell) and a vitamin-mineral-hormonal preparation has been proposed (Haubold et al. 1960); the claim that this therapy produces improvement has been refuted by Bardon (1964). White & Kaplitz (1964) evaluated the vitamin-mineral-hormonal preparation without the addition of Siccacell and noted that on the tests recorded the patients did no better than the controls.

Since the report of Gershoff et al. (1958) that Down's syndrome patients excrete a reduced amount of urinary xanthurenic acid after oral tryptophan loading, there has been a great amount of work on tryptophan absorption, transport and metabolism in this condition (see p. 125). During the course of these studies, it was suggested that certain features of the clinical phenotype in the syndrome might be related to serotonin (5-hydroxytryptamine) depletion of the central nervous system. This led to therapeutic trials of 5-hydroxytryptophan, the precursor of 5-hydroxytryptamine (Bazelon et al. 1967, Weise et al. 1974). Initial studies suggested that 5-hydroxytryptophan resulted in increased muscle tone and improved early development when started in the Down's syndrome infant. It is of interest that parents reported improvement in strabismus and tongue protrusion also. Later double-blind studies showed that 5-hydroxytryptophan did not help the infants with the syndrome. Indeed, some treated infants did worse than the untreated controls. Convulsions and electroencephalographic abnormalities occurred in the treatment group of infants (Coleman 1971, 1973).

(b) Surgical

Surgery has a place in the treatment of certain physical abnormalities associated with Down's syndrome, including cardiac and gastro-intestinal defects (see Chapter 2). As in normal persons, such procedures contribute significantly to the patient's well-being and, indeed, can be life saving. The use of cosmetic surgery has been proposed to modify the facial appearance of some individuals with the syndrome (Otermin Aguirre 1973). An attempt is being made to determine what cosmetic surgery is needed to change the facial appearance in the syndrome and to evaluate how these changes would influence the patient, his family and the community (Smith 1974). Before this type of surgery is used or could be recommended, a great deal of careful appraisal of the implications is required.

PROPHYLAXIS

A controversy has always existed concerning the degree of risk of having a second Down's syndrome child after a mother has given birth to one. This question is one that parents frequently ask after the birth of their Down's syndrome infant. In the past, some authorities have held that the occurrence of a second affected child in a family or sibship is very rare and that the risk of having a second such child is no greater than the general population risk. Under these conditions, the risk depends only upon the incidence of Down's syndrome in the mother's particular age group. Others have maintained that there is an increased risk of having a second Down's syndrome child but there has been disagreement about the amount of risk involved. Penrose (1951) analysed familial cases of Down's syndrome and showed that transmission through the mother predominated over that through the father. Moreover, when a maternal relative was affected, the maternal age at the birth of the Down's syndrome infant was decreased as was also shown by Soltan et al. (1964). In large surveys (Lahdensuu 1937, Doxiades & Portius 1938, Øster 1953, Hanhart 1960a) examples of uncle and niece, aunt and nephew and first-cousin pairs had been reported as well as sibship concentrations. Sibships containing 4 cases were reported by Babonneix & Villette (1916), Péhu & Gaté (1937) and by Turpin & Lejeune (1953). Instances of 3 cases in one sibship were reported by Fantham (1925), Benda (1946) and by van der Scheer (1919a). It was estimated that pairs of affected sibs occurred about once for every 100 single cases collected at random (Penrose 1932b).

Light has been thrown on the problem of the risk of a second affected infant by cytological diagnosis. In some families where the mother is a (Dq21q) heterozygous carrier or in others where the father is a (Gq21q) heterozygous carrier, good information is already available concerning the risk of having a second Down's syndrome child. In other types of family, for example those in which the mother is mosaic for trisomy 21 cells, or in the cases of translocation Down's syndrome individuals (either (Dq21q) or (Gq21q)) where the parents have normal chromosomes, the risk of having a second Down's syndrome infant is increased, but the degree of risk is uncertain.

It would seem unwise to be too dogmatic about these risks. In a few categories it is possible to say that the risk of having a second affected infant is serious and in others that it is insignificant. The basis of this is artificial. Roberts (1963) suggested that a bad risk is one in which the chance of the abnormal event's happening is 1 in 10 or less. A good risk would be one in which the chance would be 1 in 20 or greater. From his experience, risk figures falling between these two values occur rather infrequently.

The analysis in Chapter 12 has shown that the distribution curve for the incidence of Down's syndrome, based upon the mother's age at the time of the birth of the affected child, can be divided into two parts. One component curve (A) is similar to the incidence of births in the general population, while the other (B) shows increase with maternal age. The two curves intersect at about 34 years of age. Carter & Evans (1961) and Berg & Kirman (1961) found that the risk of having a second Down's syndrome infant mainly concerns mothers under 35 years of age; however, this was not so in a series of cases reported by Soltan et al (1964).

Table 112. Maternal Age and Type of Down's Syndrome

Source	Sporadic				Familial				Total
	Standard −34* 35+		Translocation −34 35*		Standard −34 35+		Translocation −34 35+		
Mellman (1962)	2	6	0	0	0	2	2	0	12
Hayashi (1962)	39	26	1	0	1	1	1	0	69
Sergovich (1962)	40	36	1	1	0	4	1	0	83
Chitham & MacIver (1965)	46	49	2	1	1	2	1	0	102
Penrose (1965d)	39	39	6	2	11	5	5	1	108
Totals	166	156	10	4	13	14	10	1	374
	322		14		27		11		

*Indicates maternal age group.

The proportions of standard trisomics and translocations can be seen in Table 112. This is compiled from pooled data and the Down's syndrome individuals are classified in two ways: first, as "sporadic" or "familial", where familial means that a close relative (parent, sib or collateral) is known to have Down's syndrome and, secondly, as "standard" or "translocation", where translocation means that a fusion of either D:21 or G:21 type has been found. The table is not without bias since, as in most series, the reasons for the cytological studies were not given and several cases were investigated because of suspected hereditary influence. In spite of these shortcomings, the figures probably give a fair indication of the relative proportions.

Four per cent (14/336) of sporadic cases show a translocation, but a translocation Down's syndrome individual occurs in 29 per cent (11/38) of the familial cases. In the older age group of mothers, translocation cases occur in only 3 per cent (5/175) although, in the younger age group of mothers, the occurrence is 10 per cent (20/199). In sporadic cases of Down's syndrome with a young mother the chances are about 17 to 1 (166/10) that the child's chromosomes will show a standard trisomy rather than a translocation, and the chance is increased to about 40 to 1 (156/4) if the mother is in the older age group. The most important difference is found when familial cases with young mothers are compared with familial cases with older mothers. For young mothers, the chance is about equal (13 to 10) for standard trisomy of translocation. If the mother is in the older age group the chance is 4 to 1 in favour of standard trisomy.

The simplest method of prevention arises immediately from consideration of the data on the mother's age. Since the mean age for class B is about 38½ years, about half the Down's syndrome individuals in this class are born after that age. It follows that, if no conceptions occurred after the maternal age of 37 years, half the cases in class B, that is about one-third of all cases, would be prevented from being born. The sacrifice of normal births involved would, of course, be considerable, but there would be compensatory advantages. Other age-dependent malformations would be reduced in frequency, that is, Klinefelter's syndrome, hydrocephaly and numerous conditions caused by autosomal trisomy.

GENETICAL PROGNOSIS

In those circumstances in which parents ask for advice concerning the risk of repetition and no cytological tests are possible, an empirical estimate can be used. On the basis of family records (Penrose 1956) the risk is increased by a factor of 2½, as compared with the random chance of Down's syndrome in the population. The risk for an unselected mother in the general population can be ascertained directly from surveys by Carter & MacCarthy (1951) and Collmann & Stoller (1962a) (see Table 113). The incidence in the younger age groups, where class A Down's syndrome individuals are most frequent, is much greater in the larger and more representative survey, but the figures for the older age groups agree well in the two samples. It is noteworthy that, in the general population, the risk of Down's syndrome never exceeds 1/20 and can therefore always be regarded as good. If these risks are all multiplied by 2½, however, that in the last age group would fall between 1/10 and 1/20 and could be considered relatively unfavourable.

Table 113. Absolute Risks in Different Maternal Age Groups: Incidence per 1,000 Births

Age group	Carter & MacCarthy (1951) (100 cases)		Collmann & Stoller (1962a) (1,119 cases)	
15–19	0.00		0.43	1/2,300
20–24	0.28	1/3,600	0.61	1/1,600
25–29	0.29	1/3,000	0.82	1/1,200
30–34	1.72	1/580	1.13	1/880
35–39	3.52	1/280	3.45	1/290
40–44	14.18	1/70	10.00	1/100
45–49	26.32	1/38	21.76	1/46
All	1.51	1/664	1.44	1/696

Prognostic accuracy can be greatly improved by studying the karyotype of the patient and further enhanced by investigating also the karyotypes of the parents. There are several quite different situations which can be revealed in this way. Some of them lead to definite judgments but others leave important points in doubt. The best understood and commonest situations are summarized here.

(i) *The affected child has a standard karyotype, presumed trisomic for No. 21*

(a) *Both parents have normal karyotype.* In this case the risks for future sibs are as those for parents in the general population, rising with the mother's age. In view of the possibility that gonadal mosaicism in a parent may have been present though not detected, allowance may be made for a slight additional risk. There is also the possibility of a gene being present which facilitates non-disjunction. Even so, the prognosis for all maternal ages is good.

(b) *One parent is mosaic for No. 21 trisomy.* When the mother is known to have trisomic cells, the genetic prognosis may be unfavourable. The exact risk depends upon the proportion of gonadal cells which are abnormal and it will be one-half of this value. For example, if 1/3 of the maternal gonadal cells are abnormal, the risk of Down's syndrome in a child will be 1/6. The proportion can be roughly gauged from the results of fibroblast cultures. The risk in consequence of maternal mosaicism is then added to the ordinary risk already mentioned. If the father is mosaic, the same risk factors apply as those presented for the mother, but in this situation a more favourable prognosis probably would prevail, since selective forces more likely would favour fertilization by a sperm with 23 chromosomes and monosomic-21 rather than a sperm with 24 chromosomes and disomic-21.

(ii) *The affected child has a translocation of the D:21 type*

(a) *Both parents have normal karyotypes.* On empirical grounds there is no indication that any special risk is encountered for sibs born subsequently though allowance should be made for the possibility of mosaicism for translocation in parental gonads. Thus the risks are similar to those described under (i) (a).

(b) *One parent carries the D:21 type of translocation in balanced form.* Here the risks are serious when the mother is a carrier. On a theoretical basis, approximately one-third of all the children should be translocation Down's syndrome individuals, another third carriers and one-third entirely normal. What one finds when observing a large number of these families is that fewer than one-third of the offspring have Down's syndrome. The empirical risk for the translocation female producing an infant with Down's syndrome is approximately 1:9. This reduced risk, from the theoretical value of 1:3, could possibly be accounted for by loss of Down's syndrome fetuses as spontaneous abortions. The chances of a carrier or normal karyotype in somatically normal offspring are nearly equal. The risk for standard trisomic Down's syndrome is also perhaps slightly increased. If the father carries the translocation, the risk of an affected child is much smaller, probably less than 1:40. The chances of translocation or normal karyotype in somatically normal offspring are not equal, since there is a slight increase in the number of balanced translocation carriers born. If the parent carries the translocation in mosaic form, the risks are correspondingly decreased except in rare mosaic types where the abnormal cells are effectively trisomic. In all such families the risks of standard Down's syndrome, depending upon maternal age, are relatively unimportant as compared with the direct genetical hazards. (See also Chapter 10).

(iii) *The affected child has a translocation of the 21:22 type*
(a) *Both parents have normal karyotypes.* In this situation there is some evidence which suggests that advancing paternal age may increase the risk of the birth of an affected child. Otherwise the prognosis is good, as it is for parents in the general population.

(b) *One parent carries the translocation.* In theory there are two possibilities. First, that the aberration is an isochromosome No. 21 and, secondly, that it is a fusion of chromosomes Nos 21 and 22. In the first case, the risk is the worst possible in human genetical prognosis; all children must be affected. A hint of this will be given if there have been no previous normal offspring and many miscarriages. Fluorescent staining and G-banding will identify the 21:21 translocation or isochromosome number 21. For the 21:22 translocations, the estimated risk of having an infant with Down's syndrome is approximately 1:8 to 1:10 for both carrier mothers and carrier fathers. These risk figures are high enough to predict an unfavourable prognosis. When the father carries the translocation, there may be some additional risk with advancing age (see Table 83, Chapter 10). In exceptional circumstances the carrier parent may be mosaic and then the risks will be correspondingly diminished.

(iv) *Other special situations*

There are many rare circumstances which arise in the course of prognostic work and which cannot be precisely evaluated. One of these occurs when mosaicism is diagnosed in the child and prognosis for sibs is desired. The answer depends upon whether the mosaicism is believed to have developed in an initially normal or a trisomic zygote. If the zygote started trisomic the prognosis would be the same as that if the child were non-mosaic. If mosaicism had developed in a normal zygote, the risk for subsequent sibs would be increased only by the possibility that some genetical predisposition to familial mosaicism was present.

Another situation, or group of situations, arises if the karyotype of a parent is aberrant in some way not obviously related to that in the Down's syndrome child. For example, the parent may have a D:21 type of fusion and the child a standard trisomy. The occurrence of such cases has led to the suggestion that pairing between all the acrocentric chromosomes may be in some way interrelated. Alternatively, instances can be expressions of particular genes which tend to produce chromosomal aberrations. Prognosis in such cases has to be guarded but, on the whole, it is not likely to be unfavourable.

So long as uncertainty exists concerning the exact morphology of small acrocentric autosomes prognosis in many cases will remain difficult. Variation in the satellite formation and the size of the shorter arm seems to be part of human polymorphism. How far secondary constrictions predispose to non-disjunction is, at present, not clear. Abnormalities of chromosome number 21, such as deletions, enlargement of short arms and inversions, which could lead to non-disjunction, have not had risk figures determined. Some authors (Dekaban *et al.* 1966) think the risk is increased; Sands (1969) found no increased risk.

Transmission of the extra number 21 chromosome by chromosomally normal fathers, as determined by fluorescent studies (see p. 249), have been too few to determine exact risk factors.

INDICATIONS FOR AMNIOCENTESIS

Amniocentesis done with care and appropriate precautions by an experienced physician generally appears to be safe for both the mother and the fetus. Culturing of amniotic cells for chromosomal studies is usually successful from the fluid of the first amniocentesis, though a second amniocentesis is occasionally required, and, in rare instances, repeated culturing of amniotic cells have been unsuccessful. This may be due to faulty culturing techniques or failure of cell growth may have some other basis. While spontaneous abortion occasionally follows an amniocentesis, the rate does not appear to be any higher than that for spontaneous abortions occurring in the first trimester when no amniocentesis was performed. Amniocenteses are frequently performed in the following circumstances:

1. *Chromosomal indications in the parents.* These include D:21, 21:22 and 21:21 balanced translocation carrier states, mosaicism with a trisomic cell line and, should the circumstance arise, parental standard trisomy 21 or other suspicious structural anomalies in a parental No. 21 chromosome.

2. *Maternal age.* At the present time, it is not the general practice to undertake amniocentesis, in the absence of other indications, at all maternal ages. Because of the increasing risk of having a Down's syndrome child with advancing maternal age (see p. 246), amniocentesis is usually done on "older" mothers. Some clinicians have recommended the procedure for all women from 35 years of age onwards. However, this is not universally accepted, though practically all agree, in the absence of ethical objections, that women of 40 years and over are appropriate candidates for the procedure. It must be remembered that, because of the nature of the maternal age-dependent incidence curve (see p. 248), there is a marked increase in the number of normal fetuses exposed to amniocentesis at a maternal age of 35 years as opposed to a maternal age of 40 years and over. For example, if the risk of having an infant with Down's syndrome is 1:100, at a maternal age of 40, there are three times as many normal fetuses exposed to amniocentesis at a maternal age of 35 years when the risk is less than one in 300 live births.

The general issue of maternal age and amniocentesis is, to a large extent, dependent on the resolution of the question as to when the risk of having a Down's syndrome child outweighs any risks of the amniocentesis itself, a matter which is still unsettled.

3. *Family history of Down's syndrome.* Many recommend an amniocentesis if the parents have previously had a Down's syndrome child, and fewer do so if a more distant relative was affected unless there is a specific chromosomal or maternal age indication of the kinds discussed above. Again, the issue depends substantially on the imperfect evidence of the amniocentesis risks versus the risk of a child having Down's syndrome.

4. *Psychological considerations.* A factor which should be taken into account in considering amniocentesis is the emotional state of the parents irrespective of maternal age or family history. While amniocentesis may not be biologically indicated in most circumstances, at present, on the basis of known comparative risks, there are low risk situations where the parents would like to have children but fear an initial or repeat occurrence of Down's syndrome in the family. A sympathetic appraisal of such a situation could reasonably lead to a recommendation of amniocentesis even if the risks are small.

5. *Ethical concerns.* There is currently, in many countries, vigorous and ofter heated debate about the ethics of abortion, a controversy which bears on amniocentesis. It is our view that the professional genetic counsellor, irrespective of his or her personal philosophy, has an obligation to comprehensively present the facts regarding amniocentesis to any

family in whom there may be a medical indication for undertaking it. The actual decision whether to proceed or otherwise should then rest with the family according to the dictates of their own consciences and feelings.

14. Social and Educational Considerations

The idea that persons with Down's syndrome could benefit from congenial and stimulating social environments and from special educational and training programmes is not new. As can be inferred from the case records of the Royal Earlswood institution in England, such concepts were recommended by Langdon Down and his successors from as early as 1858 onwards. Protagonists of these notions are to be found in that century and throughout the present one. Nevertheless, there has been a tendency to categorize the Down's syndrome individual in terms of a circumscribed stereotype, usually suggesting a degree of affliction not amenable to much social or educational influence.

It has come to be increasingly realized, in recent times, that such individuals vary considerably in their clinical characteristics, mental as well as physical, and that each has a personality of his own. This, combined with an improved life expectancy (see p. 239), has led in many countries to greater attention to their social and educational requirements. The consequence has been a substantial growth of new programmes and facilities designed to meet these needs. On the whole, they have reflected an emphasis on the capacities and potential of affected persons rather than on their disabilities and weaknesses. As has often been the case in the development and improvement of opportunities for the handicapped, lay associations of parents and relatives have provided a particularly significant stimulus in these directions.

SOCIAL ASPECTS

Considerable emphasis is now being placed on the advantages to the Down's syndrome child of home or home-like environments, integrated into the general community, as opposed to relative crowding and comparative isolation of many traditional institutions. Homes are, of course, not invariably good and institutions not necessarily bad; but, in general, the homely community-based circumstances referred to are usually best suited for the maximal development of the child's social potential and competence. This is particularly so when appropriate supportive professional staff (e.g. social workers, public health nurses) and ancillary services (e.g. assessment centres, social and recreational programmes) are readily available in the community.

The merits of home-like arrangements have been variously demonstrated.

For example, Tizard (1960) reported on a group of young retarded children, half of them with Down's syndrome, who were accommodated as "families" in a house. They were treated according to their mental, rather than chronological, age on patterns recently evolved for the residential care of young normal children of comparable mental age. In comparison with a matched group in the parent institution, they showed significant improvement in social and emotional behaviour, in personal independence and in verbal intelligence. Additional evidence is provided in Chapter 4 of the better prognosis for affected individuals which may be expected in suitable homes of their own.

With regard to the upbringing of the Down's syndrome child living at home, Brinkworth & Collins (1969) have provided much helpful and practical guidance to parents. They emphasized the advantages of early training. Further useful guidelines for the teaching of retarded children within the family milieu have been presented by Barnard & Powell (1972). Carr (1974) has emphasized the importance of specialized help and advice to parents in their task of raising a retarded child.

Concern is sometimes expressed about sexual relationships of Down's syndrome individuals, particularly if they are to some extent integrated as members of the community. As indicated in Chapter 10, pregnancy is a rare event in Down's syndrome females and no fully affected male is known to have fathered a child. Anxiety on this score is thus usually not well-founded and, in any case, appropriate contraceptive measures can be considered in particular circumstances if so desired. Apart from the question of possible pregnancy, there does not seem to be any particular tendency for those with the syndrome to indulge in alarming sexual activity with others. Sexual behaviour on the part of those with Down's syndrome may be viewed differently by different people, depending on personal outlooks, but, in general, individuals with the syndrome can hardly be ranked among those who may be said to constitute a sexual hazard to others. If some caution is indicated, it will most likely be required in the context of the Down's syndrome individual possibly being sinned against than sinning.

EDUCATIONAL ASPECTS

Though the Down's syndrome child generally is not well-suited for a type of education involving much of the way of abstract concepts, he or she usually can benefit from appropriate teaching of simple reading, writing and arithmetic and of many useful self-help skills. Practically orientated programmes in these spheres can contribute substantially to a certain measure of independence and a sense of well-being that often accompanies this. In affected children, as in normal ones, a wide variety of play activities (Carlson & Ginglend 1961) offer an attractive vehicle for much useful learning. The judicious encouragement of motor skills (Cratty

1969) further contributes to the educational process. Other procedures, such as speech therapy, are also applicable in particular circumstances. Molloy (1972) has provided valuable information on the planning and evaluation of training programmes, and on the application of basic learning techniques, for children with levels of retardation of the degree often found in Down's syndrome.

With the survival of an increasing proportion of persons with Down's syndrome into adulthood, special training programmes in the acquisition of productive skills, and opportunities to apply these in suitable settings, have grown in number and scope. Quite complicated tasks, even involving the use of fairly elaborate tools and machinery, can be taught in these circumstances, and it is impressive to see how well and with what satisfaction they are often performed (see Fig. 102). A great deal of information about occupational arrangements and opportunities for the retarded, much of it applicable to Down's syndrome, has been conveniently presented in a comprehensive volume edited by Stahlecker (1967). Many Down's syndrome adults can find a suitable vocational niche for themselves within the orbit of sheltered workshops. Practical guidelines for such workshop programmes have been clearly documented and well-illustrated by Zaetz (1971).

A perusal of the references quoted, and the extensive bibliographies which accompany most of them, provides an indication of the rapidly

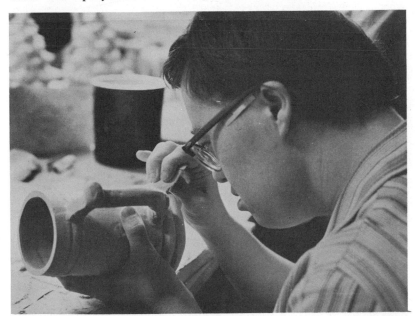

Fig. 102. Young man with Down's syndrome concentrating on task in hand. (Photograph by Boris Spremo, Toronto. Courtesy of Metropolitan Toronto Association for the Mentally Retarded.)

growing literature on the education and training of the mentally retarded, among them those with Down's syndrome, which has become available since the pioneer beginnings of books such as those of Séguin (1846, 1866). These writings range in content from observations on early pre-school educational programmes to rehabilitative measures in adulthood. Additional instructive, recently published texts of these kinds include the relevant sections of the volumes edited by Koch & Dobson (1971) and by Clarke & Clarke (1974) respectively.

GENERAL CONCLUSION

Persons with Down's syndrome vary to some extent in their capacities, but generally show considerable social and educational potential. Social competence and the acquisition of useful skills can be encouraged and developed in suitably stimulating environments with facilities designed for these purposes. Such opportunities, frequently based in the community, are becoming increasingly available in many countries.

It is perhaps not inappropriate to add a word of caution in an attempt to place these praiseworthy developments in perspective. Though much can be achieved along the lines mentioned, what may be regarded as an ultimate objective of an essentially healthy and independent life (in other words, cure) remains, at any rate in the present state of knowledge, unattainable. Nor do there appear to be realistic prospects, in the foreseeable future, in this regard. It seems more likely that the goal of prevention will come within reach rather than that of cure. Continued studies of the biological and clinical enigmas of the syndrome, of the kinds reviewed in this book, are steps in that direction.

References

Aarskog, D. (1966) A new cytogenetic variant of translocation Down's syndrome. *Cytogenetics* 5, 82.
Aarskog, D. (1969) Down's syndrome transmitted through maternal mosaicism. *Acta paediat. scand.* 58, 609.
Aase, J.M., Wilson, A.C. & Smith, D.W. (1973) Small ears in Down's syndrome: a helpful diagnostic aid. *J. Pediat.* 82, 845.
Abbott, M.E. (1924) New accessions in cardiac anomalies. I. Pulmonary atresia of inflammatory origin. II. Persistent ostium primum with mongolian idiocy. *Bull. Int. Ass. Med. Mus.* 10, 111.
Abbott, M.E. (1936) *Atlas of congenital cardiac disease.* New York: American Heart Association.
Adinolfi, M., Gardner, B. & Martin, W. (1967) Observations on the levels of γG. γA. and γM globulins, anti-A and anti-B agglutinins, and antibodies to *Escherichia coli* in Down's anomaly. *J. clin. Path.* 20, 860.
Agarwal, S.S., Blumberg, B.S., Gerstley, B.J.S., London, W.T., Sutnick, A.I. & Loeb, L.A. (1970) DNA polymerase activity as an index of lymphocyte stimulation: studies in Down's syndrome. *J. clin. Invest.* 49, 161.
Airaksinen, E.M. (1971) Platelet-rich plasma 5-hydroxy-tryptamine, urinary 5-hydroxyindole acetic acid and tryptophan ingestion in mongols. *J. ment. Defic. Res.* 15, 244.
Airaksinen, E.M. (1973) The metabolism of 5-HT in mongolism. *Abst. 3rd Congr. Int. Ass. Sci. Study Ment. Defic.* P. 12.
Akesson, H.O. & Forssman, H. (1966) A study of maternal age in Down's syndrome. *Ann. hum. Genet., Lond.* 29, 271.
Al-Aish, M.S., Dodson, E. & Plato, C.C. (1971) Down's syndrome with XYY: 48,XYY, G+. *Amer. J. Dis. Child.* 121, 444.
Alberti, A. (1904) Un caso di idiozia mongoloide. *Gior. di Psichiat. Clin. e Tecn. Manic., Ferrara,* 32, 335.
Alfi, O.S., Donnell, G.N. & Derencsenyi, A. (1971) Identification of the G chromosomes in Down's syndrome by quinacrine fluorescence microscopy. *J. Pediat.* 79, 656.
Allen, C.M. (1968) Infant mortality from congenital cardiac malformations in California, 1957-1966. *Amer. J. publ. Hlth.* 58, 1368.
Allen, G. & Baroff, G.S. (1955) Mongoloid twins and their siblings. *Acta genet. (Basel)* 5, 294.
Allison, A.C., Blumberg, B.S. & ap Rees (1958) Haptoglobin types in British, Spanish Basque and Nigerian African populations. *Nature, Lond.* 181, 824.
Alter, A.A., Lee, S.L., Pourfar, M. & Dobkin, G. (1962) Leukocyte alkaline phosphatase in mongolism: a possible chromosome marker. *J. clin. Invest.* 41, 1341.
von Ammon, F.A. (1831) Der Epicanthus. *Z. Ophthal.* 1, 535.
von Ammon, F.A. (1841) *Klinische Darstellungen der Krankheiten und Bildungsfehler des menschlichen Auges.* Berlin: G. Reimer.
von Ammon, F.A. (1860) Der Epicanthus und das Epiblepharon. Zwei Bildungsfehler der menschlichen Gesichtshaut. *J. Kinderkrank.* 34, 313.
Andersson, H., Fällström, S.P., Lundborg, P. & Roos, B.E. (1973) 5-hydroxyindoleacetic acid in children with Down's syndrome. *Acta paediat. scand.* 62, 158.

279

Andrén, L. & Hall, B. (1968) Increased curvature of the ilium: a new roentgeno-logical sign of mongoloid pelvis. *Develop. Med. Child Neurol.* 10, 781.

Anson, B.J. (1959) The aortic arch and its branches. *Cardiology,* Vol. 1. New York: McGraw-Hill Book Co.

Apert, E. (1914) Mongolism. *Le Monde Médicale,* Paris (Eng. ed.), 24, 201.

Appleton, M.D., Haab, W., Burti, U. & Casagrande, D. (1967) Quantitative evaluation of mongoloid gamma-globulins. *Amer. J. ment. Defic.* 72. 482.

Appleton, M.D., Haab, W., Hart, M.I. & Neary, J. (1966) Physical studies of mongoloid serum gamma-globulins. *Amer. J. ment. Defic.* 71, 465.

Appleton, M.D., & Pritham, G.H. (1963) Biochemical studies in mongolism. II. The influence of age and sex on the plasma proteins. *Amer. J. ment. Defic.* 67, 521.

Arakaki, D.T. & Waxman, S.H. (1970) Chromosome abnormalities in early spontaneous abortions. *J. med. Genet.* 7, 118.

Ardran, G.M., Harker, P. & Kemp, F.H. (1972) Tongue size in Down's syndrome. *J. ment. Defic. Res.* 16, 160.

Assicot, M. & Bohvon, C. (1971) Presence of two distinct catechol-O-methyltransferase activities in red blood cells. *Biochimie* 53, 871.

Astley, R. (1963) Chromosomal abnormalities in childhood, with particular reference to Turner's syndrome and mongolism. *Brit. J. Radiol.* 36, 2.

Atkins, L. & Bartsocas, C.S. (1974) Down's syndrome associated with two Robertsonian translocations, 45,XX,-15,-21+t(15q21q) and 46,XX-21,+t(21q 21q). *J. med. Genet.* 11, 306.

Atkins, L., O'Sullivan, M.A. & Pryles, C.V. (1962) Mongolism in three siblings with 46 chromosomes. *New Engl. J. Med.* 266, 631.

Aula, P., Hjelt, L. & Kauhtio, J. (1961) Chromosomal investigation in congenital malformations. *Ann. Paediat. Fenn.* 7, 206.

Aula, P., Leisti, J. & von Koskull, H. (1973) Partial trisomy 21. *Clin. Genet.* 4, 241.

Auld, R.M., Pommer, A.M., Houck, J.C. & Burke, F.G. (1959) Vitamin A absorption in mongoloid children, *Amer. J. ment. Defic.* 63, 1010.

Aung, M.H. (1973) Atlanto-axial dislocation in Down's syndrome: report of a case with spinal cord compression and review of the literature. *Bull. Los Angeles neurol. Soc.* 38, 197.

Austin, J.H.M., Preger, L., Siris, E. & Taybi, H. (1969) Short hard palate in newborn: roentgen sign of mongolism. *Radiology* 92, 775.

Babonneix, L. (1909) Contribution à l'étude anatomique de l'idiotie mongolienne. *Arch. Méd Enf.* 12, 497.

Babonneix, L. & Villette, J. (1916) Idiotie mongolienne familiale. *Arch. Méd. Enf.* 19, 478.

Back, F., Dörmer, P., Baumann, P. & Olbrich, E. (1967) Trisomy 21 or 22 in Down's syndrome? *Lancet* 1, 1228.

Báguena Candela, R., Forteza Bover, G. & Amat Aguirre, E. (1965) Un caso de mongolismo por mosaico normal/trisomia G. *Med. esp.* 54, 249.

Báguena Candela, R., Forteza Bover, G., Ortiz Hernandez, M.D. & Comin Ferrer, J. (1966) Un caso con estigmas del sindrome de Bonnevie-Ullrich y de mongolismo y cariotipo 45/XO-trisomia G. *Med. esp.* 55, 454.

Baikie, A.G. (1971) Banding patterns of metaphase chromosomes in Down's syndrome *Lancet* 2, 494.

Baikie, A.G., Loder, P.B., de Gruchy, G.C. & Pitt, D.B. (1965) Phosphohexokinase activity of erythrocytes in mongolism: another possible marker for chromosome 21. *Lancet* 1, 412.

Baird, P.A. & Miller, J.R. (1968) Some epidemiological aspects of Down's syndrome in British Columbia. *Brit. J. prev. soc. Med.* 22, 81.

Ball, J.R.B., Brackenridge, C.J., McKay, H. & Pitt, D.B. (1972) Haptoglobin distributions in Down's syndrome. *Clin. Genet.* 3, 334.

Barbour, P.F. (1902) A case of mongolian imbecility. *Arch. Pediat.* 19, 282.

Bardon, L.M.E. (1964) Siccacell treatment in mongolism. *Lancet* 2, 234.

Bargman, G.J., Neu, R.L., Powers, H.O. & Gardner, L.I. (1970) 48,XY,21+,mar+mat: a case of trisomy 21 associated with an inherited small marker chromosome. *J. med. Genet.* **7**, 99.

Barkla, D.H. (1963) Congenital absence and fusion in the deciduous dentition in mongols. *J. ment. Defic. Res.* **7**, 102.

Barkla, D.H. (1966a) Ages of eruption of permanent teeth in mongols. *J. ment. Defic. Res.* **10**, 190.

Barkla, D.H. (1966b) Congenital absence of permanent teeth in mongols. *J. ment. Defic. Res.* **10**, 198.

Barnard, K.E. & Powell, M.L. (1972) *Teaching the mentally retarded child: a family care approach.* Saint Louis: C.V. Mosby Co.

Barnes, N.P. (1923) Mongolism—importance of early recognition and treatment. *Ann. clin. Med.* **1**, 302.

Barnicot, N.A., Ellis, J.R. & Penrose, L.S. (1963) Translocation and trisomic mongol sibs. *Ann. hum. Genet., Lond.* **26**, 279.

Barnicot, N.A. & Huxley, H.E. (1965) Electron microscope observations on mitotic chromosomes. *Quart. micr. Sci.* **106**, 197.

Baron, J. (1972) Temperament profile of children with Down's syndrome. *Develop. Med. Child Neurol.* **14**, 640.

Barr, M.W. (1904) *Mental defectives: their history, treatment and training.* London: Rebman Ltd.

Bartels, H., Kruse, K. & Tolksdorf, M. (1968) Enzymes in Down's syndrome. *Lancet* **1**, 820.

Bartsch-Sandhoff, M. & Schade, H. (1973) Zwei subterminale Heterochromatin-regionen bei einer seltenen Form einer 21/21-Translokation. *Humangenetik* **18**, 329.

Bateman, A.J. (1960) Blood-group distributions to be expected in persons trisomic for the ABO gene. *Lancet* **1**, 1293.

Baumeister, A.A. & Williams, J. (1967) Relationship of physical stigmata to intellectual functioning in mongolism. *Amer. J. ment. Defic.* **71**, 586.

Bavin, J.T.R., Marshall, R. & Delhanty, J.D.A. (1963) A mongol with a 21:22 type chromosomal translocation. *J. ment. Defic. Res.* **7**, 84.

Bayley, N. (1958) Value and limitation of infant testing. *Children* **5**, 129.

Bazelon, M., Paine, R.S., Cowie, V.A., Hunt, P., Houck, J.C. & Mahanand, D. (1967) Reversal of hypotonia in infants with Down's syndrome by administration of 5-hydroxytryptophan. *Lancet* **1**, 1130.

Beach, F. (1878) On the diagnosis and treatment of idiocy, with remarks on prognosis. *Lancet* **2**, 764 and 801.

Beadle, G.W. (1932) A gene for sticky chromosomes in Zea mays. *Z. indukt. Abstamm-u. Verebslehre* **63**, 195.

Beall, G. & Stanton, R.G. (1945) Reduction in the number of mongolian defectives—a result of family limitation. *Canad. J. Pub. Hlth.* **36**, 33.

Beber, B.A. (1965) Absence of a rib in Down's syndrome. *Lancet* **2**, 289.

Becker, K.L., Burke, E.C. & Albert, A. (1963) Double autosomal trisomy (D trisomy plus mongolism). *Proc. Mayo Clin.* **38**, 242.

Beckman, L., Gustavson, K.-H. & Åkesson, H.O. (1962) Studies of some morphological traits in mental defectives. *Hereditas* **48**, 105.

Beckman, L., Gustavson, K.-H. & Norring, A. (1965) Dermal configurations in the diagnosis of the Down syndrome: an attempt at a simplified scoring method. *Acta genet., Basel* **15**, 3.

Behrman, R.E., Sigler, A.T. & Patchefsky, A.S. (1966) Abnormal hematopoieses in 2 of 3 siblings with mongolism. *J. Pediat.* **68**, 569.

Beidleman, B. (1945) Mongolism: a selective review. *Amer. J. ment. Defic.* **50**, 35.

Beley, A., Sevestre, P. & Lecuyer, R. (1958) Étude psycho-biologique comparative de 20 mongoliens et de 20 arrieres non différenciés. *Ann. méd. Psychol.* **116**, 947.

Benda, C.E. (1946) *Mongolism and cretinism.* New York: Grune & Stratton.

Benda, C.E. (1960) *The child with mongolism.* New York: Grune & Stratton.

Benda, C.E. & Bixby, E.M. (1939) Function of the thyroid and the pituitary in mongolism. *Amer. J. Dis. Child.* 58, 1240.

Benda, C.E. & Mann, G.V. (1955) The serum cholesterol and lipoprotein levels in mongolism. *J. Pediat.* 46, 49.

Benda, C.E. & Strassmann, G.S. (1965) The thymus in mongolism. *J. ment. Defic. Res.* 9, 109.

Benirschke, K., Brownhill, L., Hoefnagel, D. & Allen, F.H. (1962) Langdon Down anomaly (mongolism) with 21/21 translocation and Klinefelter's syndrome in the same sibship. *Cytogenetics* 1, 75.

Bennholdt-Thomsen, C. (1932) Über den Mongolismus und andere angeborene Abartungen in ihrer Beziehung zum hohen Alter der Mutter. *Z. Kinderheilk.* 53, 427.

Benson, P.F. (1975) Gene dosage effect in trisomy 21. *Lancet* 1, 584.

Benson, P.F. & de Jong, M. (1968) Leucocyte-hexokinase isoenzymes in Down's syndrome. *Lancet* 2, 197.

Beolchini, P.E., Bariatti, A.B. & Morganti, G. (1962) Indagini genetico-statistiche sulle fratrie di 432 soggetti mongoloidi. *Acta Genet. med. (Roma)* 11, 430.

Berg, J.M. (1958) Iris colour in mongolism. *Brit. Med. J.* 1, 563.

Berg, J.M. (1968a) Observations on thenar/first interdigital dermatoglyphic patterns in mongolism. *J. ment Defic. Res.* 12, 307.

Berg, J.M. (1968b) A study of the *td* dermal ridge-count on the human palm. *Hum. Biol.* 40, 375.

Berg, J.M. (1969) Unpublished observations.

Berg, J.M. (1975) L.S. Penrose–His contributions to mental deficiency. *Proc. 2nd Congr. int. Assoc. sci. Study ment. Defic.*, The Hague 2, 1. Warsaw: Polish Medical Publishers.

Berg, J.M., Brandon, M. & Kirman, B.H. (1959) Atropine in mongolism. *Lancet* 2, 441.

Berg, J.M, Crome, L. & France, N.E. (1960) Congenital cardiac malformations in mongolism. *Brit. Heart J.* 22, 331.

Berg, J.M., Gilderdale, S. & Way, J. (1969) On telling parents of a diagnosis of mongolism. *Brit. J. Psychiat.* 115, 1195.

Berg, J.M. & Kirman, B.H. (1959) Some aetiological problems in mental deficiency. *Brit. med. J.* 2, 848.

Berg, J.M. & Kirman, B.H. (1961) Risk of dual occurrence of mongolism in sibships. *Arch. Dis. Child.* 36, 645.

Berg, J.M., Kirman, B.H., Stern, J. & Mittwoch, U. (1961) Treatment of mongolism with pituitary extract. *J. ment. Sci.* 107, 475.

Berg, J.M. & Smith, G.F. (1971) Behaviour and intelligence in males with XYY sex chromosomes. *Proc. 2nd Congr. int. Assoc. sci. Study ment. Defic.*, Warsaw 135. Warsaw: Polish Medical Publishers.

Berg, J.M. & Stern, J. (1963) Observations on children with mongolism. *Proc. 2nd Int. Cong. ment. Retard., Vienna* 1, 367.

Bergemann, E. (1961) Manifestation familiale du karyotype triplo-X: communication préliminaire. *J. Génét. hum.* 10, 370.

Berman, J., Hultén, M. & Lindsten, J. (1967) Blood serotonin in Down's syndrome. *Lancet* 1, 730.

Bernard, J., Mathé, G. & Delorme, J.-Cl. (1954) Les leucoses des tres jeunes enfants. *Arch. Franç. Pédiat.* 12, 470.

Bernhard, W.G., Gore, I. & Kilby, R.A. (1951) Congenital leukaemia. *Blood* 6, 990.

Berry, R.J.A. & Porteus S.D. (1920) *Intelligence and social valuation.* Vineland Training School Publication No. 20.

Betlejewski, S., Jordan, J. & Walczyński, Z. (1966) Le pavillon de l'oreille chez les enfants atteints du syndrome de Down. *Ann. Paediat. (Basel)* 207, 247.

Betlejewski, S., Klajman, S. & Walczyński, Z. (1964) Radiologische Untersuchungen der Entwicklung der Nasennebenhöhlen im Down-Syndrom. *Ann. Paediat. (Basel)* **203**, 355.

Biach, P. (1909) Zur Kenntnis des Zentralnervensystems beim Mongolismus. *Dtsch. Z. Nervenheilk.* **37**, 7.

Biscatti, G. (1964) Mosaico trisomia 21/normale in una bambina con malformazioni varie e segni di mongolismo. *Pediatrica* **72**, 315.

Bishun, N.P. (1968) Normal/trisomy C mosaicism in the mother of a "mongoloid" child. *Acta paediat. scand.* **57**, 243.

Bixby, E.M. (1939) Biochemical studies in mongolism. *Amer. J. ment. Defic.* **44**, 59.

Bixby, E.M. (1940) Further biochemical studies in mongolism. *Amer. J. ment. Defic.* **45**, 201.

Bixby, E.M. (1941) Biochemical studies in mongolism. *Amer. J. ment. Defic.* **46**, 183.

Bixby, E.M. & Benda, C.E. (1942) Glucose tolerance and insulin tolerance in mongolism. *Amer. J. ment. Defic.* **47**, 158.

Blacketer-Simmonds, D.A. (1953) An investigation into the supposed difference existing between mongols and other mentally defective subjects with regard to certain psychological traits. *J. ment. Sci.* **99**, 702.

Blakeslee, A.F. (1923) Variations in the Jimson weed (*Datura stramonium*) caused by differences in the number of chromosomes. *Eugenics, Genetics and the Family. 2nd Int. Cong. Eugen.* **1**, 82.

Blank, C.E., Gemmell, E., Casey, M.D. & Lord, P.M. (1962) Mosaicism in a mother with a mongol child. *Brit. med. J.* **2**, 378.

Blank, C.E., Lord, P.M., Casey, M.D. & Laurance, B.M. (1963) Chromosome mosaicism in a mongol born to a young mother. *Cytogenetics* **2**, 76.

Bleyer, A. (1925) The occurrence of mongolism in Ethiopians. *J. Amer. med. Ass.* **84**, 1041.

Bleyer, A. (1932) The frequency of mongoloid idiocy. *Amer. J. Dis. Child.* **44**, 503.

Bleyer, A. (1934) Indications that mongoloid imbecility is a gametic mutation of degenerative type. *Amer. J. Dis. Child.* **47**, 342.

Bleyer, A. (1937) Theoretical and clinical aspects of mongolism. *J. Missouri med. Ass.* **34**, 222.

Bleyer, A. (1938) The role of advanced maternal age in mongolism: a study of 2,822 cases. *Amer. J. Dis. Child.* **55**, 79.

Bloom, A.D., Archer, P.G. & Awa, A.A. (1967) Variation in the human chromosome number. *Nature, Lond.* **216**, 487.

Blumberg, B.S. (1966) An inherited serum isoantigen in leukemia and Down's syndrome. *J. clin. Invest.* **45**, 988.

Blumberg, B.S., Gerstley, B.J.S., Hungerford, D.A., London, W.T. & Sutnick, A.I. (1967) A serum antigen (Australia antigen) in Down's syndrome, leukemia and hepatitis. *Ann. intern. Med.* **66**, 924.

Blumberg, B.S., Gerstley, B.J.S., Sutnick, A.I., Millman, I. & London, W.T. (1970) Australia antigen, hepatitis virus and Down's syndrome. *Ann. N.Y. Acad. Sci.* **171**, 486.

Blumenthal, I. & Variend, M.S. (1972) Maternal urinary oestriol excretion and fetal chromosome abnormalities. *Lancet* **2**, 1084.

Bodensteiner, J.B. & Zellweger, H. (1971a) Trisomy E/trisomy G mosaicism: a report of two cases. *Helv. paediat. Acta.* **26**, 63.

Bodensteiner, J.B. & Zellweger, H. (1971b) Mongolism preventable by amniocentesis: an appraisal of the genetic considerations. *Clin. Pediat.* **10**, 554.

Bodian, M. & Carter, C.O. (1963) Family study of Hirschsprung's disease. *Ann. hum. Genet., Lond.* **26**, 261.

Bodian, M., White, L.L.R., Carter, C.O. & Louw, J.H (1952) Congenital duodenal obstruction and mongolism. *Brit. med. J.* **1**, 77.

Bolling, D.R., Borgaonkar, D.S., Herr, H.M. & Davis, M. (1971) Evaluation of dermal patterns in Down's syndrome by predictive discrimination. II. Composite score based on the combination of left and right pattern areas. *Clin. Genet.* 2, 163.

Bonham Carter, R.E. (1962) Unpublished observation.

Bonnevie, K.J. (1924) Studies on papillary patterns of human fingers. *J. Genet.* 15, 1.

Böök, J.A., Fraccaro, M. & Lindsten, J. (1959) Cytogenetical observations in mongolism. *Acta paediat., Uppsala* 48, 453.

Boorman, K.E. (1950) An analysis of the blood types and clinical condition of 2,000 consecutive mothers and their infants. *Ann. Eugen., Lond.* 15, 120.

Borgaonkar, D.S., Bias, W.B., Chase, G.A., Sadasivan, G., Herr, H.M., Golomb, H.M., Bahr, G.F. & Kunkel, L.M. (1973a) Identification of a C6/G21 translocation chromosome by the Q-M and Giemsa banding techniques in a patient with Down's syndrome with possible assignment of Gm locus. *Clin. Genet.* 4, 53.

Borgaonkar, D.S., Bolling, D.R. & Herr, H.M. (1973b) Evaluation of dermal patterns in the diagnosis of the Down syndrome by predictive discrimination. III. Variations due to sex and ethnic background and its effect on the use of indices. *Hum. Hered.* 23, 442.

Borgaonkar, D.S., Davis, M., Bolling, D.R. & Herr, H.M. (1971) Evaluation of dermal patterns in Down's syndrome by predictive discrimination. I. Preliminary analysis based on frequencies of patterns. *Johns Hopk. med. J.* 128, 141.

Boullin, D.J. & O'Brien, R.A. (1973) The metabolism of 5-hydroxy-tryptamine by blood platelets from children with mongolism. *Biochem. Pharmacol.* 22, 1647.

Bourneville, D.M. (1902) L'idiotie du type mongolien. *Rech. Clin. Thér. Epilepsie* 22, 136.

Bourneville, D.M. (1903a) De l'idiotie mongolienne. *Arch. Neurol., Paris* 16, 252.

Bourneville, D.M. (1903b) L'idiotie mongolienne. *Prog. Méd.* 3, 117.

Bourneville, D.M. & Royer (1906) Imbecilité prononcé congénitale (type mongolien), traitement thyroidien. *Arch. Neurol., Paris* 22, 425.

Bowen, P., Chernick, B.C., Campbell, D.J. & Rouget, A. (1974) Mild characteristics of Down's syndrome with normal karyotype in cultured lymphocytes and skin fibroblasts. *Birth Defects Original Article Series* 10, No. 10, P. 42.

Boxer, L.A. & Yokoyama, M. (1972) Lymphocyte antigens in patients with Down's syndrome. *Vox Sang. (Basel)* 22, 539.

Bradway, K.P. (1937) Hysterical mutism in a mongol imbecile. *J. abnorm. soc. Psychol.* 31, 458.

Brahdy, M.B. (1927) Mongolian imbecility—report of a case in a colored girl. *Arch. Pediat.* 44, 724.

Brandt, N. (1962) Genes on the mongol chromosome? *Lancet* 2, 837.

Brandt, N., Froland, A., Mikkelsen, M., Nielsen, A. & Tolstrup, N. (1963) Galactosaemia locus and the Down's syndrome chromosome. *Lancet* 2, 700.

Breg, W.R., Cornwell, J.G. & Miller, O.J. (1962) The association of the triple-X syndrome and mongolism in two families. *Amer. J. Dis. Child.* 104, 534.

Brewis, M., Poskanzer, D.C., Rolland, C. & Miller, H. (1966) Neurological disease in an English city. *Acta Neurol. scand.* 42, Suppl. 24.

Bridges, C.B. (1916) Non-disjunction as proof of chromosome theory of heredity. *Genetics* 1, 1 and 107.

Bridges, C.B. (1923) Aberrations in chromosomal materials. *Eugenics, Genetics and the Family. 2nd Int. Cong. Eugen.* 1, 76.

Brinkworth, R. & Collins, J.E. (1969) *Improving mongol babies and introducing them to school.* Belfast: National Society for Mentally Handicapped Children.

Brismar, B. (1965) Dermatoglyphics in the hallucal area of the sole: a mother/child correlation. *Acta Genet. med. (Roma)* 14, 86.

Brøgger, A. & Gundersen, S.K. (1966) Double fertilization in Down's syndrome. *Lancet* 1, 1270.

Brøgger, A., Mohr, J., Wehn, M. & Vislie, H. (1964) Concerning translocation as a cause of mental retardation. *Int. Copenhagen Cong. Sci. Study Ment. Retard.* 1, 128.

Brooks, D.N., Wooley, H. & Kanjilal, G.C. (1972) Hearing loss and middle ear disorders in patients with Down's syndrome. *J. ment. Defic. Res.* 16, 21.

Brothers, C.R.D. & Jago, G.C. (1954) Report on the longevity and the causes of death in mongoloidism in the State of Victoria. *J. ment. Sci.* 100, 580.

Brothwell, D.R. (1960) A possible case of mongolism in a Saxon population. *Ann. hum. Genet., Lond.* 24, 141.

Brousseau, K. & Brainerd, H.G. (1928) *Mongolism: a study of the physical and mental characteristics of mongolian imbeciles.* London: Baillière, Tindall & Cox.

Brouwer, D. (1962) "Mongolian spot." *Lancet* 1, 865.

Brown, E.E., (1954) Pathogenesis of mongolism following maternal illness; role of adrenals. *Arch. Pediat.* 71, 47.

Brown, R.H. & Cunningham, W.M. (1961) Some dental manifestations of mongolism. *Oral Med.* 14, 664.

Brown, R.K., Burdick, C.O., Malone, J. & Wright, Y.M. (1967) Familial D/D translocation associated with trisomy 21: report of a case with pedigree study. *J Amer. med. Ass.* 202, 60.

Brushfield, T. (1924) Mongolism. *Brit. J. Child. Dis.* 21, 241.

Brushfield T. (1925) The plantar lines in mental defectives. *Brit. J. Child. Dis.* 22, 274.

Bryant, J.I., Emanuel, I., Huang, S., Kronmal, R. & Lo, J. (1970) Dermatoglyphics of Chinese children with Down's syndrome. *J. med. Genet.* 7, 338.

Buchan, A.R. (1962) A study of mongolism in Newcastle-upon-Tyne, 1948-1959. *Med. Offr.* 107, 51.

Buchanan, J.G. & Becroft, D.M.O. (1970) Down's syndrome and acute leukaemia: a cytogenetic study. *J. med. Genet.* 7, 67.

Buckton, K., Harnden, D.G., Baikie, A.G. & Woods, G.E. (1961) Mongolism and leukaemia in the same sibship. *Lancet* 1, 171.

Bullard, W.N. (1911) Mongolian idiocy. *Boston med. surg. J.* 164, 56.

Bumbalo, T.S., Morelewicz, H.V. & Berens, D.L. (1964) Treatment of Down's syndrome with the "u" series of drugs. *J Amer. med. Ass.* 187, 361.

Burger, P.C. & Vogel, F.S. (1973) The development of the pathologic changes of Alzheimer's disease and senile dementia in patients with Down's syndrome. *Amer. J. Path.* 73, 457.

Burgio, G.R., Severi, F., Rossoni, R. & Vaccaro, R. (1965) Mongolism and thyroid autoimmunity. *Lancet* 1, 166.

Burns, J.K. (1973) Birth-weight distribution patterns in relation to estimated duration of pregnancy in normal infants, spina bifida and Down's syndrome. *J. Physiol.* 230, 50.

Butterworth, T., Leoni, E.P., Beerman, H., Wood, M.G. & Stern, L.P. (1960) Cheilitis of mongolism. *J. invest. Derm.* 35, 347.

Cafferata, J.F. (1909) Contribution à la littérature du mongolisme. *Arch. Méd. Enf.* 12, 929.

Caffey, J. & Ross, S. (1956) Mongolism (mongoloid deficiency) during early infancy. Some newly recognized diagnostic changes in the pelvic bones. *Pediatrics* 17, 642.

Caffey, J. & Ross, S. (1958) Pelvic bones in infantile mongoloidism. *Amer. J. Roentgenol.* 80, 458.

Caldecott, C. (1909) Tuberculosis as a cause of death in mongolism. *Brit. med. J.* 2, 665.

Cannings, C. & Cannings, M.R. (1968) Mongolism, delayed fertilization and human sexual behaviour. *Nature, Lond.* 218, 481.

Cantor, G.N. & Girardeau, F.L. (1959) Rhythmic discrimination ability in mongoloid and normal children. *Amer. J. ment. Defic.* 63, 621.

Careddu, P., Tenconi, L.T. & Sacchetti, G. (1963) Transmethylation in mongols. *Lancet* 1, 828.

Carlson, B.W. & Ginglend, D.R. (1961) *Play activities for the retarded child.* New York: Abingdon Press.

Carr, D.H. (1963) Chromosome studies in abortuses and stillborn children. *Lancet* 2, 603.

Carr, D.H. (1965) Chromosome studies in spontaneous abortions. *Obstet. Gynec.* 26, 308.

Carr, J. (1970a) Mental and motor development in young mongol children. *J. ment. Defic. Res.* 14, 205.

Carr, J. (1970b) Mongolism: telling the parents. *Develop. Med. Child Neurol.* 12, 213.

Carr, J. (1974) The effect of the severely subnormal on their families. In: *Mental deficiency: the changing outlook.* 3rd ed. A.M. Clarke & A.D.B. Clarke, eds. London: Methuen & Co.

Carter, C.O. (1958) A life-table for mongols with the causes of death. *J. ment. Defic. Res.* 2, 64.

Carter, C.O. & Evans, K.A. (1961) Risks of parents who had one child with Down's syndrome (mongolism) having another child similarly affected *Lancet* 2, 785.

Carter, C.O., Evans, K.A. & Stewart, A.M. (1961) Maternal radiation and Down's syndrome (mongolism). *Lancet* 2, 1042.

Carter, C.O., Hamerton, J.L., Polani, P.E., Gunalp, A. & Weller, S.D. (1960) Chromosome translocation as a cause of familial mongolism. *Lancet* 2, 678.

Carter, C.O. & MacCarthy, D. (1951) Incidence of mongolism and its diagnosis in the newborn. *Brit. J. soc. Med.* 5, 83.

Casa, D. (1961) Allergy and mongoloidism. *Int. Arch. Allergy* 18, 108.

Caspersson, T., Gahrton, G., Lindsten, J. & Zech, L. (1970a) Identification of the Philadelphia chromosome as a number 22 by quinacrine mustard fluorescence analysis. *Exp. Cell Res.* 63, 238.

Caspersson, T., Hultén, M., Lindsten, J. & Zech, L. (1970b) Distinction between extra G-like chromosomes by quinacrine mustard fluorescence analysis. *Exp. Cell Res.* 63, 240.

Caspersson, T., Hultén, M., Lindsten, J., Therkelsen, A.J. & Zech, L. (1971a) Identification of different Robertsonian translocations in man by quinacrine mustard fluorescence analysis. *Hereditas (Lund)* 67, 213.

Caspersson, T., Lomakka, G. & Zech, L. (1971b) The 24 fluorescence patterns of the human metaphase chromosomes—distinguishing characters and variability. *Hereditas (Lund)* 67, 89.

Casteels-Van Daele, M., Proesmans, W., van den Berghe, H. & Verresen, H. (1970) Down's anomaly (21 trisomy) and Turner's syndrome (46,XXqi) in the same sibship. *Helv. paediat. Acta* 25, 412.

Cattanach, B.M. (1964) Autosomal trisomy in the mouse. *Cytogenetics* 3, 159.

Cavalli, L.L. (1945) Alcuin problemi della analisi biometrica di popolazioni naturali. *Mem. Inst. ital. Idrobiol. de Marchi* 2, 301.

Ceccarelli, G. & Torbidoni, L. (1967) Viral hepatitis and Down's syndrome. *Lancet* 1, 438.

Centerwall, S.A. & Centerwall, W.R. (1960) Study of children with mongolism reared in the home compared to those reared away from home. *Pediatrics.* 25, 678.

Chaganti, R.S.K., Morillo-Cucci, G., Degnan, M. & German, J. (1975) Mongolism by tertiary trisomy. *Lancet* 1, 698.

Chan, M.C.K. (1969) Congenital leukaemia in Down's syndrome (report of a case with spontaneous remission). *J. Singapore paediat. Soc.* 11, 137.

Chand, A. (1932) A case of mongolism in India. *Brit. J. Child. Dis.* 29, 201.

Chandler, N.W. & Gay, B.B. (1967) Congenital duodenal stenosis producing megaduodenum in a nineteen year old mongoloid. *Amer. J. Roentgenol.* 100, 113.

Chapman, C.J., Gardner, R.J.M. & Veale, A.M.O. (1973) Segregation analysis of a large t(21q22q) family. *J. med. Genet.* 10, 362.

Chapman, M.J. & Stern, J. (1964) Personal communication.

Chaptal, J., Jean, R., Bonnet, H., Emberger, J.-M., Navarro, M. & Rieu, D. (1970) Troubles hematologiques des jeunes mongoliens. *Pédiatrie* **25**, 433.

Chaptal, J., Jean, R. & Emberger, J. -M. (1965) Translocation entre deux chromosomes du groups 13-15 chez la mere d'un mongolien par trisomie 21 reguliere. *Arch. franç. Pédiat.* **22**, 35.

Chaptal, J., Jean, R., Emberger, J.-M., Navarro, M. & Mallet, H. (1966) Anomalie structurale d'un chromosome du groupe 13-15 chez un mongolien par trisomie 21 reguliere et chez sa mere. *Arch. franç. Pédiat.* **23**, 57.

Chaudhuri, A. & Chaudhuri, K.C. (1965) Chromosome mosaicism in an Indian child with Down's syndrome. *J. med. Genet.* **2**, 131.

Chen, A.T.L., Ebbin, A.J., Schimpeler, S., Heath, C.W. & Falek, A. (1969) Birth weight and mortality in Down's syndrome infants. *Soc. Biol.* **16**, 290.

Chitham, R.G. & MacIver, E. (1965) A cytogenetic and statistical survey of 105 cases of mongolism. *Ann. hum. Genet., Lond.* **28**, 309.

Chudina, A.P., Malyutina, T.S. & Pogosyants, E.E. (1966) Comparative radiosensitivity of chromosomes in cultured peripheral blood leukocytes of normal subjects and of patients with Down's syndrome. *Genetika* **4**, 51.

Clark, R.M. (1929) The mongol: a new explanation. *J. ment. Sci.* **75**, 261.

Clarke, A.M. & Clarke, A.D.B. (Ed.) (1974) *Mental deficiency: the changing outlook.* 3rd ed. London: Methuen & Co.

Clarke, C.M., Edwards, J.H. & Smallpeice, V. (1961) 21 trisomy/normal mosaicism in an intelligent child with mongoloid characters. *Lancet* **1**, 1028.

Clarke, C.M., Ford, C.E., Edwards, J.H. & Smallpeice, V. (1963) 21-trisomy/normal mosaicism in an intelligent child with some mongoloid characters. *Lancet* **2**, 1229.

Clift, M.W. (1922) Roentgenological findings in mongolism. *Amer. J. Roentgenol.* **9**, 420.

Coghlan, M.K. & Evans, P.R. (1964) Infantile eczema, asthma and hay fever in mongolism. *Guy's Hosp. Rep.* **113**, 223.

Cohen, B.H. & Lilienfeld, A.M. (1970) The epidemiological study of mongolism in Baltimore. *Ann. N.Y. Acad. Sci.* **171**, 320.

Cohen, M.M. & Davidson, R.G. (1967) Down's syndrome associated with a familial (21q-;22q+) translocation. *Cytogenetics* **6**, 321.

Cohen, M.M. & Davidson, R.G. (1972) Double aneuploidy (47,XX,21+/45,X) arising through simultaneous double non-disjunction. *J. med. Genet.* **9**, 242.

Cohen, M.M., Winer, R.A. & Shklar, G. (1960) Periodontal disease in a group of mentally subnormal children. *J. dent. Res.* **39**, 745.

Cohen, T. & Warland, B.J. (1960) Personal communication.

Coleman, M. (1971) Infantile spasms associated with 5-hydroxy-tryptophan administration in patients with Down's syndrome. *Neurology (Minneap.)* **21**, 911.

Coleman, M. (1973) *Serotonin in Down's syndrome.* New York: American Elsevier.

Collmann, R.D. & Stoller, A. (1962a) A survey of mongoloid births in Victoria, Australia, 1942–57. *Amer. J. publ. Hlth.* **52**, 813.

Collmann, R.D. & Stoller, A. (1962b) Notes on the epidemiology of mongolism in Victoria, Australia, from 1942 to 1957. *Proc. Lond. Conf. Study Ment. Defic.* **2**, 517.

Collmann, R.D. & Stoller, A. (1963a) Data on mongolism in Victoria, Australia: prevalence and life expectation. *J. ment. Defic. Res.* **7**, 60.

Collman, R.D. & Stoller, A. (1963b) A life table for mongols in Victoria, Australia. *J. ment. Defic. Res.* **7**, 53.

Collmann, R.D. & Stoller, A. (1963c) Comparison of age distributions for mothers of mongols born in high and in low birth incidence areas and years in Victoria, 1947–57. *J. ment. Defic. Res.* **7**, 79.

Comby, J. (1903) Le mongolisme. *Arch. Méd. Enf.* **6**, 746.

Comby, J. (1906) Le mongolisme infantile. *Arch. Méd. Enf.* 9, 193.
Comby, J. (1907) Nouveau cas de mongolisme infantile. *Arch. Méd. Enf.* 10, 1.
Comby, J. (1917) Idiotie mongolienne. *Arch. Méd. Enf.* 20, 505, 561 and 617.
Cone, T.E. (1954) Diabetes mellitus in a mongoloid. *J. med. Soc. N.J.* 51, 66.
Conen, P.E. & Erkman, B (1966) Combined mongolism and leukemia. Report of eight cases with chromosome studies. *Amer. J. Dis. Child.* 112, 429.
Cooper, H.L. & Hirschhorn, K. (1962) Enlarged satellites as a familial chromosome marker. *Amer. J. hum. Genet.* 14, 107.
Corcoran, P., Gerald, P.S., Diamond, L.K., Zergollern, L., Hoefnagel, D. & Benirschke, K. (1964) Gm locus on translocation chromosome? *Lancet* 1, 987.
Cordero, J. (1911) Le mongolisme infantile. *An. Soc. Med.-quir. Hosp.* (Reviewed in *Arch. Méd. Enf.* 15 (1912), 389)
Coriat L.F., Ferreyra, M.E. & Alfonso, J.F. (1971) Familial Down's syndrome. *Proc. 2nd Congr. int. Assoc. sci. Study ment. Defic., Warsaw* 603.
Cornwell, A.C. & Birch, H.G. (1969) Psychological and social development in home-reared children with Down's syndrome (Mongolism). *Amer J. ment. Defic.* 74, 341.
Court Brown, W.M. (1967) *Human population cytogenetics.* Amsterdam: North-Holland Publishing Co.
Court Brown, W.M., Harnden, D.G., Jacobs, P.A., Maclean, N. & Mantle, D.J. (1964) Abnormalities of the sex chromosome complement in man. *Spec. Rep. Ser. med. Res. Coun.* No. 305. London: H.M.S.O.
Court Brown, W.M., Jacobs, P.A. & Brunton, M. (1965) Chromosome studies on randomly chosen men and women. *Lancet* 2, 561.
Cowie, V.A. (1966) Genetic counselling. *Proc. roy. Soc. Med.* 59, 149.
Cowie, V.A. (1970) *A study of the early development of mongols.* Oxford: Pergamon Press.
Cowie, V.A. & Kahn, J. (1965) A mongol child without trisomy G. *Lancet* 2, 58.
Cox, R.P. (1965) Regulation of alkaline phosphatase in skin fibroblast cultures from patients with mongolism. *Exp. Cell Res.* 37, 690.
Crandall, B.F. & Ebbin, A.J. (1973) Trisomy 18 and 21 in two siblings. *Clin. Genet.* 4, 517.
Crandall, B.F., Weber, F., Muller, H.M. & Burwell, J.K. (1972) Identification of 21r and 22r chromosomes by quinacrine fluorescence. *Clin. Genet.* 3, 264.
Cratty, B.J. (1969) *Motor activity and the education of retardates.* Philadelphia: Lea & Febiger.
Creasy, M.R. & Crolla, J.A. (1974) Prenatal mortality of trisomy 21 (Down's syndrome). *Lancet* 1, 473
Crome, L. (1965) The Pathology of Down's disease. In *Mental deficiency.* 2nd ed. L.T. Hilliard & B.H. Kirman, eds. London: J. & A. Churchill Ltd.
Crome, L., Cowie, V. & Slater, E. (1966) A statistical note on cerebellar and brain-stem weight in mongolism. *J. ment. Defic. Res.* 10, 69.
Crookshank, F.G. (1924) *The mongol in our midst.* London: Kegan Paul, Trench & Trubner Ltd.
Cullen, J.F. (1963) Blindness in mongolism (Down's syndrome). *Brit. J. Ophthal.* 47, 331.
Cullen, J.F. & Butler, H.G. (1963) Mongolism (Down's syndrome) and keratoconus. *Brit. J. Ophthal.* 47, 321.
Cullum, L. & Liebman, J. (1969) The association of congenital heart disease with Down's syndrome (mongolism). *Amer. J. Cardiol.* 24, 354.
Cummins, H. (1936) Dermatoglyphic stigmata in mongoloid imbeciles. *Anat. Rec.* 64, 11.
Cummins, H. (1939) Dermatoglyphic stigmata in mongoloid imbeciles. *Anat. Rec.* 73, 407.
Cummins, H. (1963) Personal communication.

Cummins, H. & Midlo, C. (1943) *Finger-prints, palms and soles.* Philadelphia: The Blakiston Company.

Currarino, G. & Swanson, G.E. (1964) A developmental variant of ossification of the manubrium sterni in mongolism. *Radiology* 82, 916.

Curtis, B.H., Blank, S. & Fisher, R.L. (1968) Atlantoaxial dislocation in Down's syndrome. *J. Amer. med. Ass.* 205, 464.

Cutress, T.W. (1971a) Periodontal disease and oral hygiene in trisomy 21. *Arch. oral Biol.* 16, 1345.

Cutress, T.W. (1971b) Dental caries in trisomy 21. *Arch. oral Biol.* 16, 1329.

Cutress, T.W., Suckling, G.W. & Brown, R.H. (1971) Periodontal disease and serum citric acid levels in trisomy-21. A further study. *Arch. oral Biol.* 16, 1367.

Dallaire, L. & Fraser, F.C. (1964) Two unusual cases of familial mongolism. *Canad. J. Genet. Cytol.* 6, 540.

Dallapiccola, B., Alboni, P. & Ballerini, G. (1971) Capillary fragility in Down's syndrome. *Coagulation* 4, 217.

Dallapiccola, B. & Ricci, N. (1967) I dermatoglifi nella sindrome di Down tipica ed atipica. *Acta Genet. med. (Roma)* 16, 384.

Dalton, A.J., Crapper, D.R. & Schlotterer, G.R. (1974) Alzheimer's disease and Down's syndrome—visual retention deficits. *Cortex* 10, 366.

Danton, R.A. & Nyhan, W.L. (1966) Concentrations of uric acid in the sweat of control and mongoloid children. *Proc. Soc. exp. Biol. (N.Y.)* 121, 270.

Davidenkova, E.F., Shtilbanse, I.I., Godinova, A.M., Savelieva-Vassilieva, E.A. & Verlinskaia, D.K. (1964) The role of maternal pathology in Down's syndrome. *F. Proc. Trans. (Suppl.)* 23, 873.

Davidoff, L.M. (1928) The brain in mongolian idiocy: a report of ten cases. *Arch. Neurol. Psychiat.* 20, 1229.

Davidson, W.M. & Robertson Smith, D. (1954) A morphological sex difference in the polymorphonuclear neutrophil leucocytes. *Brit. med. J.* 2, 6.

Davies, P.A. & Smallpeice, V. (1963) The single transverse palmar crease in infants and children. *Develop. Med. Child Neurol.* 5, 491.

Day, R.W. & Miles, C.P. (1965) Familial Down's syndrome with undetected translocation. *J. Pediat.* 67, 399.

Day, R.W., Wright, S.W., Koons, A. & Quigley, M. (1963) XXX 21-trisomy and retinoblastoma. *Lancet* 2, 154.

Deaton, J.G. (1973) The mortality rate and causes of death among institutionalised mongols in Texas. *J. ment. Defic. Res.* 17, 117.

De Carvalho, S. (1963) Preliminary experimentation with specific immunotherapy of neoplastic disease in man. I. Immediate effects of hyperimmune equine gammoglobulins. *Cancer* 16, 306.

Deckers, J.F.M., Oorthuys, A.M.A. & Doesburg, W.H. (1973a) Dermatoglyphics in Down's syndrome. I: Evaluation of discriminating ability of pattern areas. *Clin. Genet.* 4, 311.

Deckers, J.F.M., Oorthuys, A.M.A. & Doesburg, W.H. (1973b) Dermatoglyphics in Down's syndrome. II: Evaluation of scoring methods. *Clin. Genet.* 4, 318.

Deckers, J.F.M., Oorthuys, A.M.A. & Doesburg, W.H. (1973c) Dermatoglyphics in Down's syndrome. III: Proposal of a simplified scoring method. *Clin. Genet.* 4, 381.

Degenhardt, K.H. & Fränz, J. (1967) Cytogenetische Untersuchungen bei Mongoloidismus und weiteren angeborenen Entwicklungsstörüngen. *Germ. med. Mth.* 7, 338.

Dekaban, A. (1965) Twins, probably monozygotic: one mongoloid with 48 chromosomes, the other normal. *Cytogenetics* 4, 227.

Dekaban, A.S., Thron, R. & Steusing, J. (1966) Chromosomal aberrations in irradiated blood and blood cultures of normal subjects and of selected patients with chromosomal abnormalities. *Radiat. Res.* 27, 50.

Dekaban, A.S. & Zelson, J. (1968) Retardation in a child with an extra submetacentric chromosome fragment and partial mongolism. *J. ment. Defic. Res.* **12**, 216.

De Mars, R. (1964) Some studies of enzymes in cultivated human cells. *Nat. Cancer Inst. Monogr.* **13**, 181.

De Mayo, A.P. Kiossoglou, K.A., Erlandson, M.E., Notterman, R.F. & German, J. (1967) A marrow chromosomal abnormality preceding clinical leukemia in Down's syndrome. *Blood* **29**, 233.

De Myer, W. & Palmer, C. (1965) Closed metopic suture with trigonocephaly in Down's syndrome. *Neurology (Minneap.)* **15**, 756.

Dent, T., Edwards, J.H. & Delhanty, J.D.A. (1963) A partial mongol. *Lancet* **2**, 484.

Denver Conference (1960) A proposed standard system of nomenclature of human mitotic chromosomes. *Lancet* **1**, 1063.

Desgeorges, P. (1905) *Contribution à l'étude de l'idiotie mongolienne.* Diss., Paris.

Diamond, E.F. & Moon, M.S. (1961) Neuromuscular development in mongoloid children. *Amer. J. ment. Defic.* **66**, 218.

Dicker, L. (1972) Dermatoglyphics and level of retardation in Down's syndrome. *Amer. J. ment. Defic.* **77**, 143.

Dicks-Mireaux, M.J. (1972) Mental development of infants with Down's syndrome. *Amer. J. ment. Defic.* **77**, 26.

Dignan, P. St. J. (1973) Polydactyly in Down's syndrome. *Amer. J. ment. Defic.* **77**, 486.

Dodge, J.A., Neill, D.W. & Scally, B.G. (1967) Low butanol-extractable-iodine levels in the serum of patients with Down's syndrome. *Lancet* **1**, 78.

Doery, J.C.G., Hirsh, J., Garson, D.M. & de Gruchy, G.C. (1968) Platelet-phosphohexokinase levels in Down's syndrome. *Lancet* **2**, 894.

Domino, G. (1965) Personality traits in institutionalized mongoloids. *Amer. J. ment. Defic.* **69**, 568.

Domino, G., Goldschmid, M. & Kaplan, M. (1964) Personality traits of institutionalized mongoloid girls. *Amer. J. ment. Defic.* **68**, 498.

Domino, G. & Newman, D. (1965) Relationship of physical stigmata to intellectual subnormality in mongoloids. *Amer. J. ment. Defic.* **69**, 541.

Donaldson, D.D. (1961) The significance of spotting of the iris in mongoloids. *Arch Ophthal.* **65**, 26.

Donnell, G.N., Ng, W.G., Bergren, W.R., Melnyk, J. & Koch, R. (1965) Enhancement of erythrocyte-galactokinase activity in Langdon-Down trisomy. *Lancet* **1**, 553.

Donner, M. (1954) An investigation into immunological reactions and antibody production in mongolism. *Ann. Med. exp. Fenn.* **32**, Supp. 9.

le Double, A.F. (1903) *Traité des variations des os du crâne de l'homme.* Paris.

Dow, R.S. (1951) A preliminary study of periodontoclasia in mongolian children at Polk State School. *Amer. J. ment. Defic.* **55**, 535.

Doxiades, L. & Portius, W. (1938) Zur Ätiologie des Mongolismus unter besonderer Berücksichtigung der Sippenbefunde. *Z. Konst.-Lehre* **21**, 384.

Doxiadis, S., Pantelakis, S. & Valaes, T. (1970) Down's syndrome and infectious hepatitis. *Lancet* **1**, 897.

Drescher, J., Halsband, H., Brunck, H.-J. & Tolksdorf, M. (1968) Abnorme Hamatopoese mit hepatosplenomegalie bei Neugeborenen mit Down-Syndrom. *Z. Kinderheilk.* **104**, 135.

Drillien, C.M. (1961) A longitudinal study of the growth and development of prematurely and maturely born children. *Arch. Dis. Childh.* **36**, 233.

Drillien, C.M. & Wilkinson, E.M. (1964a) Mongolism: when should parents be told? *Brit. med. J.* **2**, 1306.

Drillien, C.M. & Wilkinson, E.M. (1964b) Emotional stress preceding mongoloid births. *Develop. Med. Child. Neurol.* **6**, 140.

Duillo, M.T. & Serra, G. (1969) Trisomia 21 associata a mosaicismo gonosomico. *Minerva pediat.* **21**, 2196.

Duncan, P.M. (1866) *A manual for the classification, training and education of the feeble-minded, imbecile and idiotic.* London: Longmans, Green & Co.

Dunlap, J.E. (1933) Mongoloid idiocy in a negro infant. *J. Pediat.* **2**, 615.

Dunsdon, M.I., Carter, C.O. & Huntley, R.M.C. (1960) Upper end of range of intelligence in mongolism. *Lancet.* **1**, 565.

Durling, D. & Benda, C.E. (1952) Mental growth curves in untreated institutionalized mongoloid patients. *Amer. J. ment. Defic.* **56**, 578.

Dutton, G. (1959a) The physical development of mongols. *Arch. Dis. Childh.* **34**, 46.

Dutton, G. (1959b) The neutral 17-ketosteroid and 17 ketogenic steroid excretion of mongol and non-mongol mentally defective boys. *J. ment. Defic. Res.* **3**, 103.

Dzenitis, A.J. (1966) Spontaneous atlanto-axial dislocation in a mongoloid child with spinal cord compression. *J. Neurosurg.* **25**, 458.

Earl, C.J.C. (1934) The primitive catatonic psychosis of idiocy. *Brit. J. med. Psychol.* **14**, 230.

Eastham, R.D. & Jancar, J. (1969) Macrocytosis in Down's syndrome. *Lancet* **1**, 895.

Eastham, R.D., Jancar, J. & Duncan, E.H.L. (1965) Plasma viscosity in mental deficiency and Down's syndrome. *Brit. J. Psychiat.* **111**, 999.

Edgren, J., de la Chapelle, A. & Kääriäinen, R. (1966) Cytogenetic study of seventy-three patients with Down's syndrome. *J. ment. Defic. Res.* **10**, 47.

Edwards, J.H. (1963) Unpublished observations.

Edwards, J.H. (1970) The epidemiology of mongolism: experience in Birmingham. *Ann. N.Y. Acad. Sci.* **171**, 304.

Efinski, D., Duma, H., Apostolovski, B., Sofijanov, N., Ristevski, B. & Darkovski, S. (1974) Klinefelter's and Down's syndrome in an adolescent with abnormal EEG. *Clin. Genet.* **5**, 81.

Egozcue, J. (1971) Banding patterns of metaphase chromosomes in Down's syndrome. *Lancet* **2**, 662.

Ehrhart, H., Hörmann, W. & Armbröster, E. (1969) Untersuchungen über den Leukocytenstoffwechsel IV. Vergleichende quantitative Bestimmungen von NAD und ATP isolierten Leukocyten und Erythrocyten chronischer und akuter menschlicher Leukämien. *Klin. Wschr.* **47**, 830.

Eicher, E.M. (1973) Translocation trisomic mice: production by female but not male translocation carriers. *Science* **180**, 81.

Eissler, R. & Longenecker, L.P. (1962) The common eye findings in mongolism. *Amer. J. Ophthal.* **54**, 398.

Ek, J.I., Falk, V., Bergman, S. & Reitalu, J. (1961) A male mongoloid with 46 chromosomes. *Lancet* **2**, 526.

El-Alfi, O.S., Smith, P.M. & Biesele, J.J. (1964) Chromosomal breaks in human leucocyte cultures induced by an agent in the plasma of infectious hepatitis patients. *Hereditas* **52**, 285.

Eliachar, E., Ratel, J. & Polet, C. (1958) Erytholeucomyelose et mongolisme. *Sem. Höp. Paris* **34**, 247.

Ellingson, R.J., Eisen, J.D. & Ottersberg, G. (1973) Clinical electroencephalographic observations on institutionalized mongoloids confirmed by karyotype. *Electroenceph. clin. Neurophysiol.* **34**, 193.

Ellingson, R.J., Menolascino, F.J. & Eisen, J.D. (1970) Clinical-EEG relationships in mongoloids confirmed by karyotype. *Amer. J. ment. Defic.* **74**, 645.

Ellis, J.R. (1962) Unpublished observations.

Ellis. J.R. & Penrose, L.S. (1960) Unpublished observations.

Ellis, W.G., McCulloch, J.R. & Corley, C.L. (1974) Presenile dementia in Down's syndrome: ultrastructural identity with Alzheimer's disease. *Neurology (Minneap.)* **24**, 101.

Emanuel, B., Padorr, M.P. & Swenson, O. (1965) Mongolism associated with Hirschsprung's disease. *J. Pediat.* **66**, 437.

Emanuel, I., Huang, S.-W. & Yeh, E.-K. (1968) Physical features of Chinese children with Down's syndrome. *Amer. J. Dis. Child.* 115, 461.

Emanuel, I., Sever, L.E., Milham, S. & Thuline, H.C. (1972) Accelerated ageing in young mothers of children with Down's syndrome. *Lancet,* 2, 361.

Emberger, J. (1967) Etude cytogénétique de 78 trisomies 21. *J. Méd. Montpellier* 2, 33.

Engel, R.R., Hammond, D., Eitzman, D.V., Pearson, H. & Krivit, W. (1964) Transient congenital leukemia in 7 infants with mongolism. *J. Pediat.* 65, 303.

Engel, W., Reinwein, H., Müller, I. & Kunze, G. (1970) Chromosomenbefunde bei 365 Patienten mit Down-Syndrom oder Verdacht auf Down-Syndrom. *Humangenetik,* 8, 307.

Engler, M. (1949) *Mongolism (peristatic amentia).* Bristol and London: John Wright & Son Ltd.

Erbs, R.C. & Smith, G.F. (1962) Unpublished observations.

Erdtmann, B., de Freitas, A.G., de Souza, R.P. & Salzano, F.M. (1971) Klinefelter's syndrome and G trisomy. *J. med. Genet.* 8, 364.

Erne, H. (1953) *Uber das Papillarleistensystem und die Palmarfurchen in Familien mit einem oder mehreren Fällen von Mongolismus und ein Beitrag zum Problem der Vierfingerfurche.* M.D. Thesis, Zürich.

Esen, F.M. (1957) Congenital heart malformations in mongolism with special reference to ostium atrioventriculare commune. *Arch. Pediat.* 74, 243.

Esquirol, J.E.D. (1838) *Des maladies mentales considerés sous les rapports médical, hygiénique et médico-légal.* 2 vols. *Paris: Baillière.*

Evans, D.I.K. & Steward, J.K. (1972) Down's syndrome and leukaemia. *Lancet* 2, 1322.

Evans, E.P., Ford, C.E., Chaganti, R.S.K., Blank, C.E. & Hunter, H. (1970) XY spermatocytes in an XYY male. *Lancet* 1, 719.

Evans, H.J. & Adams, A. (1973) X-ray-induced chromosome aberrations in human lymphocytes irradiated in vitro: the influence of exposure conditions, genotype and age on aberration yields. In *Advances in radiation research (Proc. Fourth Int. Congr. Radiat. Res., 1970).* J.F. Duplan & A. Chapiro, eds. New York: Gordon & Breach, Science Publishers Inc.

Evans, P.R. (1950) Cardiac anomalies in mongolism. *Brit. Heart J.* 12, 258.

van Eys, J. & Flexner, J.M. (1969) Transient spontaneous remission in a case of untreated congenital leukemia. *Amer. J. Dis. Child.* 118, 507.

Fabia, J. (1969) Illegitimacy and Down's syndrome. *Nature, Lond.* 221, 1157.

Fabia, J. & Drolette, M. (1970a) Life tables up to age 10 for mongols with and without congenital heart defect. *J. ment. Defic. Res.* 14, 235.

Fabia, J. & Drolette, M. (1970b) Malformations and leukemia in children with Down's syndrome. *Pediatrics* 45, 60.

Falls, H.F. (1970) Ocular changes in mongolism. *Ann. N.Y. Acad. Sci.* 171, 627.

Fanconi, G. (1939) Die Mutationstheorie des Mongolismus. *Schweiz. med. Wschr.* 20, 995.

Fang, T.C. (1950) The third interdigital patterns on the palms of the general British population, mongoloid and non-mongoloid mental defectives. *J. ment. Sci.* 96, 780.

Fantham, H.B. (1925) Some factors in eugenics, together with notes on some South African cases. *S. Afr. J. Sci.* 22, 400.

Farquhar, J.W. (1962) Diabetic children in Scotland and the need for care. *Scot. med. J.* 7, 119.

Fennell, C.H. (1904) Mongolian imbecility. *J. ment. Sci.* 50, 32.

Ferguson-Smith, M.A. & Handmaker, S.D. (1961) Observations on the satellited chromosomes. *Lancet* 1, 638.

Ferguson-Smith, M.E., Ferguson-Smith, M.A., Nevin, N.C. & Stone, M. (1971) Chromosome analysis before birth and its value in genetic counselling. *Brit. med. J.* 4, 69.

Ferrier, S. (1964) Enfant mongolien–parent mosaïque. *J. Génét. hum.* **13**, 315.

Fialkow, P.J. (1964) Autoimmunity: a predisposing factor to chromosomal aberrations. *Lancet* **1**, 474.

Fialkow, P.J. (1970) Thyroid autoimmunity and Down's syndrome. *Ann. N.Y. Acad. Sci.* **171**, 500.

Fialkow, P.J., Martin, G.M. & Sprague, C.A. (1973). Replicative life-span of cultured skin fibroblasts from young mothers of subjects with Down's syndrome: failure to detect accelerated ageing. *Amer. J. hum. Genet.* **25**, 317.

Fialkow, P.J., Thuline, H.C., Hecht, F. & Bryant, J. (1971) Familial predisposition to thyroid disease in Down's syndrome: controlled immunoclinical studies. *Amer. J. hum. Genet.* **23**, 67.

Fialkow, P.J., Uchida, I., Hecht, F. & Motulsky, A.G. (1965) Increased frequency of thyroid autoantibodies in mothers of patients with Down's syndrome. *Lancet* **2**, 868.

Fielding, D.W. & Walker, S. (1972) Dyzygotic twins with Down's syndrome. *Arch. Dis. Childh.* **47**, 971.

Finch, R.A., Böök, J.A., Finley, W.H., Finley, S.C. & Tucker, C.C. (1966) Meiosis in trisomic Down's syndrome. *Ala. J. med. Sci.* **3**, 117.

Finley, W.H., Finley, S.C., Hardy, J.P. & McKinnon, T. (1968) Down's syndrome in mother and child. *Obstet. Gynec.* **32**, 200.

Finley, W.H., Finley, S.C., Rosecrans, C.J. & Tucker, C.C. (1966) Normal/21-trisomy mosaicism: report of four cases and review of the subject. *Amer. J. Dis. Child.* **112**, 444.

Fisher, D.A., Oddie, T. & Wait, J.C. (1964) Thyroid function tests. *Amer. J. Dis. Child.* **107**, 282.

Fisher, R.A. (1936) The use of multiple measurements in taxonomic problems. *Ann. Eugen, Lond.* **7**, 179.

Fishler, K., Share, J. & Koch, R. (1964) Adaptation of Gesell developmental scales for evaluation of development in children with Down's syndrome (mongolism). *Amer. J. ment. Defic.* **68**, 642.

Fitzgerald, P.H. & Lycette, R.R. (1961) Mosaicism in man involving the autosome associated with mongolism. *Heredity* **16**, 509.

Fluck, E.R. & Pritham, G.H. (1964) Biochemical studies in mongolism III. Structures of gamma globulins from mongoloid blood. *Amer. J. ment. Defic.* **69**, 31.

Fonkalsrud, E.W., de Lorimier, A.A. & Hays, D.M. (1969) Congenital atresia and stenosis of the duodenum. *Pediatrics* **43**, 79.

Forabosco, A., Dutrillaux, B., Toni, G. & Lejeune, J. (1973) Enfant trisomique 21 libre et translocation t(14q22q) maternelle. *Ann. Génét.* **16**, 57.

Ford, C.E. (1960a) Human cytogenetics: its present place and future possibilities. *Amer. J. hum. Genet.* **12**, 104.

Ford, C.E. (1960b) Chromosomal abnormality and congenital malformation. *CIBA Found. Symp. Congenital Malformations*, p. 32. London: J. & A. Churchill Ltd.

Ford, C.E. (1967) Discussion in *Mongolism—Ciba Foundation Study Group No. 25*, p. 71. London: J. & A. Churchill Ltd.

Ford, C.E. & Hamerton, J.L. (1956) The chromosomes of man. *Nature, Lond.* **168**, 1020.

Ford, C.E., Hamerton, J.L. & Sharman, G.B. (1957) Chromosome polymorphism in the common shrew. *Nature, Lond.* **180**, 392.

Ford, C.E., Jones, K.W., Miller, O.J., Mittwoch, U., Penrose, L.S., Ridler, M. & Shapiro, A. (1959a) The chromosomes in a patient showing both mongolism and the Klinefelter syndrome. *Lancet* **1**, 709

Ford, C.E., Polani, P.E., Briggs, J.H. & Bishop, P.M.F. (1959b) A presumptive human XXY/XX mosaic. *Nature, Lond.* **183**, 1030.

Ford Walker, N. (1945) Personal communication.

Ford Walker, N. (1957) The use of dermal configurations in the diagnosis of mongolism. *J. Pediat.* **50**, 19 and 27.

Ford Walker, N. (1958) The use of dermal configurations in the diagnosis of mongolism. *Pediat. Clin. N. Amer.* (May), p. 531.

Ford Walker, N., Carr, D.H., Sergovich, F.R., Barr, M.L. & Soltan, H.C. (1963) Trisomy−21 and 13−15/21 translocation chromosome patterns in related mongol defectives. *J. ment. Defic. Res.* 7, 150.

Ford Walker, N. & Johnson, H. McC. (1964) Comparative studies of the dermatoglyphics of Italian patients with Down's syndrome. *Proc. Int. Copenhagen Cong. Sci. Study Ment. Retard.* 2, 767.

Forssman, H. (1965) Personal communication.

Forssman, H. & Åkesson, H.O. (1965a) Mortality in patients with Down's syndrome. *J. ment. Defic. Res.* 9, 146.

Forssman, H. & Åkesson, H.O. (1965b) Personal communication.

Forssman, H. & Åkesson, H.O. (1966) Consanguineous marriages and mongolism. *Mongolism—Ciba Foundation Study Group No. 25*, p. 23. London: J. & A. Churchill Ltd.

Forssman, H. & Åkesson, H.O. (1967) Note on mortality in patients with Down's syndrome. *J. ment. Defic. Res.* 11, 106.

Forssman, H. & Lehmann, O. (1961) Translocation-carrying phenotypically normal males and the Down's syndrome. *Lancet* 1, 1286.

Forssman, H., Lehmann, O. & Thysell, E. (1961) Reproduction in mongolism: chromosome studies and re-examination of a child. *Amer. J. ment. Defic.* 65, 495.

Forssman, H. & Thysell, T. (1957) A woman with mongolism and her child. *Amer. J. ment. Defic.* 62, 500.

Forteza Bover, G. & Báguena Candela, R. (1965) Citogenetica de las oligofrenias. *Med. esp.* 53, 357.

Fortune, T.A. (1962) Mentally handicapped children: the parents' view. *Lancet* 1, 161.

Fowler, I. & Hollingsworth, D.R. (1973) Response to stimulation in vitro of lymphocytes from patients with Down's syndrome. *Proc. Soc. exp. Biol. (N.Y.)* 144, 475.

Foxton, J.R.V., Pitt, D., Wiener, S., Brasch, J. & Ferguson, J. (1965) Reproduction in a female with Down's syndrome. *Aust. Paediat. J.* 1, 176.

Fraccaro, M., Kaijser, K. & Lindsten, J. (1960) Chromosomal abnormalities in father and mongol child. *Lancet* 1, 724.

Fraccaro, M., Tiepolo, L., Lindsten, J., Hultén, M., Linné, T. & Andrews, D. (1967) DNA replication patterns of chromosomes numbers 21-22 in female mosaic mongols. *Mongolism—Ciba Foundation Study Group No. 25*, p. 62. London: J. & A. Churchill, Ltd.

Franchi, L., Mandl, A.M. & Zuckerman, S. (1962) *The ovary.* London: Academic Press.

Francis, S.H. (1970) Behavior of low-grade institutionalized mongoloids: changes with age. *Amer. J. ment. Defic.* 75, 92.

Francis, S.H. (1971) The effects of own-home and institution rearing on the behavioural development of normal and mongol children. *J. Child Psychol.* 12, 173.

Fraser, J. & Mitchell, A. (1876) Kalmuck idiocy: report of a case with autopsy with notes on 62 cases by A. Mitchell. *J. ment. Sci.* 22, 161.

Freier, S. (1962) "Mongolian spot." *Lancet* 1, 49.

Friedman, A. (1955) Radioiodine in children with mongolism. *Pediatrics* 16, 55.

Friedman, J.M., Sternberg, W.H., Varela, M. & Barclay, D.L. (1970) Trisomy-21 in mother and child—report of a case. *Obstet. Gynec.* 36, 731.

Friedrich, U. & Nielsen, J. (1973) Chromosome studies in 5,049 consecutive newborn children. *Clin. Genet.* 4, 333.

Fuchs-Mecke, S. & Passarge, E. (1972) Kinder von Müttern mit Down-Syndrom (Mongolismus). *Dtsch. med. Wschr.* 97, 338.

Fujiwara, S. (1973) Studies of lymphoblastoid cell lines derived from Down's syndrome. 1. Establishment of lymphoblastoid cell lines and their characteristics. *Jap. J. clin. Hemat.* 14, 868.

Fujiwara, S. (1974) Studies of lymphoblastoid cell lines derived from Down's syndrome. 2. Long-term karyological analyses of lymphoblastoid cell lines. *Jap. J. clin. Hemat.* 15, 598.

Fuller, R.W., Luce, M. & Mertz, E.T. (1962) Serum uric acid in mongolism. *Science* 137, 868.

Fulton, R.T. & Lloyd, L.L. (1968) Hearing impairment in a population of children with Down's syndrome. *Amer. J. ment. Defic.* 73, 298.

Gagnon, J., Katyk-Longtin, N., de Groot, J.A. & Barbeau, A. (1961) Double trisomie autosomique á 48 chromosomes (21 + 18). *Un. Méd. Can.* 90, 1220.

Gall, J., Garn, S.M., Harper, M. & Stimson, C.W. (1970) Non-random chromosome losses in Down's syndrome. *Nature, Lond.* 227, 499.

Galbraith, P.R. & Valberg, L.S. (1966) Granulopoiesis in Down's syndrome. *Pediatrics* 37, 108.

Galton, F. (1892) *Finger-prints.* London: Macmillan & Co.

Galton, F. (1895) *Finger-print directories.* London: Macmillan & Co.

Gardiner, P.A. (1967) Visual defects in cases of Down's syndrome and in other mentally handicapped children. *Brit. J. Ophthal.* 51, 469.

Gardner, R.J.M., Veale, A.M.O., Parslow, M.I., Becroft, D.M.O., Shaw, R.L., Fitzgerald, P.H., Hutchings, H.E., McCreanor, H.R., Wong, J., Eiby, J.R., Howarth, D.A., & Whyte, S.E. (1973) A survey of 972 cytogenetically examined cases of Down's syndrome. *N.Z. med. J.* 78, 403.

Garn, S.M., Gall, J.C. & Nagy, J.M. (1972) Brachymesophalangia-5 without cone-epiphysis mid-5 in Down's syndrome. *Amer. J. phys. Anthrop.* 36, 253.

Garrod, A.E. (1894) On the association of cardiac malformations with other congenital defects. *St. Barth. Hosp. Rep.* 30, 53.

Garrod, A.E. (1898) Case illustrating the association of congenital heart disease with the mongolian type idiocy. *Trans. clin. Soc. Lond.* 31, 316.

Garrod, A.E. (1899) Cases illustrating the association of congenital heart disease with "mongolian form of idiocy" *Trans. clin. Soc. Lond.* 32, 6.

Garrod, A.E. & Langmead, F. (1906) A case of associated congenital malformations, including transposition of viscera. *Trans. clin. Soc. Lond.* 39, 131.

Garson, O.M., Baikie, A.G., Pitt, D.B. & Newmann, N.M. (1970) Down's syndrome with translocation-en-tandem: a report of two unrelated cases. *Aust. Paediat. J.* 6, 53.

Gates, R. R. (1908) A study of reduction in *Oenothera rubrinervis. Bot. Gaz.* 46, 1.

Gayton, W.F. & Walker, L. (1974) Down's syndrome: informing the parents. A study of parental preferences. *Amer. J. Dis. Child.* 127, 510.

Gekiauskas, M.A. & Cohen, M.M. (1970) Mesiodistal crown diameters of permanent teeth in Down's syndrome (mongolism). *Amer. J. ment. Defic.* 14, 563.

van Gelderen, H.H. & Dooren, L.J. (1963) Somatosexual maturation in mentally deficient children. *Acta paediat.* 52, 557.

van Gelderen, H.H. & Hustinx, T.W.J. (1961) Combinatie van het Klinefelter-syndrom met mongolisme. *Ned. T. Geneesk.* 105, 1925.

Geneva Conference (1966) Standardization of procedures for chromosome studies in abortion. *Cytogenetics* 5, 361.

Gerald, B.E. & Silverman, F.C. (1965) Normal and abnormal interorbital distances, with special reference to mongolism. *Amer. J. Roentgenol.* 95, 154.

Gerald, P.S. (1963) Unpublished observations.

Gerard, Y., Ségal, Ph. & Bedoucha, J.-S. (1971) l'instabilité de l'atlas sur l'axis dans le mongolisme. *Presse méd.* 79, 573.

Gerbie, A.B., Nadler, H.L. & Gerbie, M.V. (1971) Amniocentesis in genetic counselling: safety and reliability in early pregnancy. *Amer. J. Obstet. Gynec.* 109, 765.

Germain, D., Monnet, P., Roux, J.-F., Salle, B., Rosenberg, D., Berger, Cl. & David, M. (1967) Les leucoblastoses transitories de la trisomie 2l. (A propos d'une observation). *Ann. Pédiat.* 43, 504.

German, J. (1968) Mongolism, delayed fertilization and human sexual behaviour. *Nature, Lond.* 217, 516.

German, J.L. & Bearn, A.G. (1962) Personal communication.

German, J.L., deMayo, A.P. & Bearn, A.G. (1962) Inheritance of an abnormal chromosome in Down's syndrome (mongolism) with leukemia. *Amer. J. hum. Genet.* 14, 31.

Gershoff, S.N., Hegsted, D.M. & Trulson, M.F. (1958) Metabolic studies of mongoloids. *Amer. J. clin. Nutr.* 6, 526.

Gertner, M., Hsu, L.Y.F., Martin, J. & Hirschhorn, K. (1970) The use of amniocentesis for prenatal genetic counseling. *Bull. N.Y. Acad. Med.* 46, 916.

Geyer, H. (1939) *Zur Atiologie der mongoloiden Idiotie.* Leipzig: Georg Thieme Verlag.

Giannelli, F., Hamerton, J.L. & Carter, C.O. (1965) Cytogenetics of Down's syndrome (mongolism). II. The frequency of interchange trisomy in patients born at a maternal age of less than 30 years. *Cytogenetics* 4, 186.

Gibson, D. & Frank, H.F. (1961) Dimensions of mongolism. I. Age limits for cardinal mongol stigmata. *Amer. J. ment. Defic.* 66, 30.

Gibson, D. & Gibbins, R.J. (1958) The relation of mongolian stigmata to intellectual status. *Amer. J. ment. Defic.* 63, 345.

Gibson, D. & Pozsonyi, J. (1965) Morphological and behavioral consequences of chromosome subtype in mongolism. *Amer. J. ment. Defic.* 69, 801.

Gifford, H. (1928) The "mongolian" eye. *Amer. J. Ophthal.* 11, 887.

Gilbert, H.D., Smith, R.E., Barlow, M.H. & Mohr, D. (1973) Congenital upper eyelid eversion and Down's syndrome. *Amer. J. Ophthal.* 75, 469.

Giraud, F., Hartung, M., Mattei, J.F. & Mattei, M.G. (1974) t(7q-;21q+) et trisomie 21 familiale. *Ann. Génét.* 17, 49.

Giraud, P., Bernard, R., Stahl, A., Giraud, F., Hartung, M. & Lebeuf, M. (1963) Mosaique chromosomique chez un mongolienne avec un Q.I. a 0.85. *Pédiatrie* 18, 753.

Glanville, E.V. (1964) Mongolism: a clue to the source of the accessory chromosome? *Lancet* 2, 1065.

Glogowska, I. (1969) Mozaika 47/48 u pacjenta z zespolem Downa. *Neurol. Neurochir. Pol.* 3, 263.

Glovsky, L. (1966) Audiological assessment of a mongoloid population. *Trng. Schl. Bull.* 63, 27.

Goddard, H.H. (1914) *Feeble-mindedness, its causes and consequences.* New York: Macmillan Co.

Goodman, H.O. & Thomas, J.J. (1966) ABO frequencies in mongolism. *Ann. hum. Genet., Lond.* 30, 43.

Gordon, A.M. (1944) Some aspects of sensory discrimination in mongolism. *Amer. J. ment. Defic.* 49, 55.

Gordon, M.C., Sinha, S.K. & Carlson, S.D. (1971) Antibody responses to influenza vaccine in patients with Down's syndrome. *Amer. J. ment. Defic.* 75, 391.

Gordon, R.G. & Roberts, J.A.F. (1938) Paraplegia and mongolism in twins. *Arch. Dis. Childh.* 13, 79.

Goring, C. (1913) *The English convict. A statistical study.* London: H.M.S.O.

Gosman, S.D. (1951) Facial development in mongolism. *Amer. J. Orthodont.* 37, 332.

Graivier, L. & Sieber, W.K. (1966) Hirschsprung's disease and mongolism. *Surgery* 60, 458.

Gray, J.E., Mutton, D.E. & Ashby, D.W. (1962) Pericentric inversion of chromosome 21: a possible further cytogenic mechanism in mongolism. *Lancet* 1, 21.

Greenberg, R.C. (1964) Some factors in the epidemiology of mongolism. *Proc. Int. Copenhagen Cong. Sci. Study ment. Retard.* 1, 200.

Greene, E.L., Shenker, R. & Karelitz, S. (1968) Serum protein fractions in patients with Down's syndrome (mongolism). *Amer. J. Dis. Child.* 115, 599.

Gregory, L., Williams, R. & Thompson, E. (1972) Leucocyte function in Down's syndrome and acute leukaemia. *Lancet* 1, 1359.

Greig, D.M. (1927) Skulls of mongolian imbeciles. *Edinb. med. J.* 34, 253 and 321.

Greulich, W.W. (1973) A comparison of the dysplastic middle phalanx of the fifth finger in mentally normal caucasians, mongoloids, and negroes with that of individuals of the same racial groups who have Down's syndrome. *Amer. J. Roentgenol.* 118, 259.

von Greyerz-Gloor, R.D., Auf der Maur, P. & Bergemann, E. (1969a) Zytogenetische und phänomenologische Untersuchungen an 272 Mongoloiden des Kantons Bern. *Schweiz. med. Wschr.* 99, 1151.

von Greyerz-Gloor, R.D., Auf der Maur, P. & Riedwyl, H. (1969b) Beurteilung des diagnostichen Wertes der Finger–und Handleistenmerkmale von Mongoloiden unter Anwendung einer Diskriminanz analyse. *Humangenetik.* 8, 195.

Griffiths, A.W. & Behrman, J. (1967) Dark adaptation in mongols. *J. ment. Defic. Res.* 11, 23.

Griffiths, A.W., Rundle, A.T. & Stewart, A. (1965) Liver function and hepatitis in mongolism. *Amer. J. ment. Defic.* 69, 805.

Griffiths, A.W. & Sylvester, P.E. (1967) Mongols and non-mongols compared in their response to active tetanus immunisation. *J. ment. Defic. Res.* 11, 263.

Gripenberg, U. & Airaksinen, E. (1964) A D/F translocation in a case of regular trisomy 21 Down's syndrome. *Cytogenetics* 3, 219.

Gripenberg, U., Elfving, J. & Gripenberg, L. (1972) A 45,XX,21-child: attempt at a cytological and clinical interpretation of the karyotype. *J. med. Genet.* 9, 110.

Gross, F. (1959) Hochgradige angeborene Duodenalstenose bei einem 18 jährigen mongoloiden Idioten. *Med. Mschr.* 13, 507.

Grosse, K.P., Hopfengartner, F. & Schwanitz, G. (1971) Doppelte aneuploidie: 46,XX/45,XO/47,XX,G+. Kasuistische mitteilung. *Humangenetik,* 13, 333.

Grotz, R.T., Henderson, N.D. & Katz, S. (1972) A comparison of the functional and intellectual performance of phenylketonuric, anoxic and Down's syndrome individuals. *Amer. J. ment. Defic.* 76, 710.

de Grouchy, J., Emerit, I., de Gennes, J.-L. & Vernant, P. (1965a) Syndrome de Klinefelter chez un garçon trisomique 21 agé de six ans. *Presse Med.* 73, 1209.

de Grouchy, J., Frézal, J., Britan, A., Jammett, M. & Lamy, M. (1965b) Remaniement d'un chromosome X, 6-12 chez un trisomique 21. *Ann. Génét.* 8, 67.

de Grouchy, J. & Roubin, M. (1965) Cinq cas de translocation dans un echantillon de 57 trisomiques 21. *Ann. Génét.* 8, 65.

de Grouchy, J., Royer, P. & Frézal, J. (1970) 21p-maternal en double exemplaire chez un trisomique 21. *Ann. Génét.* 13, 52.

de Grouchy, J., Thieffry, S., Arthuis, M., Gerbaux, J., Poupinet, S., Salmon, Ch. & Lamy, M. (1964) Chromosome marqueurs familiaux et aneuploidie. Rôle possible de l'interaction chromosomique. *Ann. Génét.* 7, 76.

Grove, L. & Rasmussen, E. (1950) Congenital atresia of the small intestine, with report of cases. *Ann. Surg.* 131, 869.

Grüneberg, H. (1963) *The pathology of development: a study of inherited skeletal disorders in animals.* Oxford: Blackwell Scientific Publications.

Grunnet, I., Howitz, J., Reymann, F. & Schwartz, J. (1970) Vitiligo and pernicious anemia. *Arch Derm. Syph. (Chic.)* 101, 82.

Gruter, V.B., Trapp, A.L. & Sanger, V.L. (1965) A lymphocytosis-stimulating substance in mongoloid plasma. *Nature, Lond.* 207, 306.

Gustavson, K.-H. (1962) Chromosomal translocation in a mongoloid girl with some atypical features. *Acta paediat., Uppsala* 51, 337.

Gustavson, K.-H. (1964) *Down's syndrome: a clinical and cytogenetical investigation.* Uppsala: Almquist & Wiksell.

Gustavson, K.-H., Atkins, L. & Patricks, I. (1964) Diverse chromosomal anomalies in two siblings. *Acta paediat., Uppsala* 53, 371.

Gustavson, K.-H. & Ek, J.I. (1961) Triple stem-line mosaicism in mongolism. *Lancet* 2, 319.

Gustavson, K.-H., Wetterberg, L., Bäckström, M. & Ross, S.B. (1973) Catechol-O-methyltransferase activity in erythrocytes in Down's syndrome. *Clin. Genet.* 4, 279.

Haberland, C. (1969) Alzheimer's disease in Down's syndrome: clinical-neuropathological observations. *Acta neurol. belg.* 69, 369.

Haberland, C. (1970) Subacute sclerosing panencephalitis in Down's syndrome. *J. ment. Defic. Res.* 14, 106.

Haberlandt, W.F. & Wunderlich, C. (1972) Down-Syndrom mit ganz Uberwiegend normalen karyotyp in der Lymphocytenkultur, aber ausgeprägter G-Trisomie in der Fibroblastenkultur. *Ärztl. Fschg.* 26, 309.

Halbertsma, T. (1923) Mongolism in one of twins and the etiology of mongolism. *Amer. J. Dis. Child.* 25, 350.

Haldane, J.B.S. (1952) Simple tests for bimodality and bitangentiality. *Ann. Eugen., Lond.* 16, 359.

Haldane, J.B.S. (1956) The estimation and significance of the logarithm of a ratio of frequencies. *Ann. hum. Genet., Lond.* 20, 309.

Halevi, H.S. (1967) Congenital malformations in Israel. *Brit. J. prev. soc. Med.* 21, 66.

Halikowski, B., Armata, J., Depowski, M. & Kurowska-Taylor, A. (1968) A case of acute blood disease in an infant with Down's syndrome. *Pediat. pol.* 43, 1157.

Hall, B. (1962) Down's syndrome (mongolism) with normal chromosomes. *Lancet* 2, 1026.

Hall. B. (1964) *Mongolism in newborns: a clinical and cytogenetic study.* Lund: Berlingska Boktryckeriet.

Hall, B. (1966) Follow-up investigation of new-born mongoloids with respect to growth retardation. *Hereditas (Lund)* 56, 99.

Halloran, K.H., Breg, W.R. & Mahoney, M.J. (1974) 21 monosomy in a retarded female infant. *J. med. Genet.* 11, 386.

Hamerton, J.L. (1962) Cytogenetics of mongolism. *Chromosomes in medicine.* London: National Spastics Society Medical and Educational Unit and W. Heinemann Medical Books.

Hamerton, J.L. (1968) Robertsonian translocations in man: evidence for prezygotic selection. *Cytogenetics* 7, 260.

Hamerton, J.L. (1971a) *Human cytogenetics.* Vol. 1: *General cytogenetics;* Vol. II: *Clinical cytogenetics.* New York & London; Academic Press Inc.

Hamerton, J.L. (1971b) Banding patterns of metaphase chromosomes in Down's syndrome. *Lancet* 2, 709.

Hamerton, J.L., Briggs, S.M., Giannelli, F. & Carter, C.O. (1961a) Chromosome studies in detection of parents with high risk of second child with Down's syndrome. *Lancet* 2, 788.

Hamerton, J.L., Cowie, V., Giannelli, F., Briggs, S.M. & Polani, P.E. (1961b) Differential transmission of Down's syndrome (mongolism) through male and female translocation carriers. *Lancet* 2, 956.

Hamerton, J.L., Giannelli, F. & Carter, C.O. (1963) A family showing transmission of a D/D translocation in a case of regular 21 trisomy syndrome. *Cytogenetics* 2, 194.

Hamerton, J.L., Giannelli, F. & Polani, P.E. (1965) Cytogenetics of Down's syndrome (mongolism). I. Data on a consecutive series of patients referred for genetic counselling and diagnosis. *Cytogenetics* 4, 171.

Hamerton, J.L., Jagiello, G.M. & Kirman, B.H. (1962) Sex chromosome abnormalities in a population of mentally defective children. *Brit. med. J,* 1, 220

Hamerton, J.L. & Steinberg, A.G. (1962) Progeny of D/G translocation heterozygote in familial Down's syndrome. *Lancet* 1, 1407.

Hamm, C.W., Solomon, I. & Robertson, W.O. (1963) Personal communication.

Hamolsky, M.W., Stein, M. & Freedberg, A.S. (1957) Thyroid hormone-plasma-protein complex in man. II. New *in vitro* method for study of "uptake" of labelled hormonal components by human erythrocytes. *J. clin. Endocr.* 17, 33.

Hanhart, E. (1944) Neue familiäre Fälle von mongoloiden Schwachsinn als Beweis für die Mitwirkung von Erbfaktoren. *Arch. J. Klaus Stift.* 19, 549.

Hanhart, E. (1960a) 800 Fälle von Mongoloidismus in konstitutioneller Betrachtung. *Arch. J. Klaus Stift.* 35, 1.

Hanhart, E. (1960b) Mongoloide Idiotie bei Mutter und zwei Kindern aus Inzesten. *Acta genet. med. (Roma)* 9, 112.

Hanhart, E., Delhanty, J.D.A. & Penrose, L.S. (1961) Trisomy in mother and child. *Lancet* 1, 403.

Harlap, S. (1974) A time-series analysis of the incidence of Down's syndrome in West Jerusalem. *Amer. J. Epidem.* 99, 210.

Harnden, D.G., Court Brown, W.M., Bond, J. & Mantle, D.J. (1964) Sex chromosome abnormalities in newborn babies. *Lancet* 1, 286.

Harnden, D.G., Miller, O.J. & Penrose, L.S. (1960) The Klinefelter-mongolism type of double aneuploidy. *Ann. hum. Genet., Lond.* 24, 165.

Harris, H., Robson, E.B. & Siniscalco, M. (1959) Genetics of plasma protein variants. *Ciba Found. Symp. Biochemistry of Human Genetics,* p. 151. London: J. & A. Churchill Ltd.

Harris, R., Timson, J. & Wentzel, J. (1969) The HL-A leucocyte system in Down's syndrome. *Transplant. Proc.* 1, 122.

Harris, W.S. & Goodman, R.M. (1968) Hyperactivity to atropine in Down's syndrome. *New Engl. J. Med.* 279, 407.

Hashem, N. & Sakr, R. (1963) Mongolism among Egyptian children. *Proc. 2nd Int. Cong. ment. Retard., Vienna* 1, 387.

Haubold, H., Loew, W. & Haefele-Niemann, R. (1960) Moglichkeiten und Grenzen einer Nachreifungsbehandlung entwicklungsgehemmter, inbesonderes mongoloider Kinder. *Landarzt* 36, 378.

Hauschka, T.S., Hasson, J.E., Goldstein, M.N., Koepf, G.F. & Sandberg, A.A. (1962) An XYY man with progeny indicating familial tendency to non-disjunction. *Amer. J. hum. Genet.* 14, 22.

Hayakawa, H., Matsui, I., Higurashi, M. & Kobayashi, N. (1968) Hyperblastic response to dilute P.H.A. in Down's syndrome. *Lancet* 1, 95.

Hayashi, T. (1962) Personal communication.

Hayashi, T. (1963) Karyotyping analysis of 83 cases of Down's syndrome in Harris County, Texas. *Tex. Rep. Biol. Med.* 31, 28.

Hayashi, T., Hsu, T.C. & Chao, D. (1962) A case of mosaicism in mongolism. *Lancet* 1, 218.

Hayles, A.B., Hinrichs, W.L. & Tauxe, W.N. (1965) Thyroid disease among children with Down's syndrome (mongolism.) *Pediatrics* 36, 608.

Haynes, S.G., Gibson, J.B. & Kurland, L.T. (1974) Epidemiology of neural-tube defects and Down's syndrome in Rochester, Minnesota, 1935-1971. *Neurology (Minneap.)* 24, 691.

Hecht, F., Bryant, J.S., Gruber, D. & Townes, P.L. (1964) The nonrandomness of chromosomal abnormalities: association of trisomy 18 and Down's syndrome. *New Engl. J. Med.* 271, 1081.

Hecht, F., Bryant, J.S., Motulsky, A.G. & Giblett, E.R. (1963) The No. 17–18 (E) trisomy syndrome. *J. Pediat.* 63, 605.

Hecht, F., Case, M.P., Louvrien, E.W., Higgins, J.V., Thuline, H.C. & Melnyk, J. (1968) Nonrandomness of translocations in man: Preferential entry of chromosomes into 13-15/21 translocations. *Science* 161, 371.

Hecht, F., Delay, M., Seely, J.R. & Stoddard, G.R. (1970) Meiotic evidence in Down's syndrome for 21/21 chromosome translocation or isochromosome. *J. Pediat.* 76, 298.

Hecht, F., McCaw, B.K., Howard, P.N., Stoddard, G. & Seely, J.R. (1973) 21/21 translocation: correlation of banding with meiotic results. *Humangenetik,* 20, 269.

Hecht, F., Nievaard, J.E., Duncanson, N., Miller, J.R., Higgins, J.V., Kimberling, W.J., Walker, F.A., Smith, G.S., Thuline, H.C. & Tischler, B. (1969) Double aneuploidy: the frequency of XXY in males with Down's syndrome. *Amer. J. hum. Genet.* 21, 352.

Hedberg, E., Holmdahl, K., Pehrson, S. & Zackrisson, U. (1963) On relationships between maternal conditions during pregnancy and congenital malformations: preliminary report. *Acta paediat. (Uppsala)* 52, 353.

Hefke, H.W. (1940) Roentgenologic study of anomalies of the hand in one hundred cases of mongolism. *Amer. J. Dis. Child.* 60, 1319.

Heiner, D.C., Sears, J.W. & Kniker, W.T. (1962) Multiple precipitins to cow's milk in chronic respiratory disease. *Amer. J. Dis. Child.* 103, 634.

Hellmann, P. (1909) Anatomische Studien über das Mongolengehirn. *Arch. Kinderheilk.* 49, 329.

Henderson, S.A. & Edwards, R.G. (1968) Chiasma frequency and maternal age in mammals. *Nature, Lond.* 218, 22.

Herring, R.M., Phillips, J., Goodman, H.O. & King, J.S. (1967) Enzymes in Down's syndrome. *Lancet* 1, 1157.

Herrman, C. (1905) Important differential points in the diagnosis of sporadic cretinism, mongolism, achondroplasia and rachitis. *Arch. Pediat.* 22, 493.

Herrman, C. (1925) Mongolian imbecility as an anthropologic problem. *Arch. Pediat.* 42, 523.

Higurashi, M., Matsui, I., Nakagome, Y. & Naganuma, M. (1969) Down's syndrome: chromosome analysis in 321 cases in Japan. *J. med. Genet.* 6, 401.

Hiles, D.A., Hoyme, S.H. & McFarlane, F. (1974) Down's syndrome and strabismus. *Amer. orthopt. J.* 24, 63.

Hill, W.B. (1908) Mongolism and its pathology: an analysis of eight cases. *Quart. J. Med.* 2, 49.

Himwich, H.E. & Fazekas, J.F. (1940) Cerebral metabolism in mongolian idiocy and phenylpyruvic amentia. *Arch. Neurol. Psychiat.* 44, 1213.

Himwich, H.E., Fazekas, J.F. & Nesin, S. (1940) Brain metabolism in mongolian idiocy and phenylpyruvic oligophrenia. *Amer. J. ment Defic.* 45, 37.

Hinden, E. (1961) Personal communication.

Hirning, L.C. & Farber, S. (1934) Histologic study of the adrenal cortex in mongolism. *Amer. J. Path.* 10, 435.

Hirsch, W., Bender, K., Mayerova, A., Riehm, H., Ritter, H. & Tariverdian, G. (1974) Down's syndrome in twins with discordant HL-A phenotypes. *Humangenetik* 21, 255.

Hirsch, W., Leichsenring, G. & Lüers, Th. (1967) Klinische und Hautleisten-Befunde bei Down-Syndrom mit Chromosomenmosaik (Mosaik-Mongolismus) *Mschr. Kinderheilk.* 115, 516.

Hirschhorn, K., Cooper, H.L. & Meyer, L.M. (1961) *2nd Int. Conf. Hum. Genet., Rome 1961.* Amsterdam: Excerpta Medica Foundation.

Hjorth, B. (1907) On the etiology of mongolism. *J. ment. Sci.* 53, 182.

Hoffman-Credner, D. & Zweymüller, E. (1957) Radiologunsuchungen der Schilddrüsenfunktion bei Zerebral-gestörten Kindern. *Wien. klin. Wschr.* 69. 60.

Holland, W.W., Doll, R. & Carter, C.O. (1962) Mortality from leukaemia and other cancers among patients with Down's syndrome (mongols) and among their parents *Brit. J. Cancer* 16, 177.

Hollien, H. & Copeland, R.H. (1965) Speaking fundamental frequency (SFF) characteristics of mongoloid girls. *J. Speech Dis.* **30,** 344.

Holmgren, G. & Ånséhm, S. (1971) The trisomy 21 and the trisomy 17−18 syndromes in siblings. *Hum. Hered.* **21,** 577.

Holt, S.B. (1951) A comparative quantitative study of the finger-prints of mongol imbeciles and normal individuals. *Ann. Eugen., Lond.* **15,** 355.

Holt, S.B. (1959) The correlations between ridge-counts on different fingers estimated from a population sample. *Ann. hum. Genet., Lond.* **23,** 459.

Holt, S.B. (1961) Quantitative genetics of finger-print patterns. *Brit. med. Bull.* **17,** 247.

Holt, S.B. (1964a) Finger-print patterns in mongolism. *Ann. hum. Genet., Lond.* **27,** 279.

Holt, S.B. (1964b) Current advances in our knowledge of the inheritance of variations in finger prints. *Proc. Int. Conf. hum. Genet., Rome* **3,** 1450.

Holt, S.B. (1968) *The genetics of dermal ridges.* Springfield: Charles C. Thomas.

Holt, S.B. (1970) Dermatoglyphics in mongolism. *Ann. N.Y. Acad. Sci.* **171,** 602.

Honda, F., Punnett, H.H., Charney, E., Miller, G. & Thiede, A. (1964) Serial cytogenetic and hematologic studies on a mongol with trisomy-21 and acute congenital leukemia. *J. Pediat.* **65,** 880.

Hongell, K. & Airaksinen, E. (1972) A Gq deletion in a girl with Down's syndrome. *Hum. Hered.* **22,** 80.

Hongell, K., Gripenberg, W. & Iivanainen, M. (1972) Down's syndrome: incidence of translocation in Finland. *Hum Hered.* **22,** 7.

Hook, E.B. & Engel, R.R. (1964) Leucocyte life-span, leucocyte alkaline phosphatase and the 21st chromosome. *Lancet* **1,** 112.

Horns, J.W. & O'Louglin, B.J. (1965) Multiple manubrial ossification centers in mongolism. *Amer. J. Roentgenol.* **93,** 395.

Horrobin, J.M. & Rynders, J.E. (1974) *To give an edge: a guide for new parents of Down's syndrome (mongoloid) children.* Minneapolis: Colwell Press Inc.

Howells, W.W. (1957) The cranial vault: factors of size and shape. *Amer. J. phys. Anthrop.* **15,** 19.

Hoyle, C.M. & Franklin, A.W. (1954) Incidence of the third fontanelle: relation to mongolism. *Lancet* **1,** 437.

Hsia, D.Y.-Y., Inouye, T., Wong, P. & South, A. (1964) Studies on galactose oxidation in Down's syndrome. *New Engl. J. Med.* **270,** 1085.

Hsia, D.Y.-Y., Justice, P., Smith, G.F. & Dowben, R.M. (1971) Down's syndrome: a critical review of the biochemical and immunological data. *Amer. J. Dis. Child.* **121,** 153.

Hsu, L.Y.F., Dubin, E.C., Kerenyi, T. & Hirschhorn, K. (1973) Results and pitfalls in prenatal cytogenetic diagnosis. *J med. Genet.* **10,** 112.

Hsu, L.Y.F., Gertner, M., Leiter, E. & Hirschhorn, K. (1971a) Paternal trisomy 21 mosaicism and Down's syndrome. *Amer. J. hum. Genet.* **23,** 592.

Hsu, L.Y.F., Hirschhorn, K., Goldstein, A. & Barcinski, M.A. (1970a) Familial chromosomal mosaicism, genetic aspects. *Ann. hum. Genet., Lond.* **33,** 343.

Hsu, L.Y., Schwager, A.J., Nemhauser, I. & Sobel, E.H. (1965) A case of double autosomal trisomy with mosaicism: 48/XX (trisomy 18+21) and 46/XX. *J. Pediat.* **66,** 1055.

Hsu, L.Y.F., Shapiro, L.R., Gertner, M., Lieber, E. & Hirschhorn, K. (1971b) Trisomy 22: a clinical entity. *J. Pediat.* **79,** 12.

Hsu, L.Y.F., Shapiro, L.R. & Hirschhorn, K. (1970b) Meiosis in an XYY male. *Lancet* **1,** 1173.

Huang, S.-W., Emanuel, I., Lo, J., Liao, S.-K. & Hsu, C.-C. (1967) A cytogenetic study of 77 Chinese children with Down's syndrome. *J. ment. Defic. Res.* **11,** 147.

Huët, G.J. (1932) Uber eine bisher unbekannte familiäre Anomalie der Leukocyten. *Klin. Wschr.* **11,** 1264.

Hug, E. (1951) Das Geschlechtsverhältnis beim Mongolismus. *Ann. Paediat.* 177, 31.

Hultén, M. (1970) Meiosis in XYY men. *Lancet* 1, 717.

Hultén, M. & Lindsten, J. (1970) The behaviour of structural aberrations at male meiosis. Information from man. In *Human population cytogenetics.* P.A. Jacobs, W.H. Price & P. Law, eds., p. 22. Edinburgh: Pfizer Medical Monographs (5).

Hultgren, E.O. (1915) Studien über die Häufigkeit der mongoloiden Idiotie in schwedischen Anstalten für Schwachsinnige und über die Atiologie dieser Krankheit. *Nord. Med. Ark.* 48, 1.

Hungerford, D.A., Mellman, W.J., Balaban, G.B., La Badie, G.V., Messatzzia, L.R. & Haller, G. (1970) Chromosome structure and function in man. III. Pachytene analysis and identification of the supernumerary chromosome in a case of Down's syndrome (mongolism). *Proc. nat. Acad. Sci. (Wash.)* 67, 221.

Hunt, N. (1967) *The world of Nigel Hunt—the diary of a mongoloid youth.* Beaconsfield, England: Darwen Finlayson Ltd.

Hustinx, T.W.J. (1963) Two cases of Down's syndrome with a translocation. *Human Chromosome Newsletter* (personal communication).

Hustinx, T.W.J. (1966) *Cytogenetisch onderzoek bij enige families.* Thesis, University of Nijmegen.

Hustinx, T.W.J., Eberle, P., Geerts, S.J., ten Brink, J. & Woltring, L.M. (1961) Mongoloid twins with 48 chromosomes. *Ann. hum. Genet., Lond.* 25, 111.

Hutton, A.C. & Smith, G.F. (1964) Haptoglobins and transferrins in patients with Down's syndrome. *Ann. hum. Genet., Lond.* 27, 413.

Hyatt, H.W. (1962) Neonatal duodenal obstruction caused by annular pancreas in two mongoloid children. *J. Amer. med. Ass.* 180, 1128.

Igersheimer, J. (1951) The relationship of lenticular changes to mongolism. *Trans. Amer. ophth. Soc.* 49, 595.

Iinuma, K., Nakagome, Y. & Matsui, I. (1973) 21 trisomy and prenatally diagnosed XXY in two consecutive pregnancies. *Hum. Hered.* 23, 467.

Ikin, E.W., Prior, A.M., Race, R.R. & Taylor, G.L. (1939) The distributions in the $A_1 A_2$ BO blood groups in England. *Ann. Eugen., Lond.* 9, 409.

Ilbery, P.L.T., Lee, C.W.G. & Winn, S.M. (1961) Incomplete trisomy in a mongoloid child exhibiting minimal stigmata. *Med. J. Aust.* 2, 182.

Illing, G. (1939) Beiträge zum Krankheitsbild der mongoloiden Idiotie. *Mschr. Kinderheilk.* 78, 353.

Illingworth, R.S. (1960) *The development of the infant and young child.* Edinburgh and London: E. & S. Livingstone Ltd.

Ingalls, T.H. (1947) Pathogenesis of mongolism. *Amer. J. Dis. Child.* 73, 279.

Ingalls, T.H. (1972) Maternal health and mongolism. *Lancet* 2, 213.

Ingalls, T.H. & Butler, R.L. (1953) Mongolism—implications of the dental anomalies. *New Engl. J. Med.* 248, 511.

Ingalls, T.H. & Henry, T.A. (1968) Trisomy and D/G translocation mongolism in brothers. *New Engl. J. Med.* 278, 10.

Ireland, W.W. (1877) *Idiocy and imbecility.* London: J. & A. Churchill.

Izakovic, V. & Getlik, A. (1969) Mozaika 46,XX/47,XX,G+ u matky dietata s Downovym syndromom trizomiou G_1. *Cs. Pediat.* 24, 698.

Jackim, E., Wortis, J. & Adesman, J. (1961) Triiodothyronine uptake by erythrocytes in mongolism. *Proc. Soc. exp. Biol. N.Y.* 107, 401.

Jackson, E.W., Turner, J.H., Klauber, M.R. & Norris, F.D. (1968) Down's syndrome: variation of leukemia occurrence in institutionalized populations. *J. chron. Dis.* 21, 247.

Jacobi, H.G. & Rogatz, J.L. (1949) Diabetes mellitus associated with mongolism: a case of a child two years of age. *Amer. J. Dis. Child.* 77, 659.

Jacobs, P.A. (1965) Personal communication.

Jacobs, P.A. (1968) Personal communication.

Jacobs, P.A., Baikie, A.G., Court Brown, W.M. & Strong, J.A. (1959) The somatic chromosomes in mongolism. *Lancet* 1, 710.

Jacobs, P.A. & Strong, J.A. (1959) A case of human intersexuality having possible XXY sex-determining mechanism. *Nature, Lond.* 183, 302.

Jaensch, W. (1930) Die Hautkapillarmikroskopie. *Z. ärzl. Fortbild.* 27, 323.

Jagiello, G. & Taylor, M.B. (1965) Chromosomal studies of two cases of trisomy-21 Down's syndrome with hyperthyroidism. *Amer. J. ment. Defic.* 69, 645.

James, W.H. (1970) Curve fitting, maternal age and mongolism. *Hum. Hered.* 20, 417,

Jansen, M. (1921) *Feebleness of growth and congenital dwarfism.* Oxford: Medical Publications.

Jelgersma, H.C. (1962) Seniele dementie bij mongolisme. *Ned. T. Geneesk.* 106, 2114.

Jelgersma, H.C. (1963) On the tuberflocculi in mongolian idiocy. *Psychiat. Neurol. Neurochir.* 66, 131,

Jenkins, R.L. (1933) Etiology of mongolism. *Amer. J. Dis. Child.* 45, 506.

Jensen, G.M., Cleal, J.F. & Yips, A.S.G. (1973) Dentoalveolar morphology and developmental changes in Down's syndrome (trisomy 21). *Amer. J. Orthodont.* 64, 607.

Jeremy, H.R. (1921) Cataracts in a mongolian idiot. *Brit. J. Child. Dis.* 18, 34.

Jérôme, H. (1962) Anomalies du métabolisme du tryptophane dans la maladie mongolienne. *Bull. Mem. Soc. méd. Hôp. Paris* 113, 168.

Jérôme, H. & Kamoun, P. (1970) Platelet binding of serotonin. *Ann. N.Y. Acad. Sci.* 171, 543.

Jérôme, H., Lejeune, J. & Turpin, R. (1960) Etude de l'excretion urinaire de certains métabolites du tryptophane chez les enfants mongoliens. *C.R. Acad. Sci.* 251, 474.

Jervis, G.A. (1942) Recent progress in the study of mental deficiency mongolism—a review of the literature of the last decade. *Amer. J. ment. Defic.* 46, 467.

Jervis, G.A. (1948) Early senile dementia in mongoloid idiocy. *Amer. J. Psychiat.* 105, 102.

Johnson, C.D. & Barnett, C.D. (1961) Relationship of physical stigmata to intellectual status in mongoloids. *Amer. J. ment. Defic.* 66, 435.

Johnson, N.P. & Young, M.A. (1963) Periodontal disease in mongols. *J. Periodont.* 34, 41.

Johnson, N.P., Young, M.A. & Gallios, J.A. (1960) Dental caries experience of mongoloid children. *J. dent. Child.* 27, 292.

Johnson, R.C. & Abelson, R.B. (1969a) Intellectual, behavioral, and physical characteristics associated with trisomy, translocation and mosaic types of Down's syndrome. *Amer. J. ment. Defic.* 73, 852.

Johnson, R.C. & Abelson, R.B. (1969b) The behavioral competence of mongoloid and non-mongoloid retardates. *Amer. J. ment. Defic.* 73, 856.

Johnston, A.W. (1961) The chromosomes in a child with mongolism and acute leukemia. *New Engl. J. Med.* 264, 591.

Johnston, A.W. & Jaslow, R.I. (1963) Children of mothers with Down's syndrome. *New Engl. J. Med.* 269, 439.

Johnston, A.W. & Petrakis, J.K. (1963) Mongolism and Turner's syndrome in the same sibship. *Ann. hum. Genet., Lond.* 26, 407.

Jones, R. (1890) The mouth in backward children of mongolian type. *J. ment. Sci.* 36, 187.

Jørgensen, P.I. & Trolle, D. (1972) Low urinary oestriol excretion during pregnancy in women giving birth to infants with Down's syndrome. *Lancet* 2, 782.

Joseph, M. & Dawburn, C. (1970) *Measurement of the facies: a study in Down's syndrome.* Spastics International Medical Publications Research Monograph No. 3. London: Heinemann Ltd.

Juberg, R.C. & Davis, L.M. (1970) Etiology of nondisjunction: lack of evidence for genetic control. *Cytogenetics* 9, 284.

Juberg, R.C. & Jones. B. (1970) The Christchurch chromosome (Gp-). Mongolism, erytholeukemia and an inherited Gp- chromosome (Christchurch). *New Eng. J. Med.* 282, 292.

Julku, M, Kivalo, E. & Paatero, Y.V. (1962) Tutkimus mongoloidien leukojen ja hampaisten rakenteesta. *Suom. Hammastääk. Toim* 58, 4.

Kääriäinen, R. & Dingman, H.F. (1961) The relationship of the degree of mongolism to the degree of subnormality. *Amer. J. ment. Defic.* 66, 438.

Kaback, M.M. & Bernstein, L.H. (1970) Biologic studies of trisomic cells growing *in vitro. Ann. N.Y. Acad. Sci.* 171, 526.

Kaczmarczyk, T. (1964) Przyczynek do niektorych zagadinien stomatologicznych u dzieci z zespolem Downa. *Czas. Stomat.* 17, 433.

Kadotani, T., Ohama, K. & Makino, S. (1970a) A case of 21-trisomic Down's syndrome from the triplo-X mother. *Proc. Jap. Acad.* 46, 709.

Kadotani, T., Ohama, K., Takahara, H., Nagai, I., Shimizu, B. & Makino, S. (1970b) A case of Down's syndrome associated with G/G translocation. *Proc. Jap. Acad.* 46, 858.

Kahn, J. & Abe, K. (1969) Consistent and variable chromosome anomalies in parents of children with Down's syndrome. *J med. Genet.* 6, 137.

Kajii, T., Ohama, K., Niikawa, N., Ferrier, A. & Avirachan, S. (1973) Banding analysis of abnormal karyotypes in spontaneous abortion. *Amer. J. hum. Genet.* 25, 539.

Kaplan, B.J. (1955) Mongolism in the Bantu, including a case report. *S. Afr. med. J.* 29, 1041.

Kaplan, S., Li, C.C., Wald, N. & Borges, W. (1964) ABO frequencies in mongols. *Ann. hum. Genet., Lond.* 27, 405.

Kashgarian, M. & Rendtorff, R.C. (1969) Incidence of Down's syndrome in American Negroes. *J. Pediat.* 74, 468.

Kassowitz, M. (1902) Infantiles Mÿxödem, Mongolismus und Mikromelie. *Wien, med. Wschr.* 52, 1202, 1256 and 1301.

Kato, K. (1935) Leucocytes in infancy and childhood. *J. Pediat.* 7, 7.

Kaufmann, H.J. & Taillard, W.F. (1961) Pelvic abnormalities in mongols. *Brit. med. J.* 1, 948.

Kearns, J.E. & Hutson, W.F. (1951) Use of radioactive iodine studies in congenital thyroid aplasia; differentiation between mongoloid and cretinoid child at birth. *Quart. Bull. Northw. Univ. med. Sch.* 25, 270.

Keay, A.J. (1958) The significance of twins in mongolism in the light of new evidence. *J. ment. Defic. Res.* 2, 1.

Kedziora, J., Hübner, H., Kanski, M., Jeske, J. & Leyko, W. (1972) Efficiency of the glycolytic pathway in erythocytes of children with Down's syndrome. *Pediat. Res.* 6, 10.

Keegan, D.L., Pettigrew, A. & Parker, Z. (1974) Psychosis in Down's syndrome treated with amitriptyline. *Canad. med. Ass. J.* 110, 1128.

Keele, D.K., Richards, C., Brown, J. & Marshall, J. (1969) Catecholamine metabolism in Down's syndrome. *Amer. J. ment. Defic.* 74, 125.

Keith, J.D., Rowe, R.D. & Vlad, P. (1958) *Heart disease in infancy and childhood.* London: Macmillan Co.

Kelch, R.P., Franklin, M. & Schmickel, R.D. (1971) Group G deletion syndromes. *J. med. Genet.* 8, 341.

Kerkay, J., Zsako, S. & Kaplan, A.R. (1971) Immunoelectrophoretic serum patterns associated with mothers of children affected with the G_1-trisomy syndrome (Down's syndrome). *Amer. J. ment. Defic.* 75, 729.

Kersting, D.W. & Rapaport, I.F. (1958) A clinopathologic study of the skin in mongolism. *Arch. Derm. (Chic.)* 77, 319.

Kerwood, L.A., Lang-Brown, H. & Penrose L.S. (1954) The interpupillary distance in mentally defective patients. *Hum. Biol.* 26, 313.

Keynes, G. (1932) Blood grouping in mongolian imbeciles. *Lancet* 1, 480.

Kiil, V. (1948) Frontal hair direction in mentally deficient individuals, with special reference to mongolism. *J. Hered.* **39**, 281.

Kilcoyne, R.F. & Taybi, H. (1970) Conditions associated with congenital megacolon. *Amer. J. Roentgenol.* **108**, 615.

King, M.J., Gillis, E.M. & Baikie, A.G. (1962) The polymorph alkaline phosphatase in mongolism. *Lancet* **2**, 661.

Kiossoglou, K.A., Garrison, M., Walker, A. & Wolman, I.J. (1963a) The leukocyte, differential and polymorphonuclear lobe counts in mongols and in "organic" mental retardation. *J. ment. Defic. Res.* **7**, 69.

Kiossoglou, K., Rosenbaum, E., Mitus, W.J. & Dameshek, W. (1963b) Multiple chromosome aberrations in Down's syndrome associated with twinning and acute granulocytic leukaemia. *Lancet* **2**, 944.

Kirman, B.H. (1951) Epilepsy in mongolism. *Arch. Dis. Childh.* **26**, 501.

Kirman, B.H. (1953) The backward baby. *J. ment. Sci.* **99**, 531.

Kisling, E. (1966) *Cranial morphology in Down's syndrome: a comparative roentgencephalometric study in adult males.* Copenhagen: Munksgaard.

Kisling, E. & Krebs, G. (1963) Paradontale forhold hos voksne patienter med Down's syndrom. *Tandlaegebladet* **67**, 101.

Kjessler, B. & de la Chapelle, A. (1971) Meiosis and spermatogenesis in two postpubertal males with Down's syndrome: 47,XY,G+. *Clin. Genet.* **2**, 50.

Kleisner, E.H., Galan, H.M. & Vasquez, H.J. (1966) Chromosome analysis of 16 mongol patients. *Human Chromosome Newsletter* **19**, 23. (personal communication.

Kluge, W. (1959) Leucocytic shift to the left in mongolism, with observations on segmentation inhibition and the Pelger-Huët anomaly. *J. ment. Defic. Res.* **3**, 56.

Koch, G. (1973) *Down-syndrom—Mongolismus.* Erlangen: Hogl.

Koch, R. & Dobson, J.C. (Ed.) (1971) *The mentally retarded child and his family: a multidisciplinary handbook.* New York: Brunner/Mazel.

Koch, R., Share, J. & Graliker, B. (1965) The effects of cytomel on young children with Down's syndrome (mongolism): a double-blind longitudinal study. *J. Pediat.* **66**, 776.

Koch, R., Share, J., Webb, A. & Graliker, B.V. (1963) The predictability of Gesell developmental scales in mongolism. *J. Pediat.* **62**, 93.

Kogon, A., Kronmal, R. & Peterson, D.R. (1968) The relationship between infectious hepatitis and Down's syndrome. *Amer. J. publ. Hlth.* **58**, 305.

Kohn, G., Taysi, K., Atkins, T.E. & Mellman, W.J. (1970) Mosaic mongolism. I. Clinical correlations. *J. Pediat.* **76**, 874.

Koivikko, A. (1970) Ventriculoradial dysplasia in a mongoloid infant. *Ann. clin. Res.* **2**, 79.

Komoto, J. (1892) The mongolian eye. *J. Amer. med. Ass.* **18**, 361.

Kontras, S.B., Currier, G.J., Cooper, R.F. & Ambuel, J.P. (1966) Maternal transmission of a 21/1 translocation associated with Down's syndrome. *J. Pediat.* **69**, 635.

Kouvalainen, K. & Österlund, K. (1967) Placental weights in Down's syndrome. *Ann. Med. exp. Fenn.* **45**, 320

Kovalesky, P. (1906) Type mongol de l'idiotie. *Ann. Méd. Psych.* **4**, 431.

Kreezer, G.L. (1939) Research in progress upon the electroencephalogram in mental deficiency. *Proc. Amer. Ass. Ment. Defic.* **44**, 120.

Kretschmer, R.R., López-Osuna, M., de la Rosa, L. & Armendares, S. (1974) Leukocyte function in Down's syndrome: quantitative NBT reduction and bactericidal capacity. *Clin. Immun. Immunopath.* **2**, 449.

Krivit, W. & Good, R.A. (1956) The simultaneous occurrence of leukemia and mongolism. Report of four cases. *Amer. J. Dis. Child.* **91**, 218.

Krivit, W. & Good, R.A. (1957) Simultaneous occurrence of mongolism and leukemia. Report of a nation wide survey. *Amer. J. Dis. Child.* **94**, 289.

Krmpotic, E. & Hardin, M.B. (1971) Secondary nondisjunction causing regular trisomy 21 in the offspring of the mosaic trisomy 21 mother. *Amer. J. Obstet. Gynec.* 110, 589.

Krone, W. & Brunschede, H. (1965) UDPG-4-epimerase activity in human fibroblasts in cell culture. *Humangenetik* 2, 192.

Krone, W., Wolf, U., Goedde, H.W. & Baitsch, H. (1964) Enhancement of erythrocyte-galactokinase activity in Langdon-Down trisomy, *Lancet* 2, 590.

Kučera, J. (1969) Age at walking, age at eruption of deciduous teeth and response to ephedrine in children with Down's syndrome. *J. ment. Defic. Res.* 13, 143.

Kučera, J. (1971) Infectious hepatitis and Down's syndrome. *Lancet* 1, 549.

Kučerova, M. (1967) Comparison of radiation effects *in vitro* upon chromosomes of human subjects. *Acta radiol.* 6, 441.

Kugel, R.B. & Reque, D. (1961) A comparison of mongoloid children. *J. Amer. med. Ass.* 175, 959.

Kung, F., Smith, G.F. & Helmken, J. (1970) Erythroleukemia and mongolism. Unpublished observations.

Kuni, C.C. (1973) Extra-adrenal pheochromocytoma with metastasis in Down's syndrome. *J. Pediat.* 83, 835.

Kurland, G.S., Fishman, J., Hamolsky, M.W. & Freedberg, A.S. (1957) Radioisotope study of thyroid function in 21 mongoloid subjects including observations in seven parents. *J. clin. Endocr.* 17, 552.

Lahdensuu, S. (1937) Über Vorkommen und Ätiologie der Idiota mongoloidea im Lichte des in Finnland gesammelten Materials. *Acta paediat., Stockh.* 21, 256.

Lahey, M.E., Beier, F.R. & Wilson, J.F. (1963) Leukemia in Down's syndrome. *J. Pediat.* 63, 189.

La Marche, P.H., Heisler, A.B. & Kronemer, N.S. (1967) Disappearing mosaicism. *R.I. med. J.* 50, 184.

Lander, E., Forssman, H. & Åkesson, H.O. (1964) Season of birth and mental deficiency. *Acta genet. (Basel)* 14, 265.

Landsteiner, K. & Levine, P. (1929) On the racial distribution of some agglutinable structures of human blood. *J. Immunol.* 16, 123.

Lang-Brown, H., Lawler, S.D. & Penrose, L.S. (1953) The blood typing of cases of mongolism, their parents and sibs. *Ann. Eugen., Lond.* 17, 307.

Langdon Down, J. (1866) Observations on an ethnic classification of idiots. *Clin. Lectures and Reports, London Hospital* 3, 259.

Langdon Down, J. (1887) *Mental affections of childhood and youth.* London: J. & A. Churchill.

Langdon-Down, R.L. (1909) Discussion following Shuttleworth's paper. *Brit. med. J.* 2, 665.

Lange, C.F., Justice, P. & Smith, G.F. (1974) Milk precipitins in mongolism. *Chem. Path. Pharm.* 7, 605.

Lanman, J.H., Sklarin, B.S., Cooper, H.L. & Hirschhorn, K. (1960) Klinefelter's syndrome in a ten-month-old mongolian idiot: report of a case with chromosome analysis. *New Engl. J. Med.* 263, 887.

Lanman, T.H. (1949) Discussion on intestinal obstruction. *Ann. Surg.* 130, 509.

Lashof, J.C. & Stewart, A. (1965) Oxford survey of childhood cancers. Progress report III: leukaemia and Down's syndrome. *Mth. Bull. Minist. Hlth. (Lond.)* 24, 136.

Lassen, N.A., Christensen, S., Hoedt-Rasmussen, K. & Stewart, B.M. (1966) Cerebral oxygen consumption in Down's syndrome. *Arch. Neurol. (Chic.)* 15, 595.

Laurent, C. & Robert, J.M. (1966) Ségrégation d'une translocation D/G "en tandem" sur trois générations. *Ann. Génét.* 9, 134.

Laurent, C. & Robert, J.M. (1968) Translocation t(2q-;21q+) sur trois générations. *Ann. Génét.* 11, 28.

Lawler, S.D. (1962) Genes on the mongol chromosome. *Lancet* 2, 837.

Lawrence, R.D. (1942) Three diabetic mongol idiots. *Brit. med. J.* 1, 695.

Laxova, R., McKeown, J.A., Saldaña, P. & Timothy, J.A.D. (1971) A case of XYY Down's syndrome confirmed by autoradiography. *J. med. Genet.* 8, 215.

Layzer, R.B. & Epstein, C.J. (1972) Phosphofructokinase and chromosome 21. *Amer. J. hum. Genet.* 24, 533.

Leck, I. (1966) Incidence and epidemicity of Down's syndrome. *Lancet* 2, 457.

Lee, L.G. & Jackson, J.F. (1972) Diagnosis of Down's syndrome: clinical vs. laboratory. *Clin. Pediat.* 11, 353.

Lehmann, O. & Forssman, H. (1960) Klinefelter's syndrome and mongolism in the same person. *Acta paediat., Uppsala* 49, 536.

Lehmann, O. & Forssman, H. (1962) Chromosome studies in eleven families with mongolism in more than one member. *Acta paediat., Stockh.* 51, 180.

Leibovitz, A. & Yannet, H. (1942) The production of humoral antibodies by the mongolian. *Amer. J. ment. Defic.* 46, 304.

Lejeune, J. (1964) The 21 trisomy—current stage of chromosomal research. *Progress in Medical genetics* 3. New York: Grune & Stratton.

Lejeune, J. (1966) Aberrations chromosomiques et cancer. *Proc. 9th Int. Cancer Congr., Tokyo.* p. 71.

Lejeune, J., Berger, R., Haines, M., Lafourcade, J., Vialatte, J., Satge, P. & Turpin, R. (1963) Constitution d'une clone á 54 chromosomes au cours d'une leucoblastose chez une enfant mongolienne. *C.R. Acad. Sci.* 256, 1195.

Lejeune, J., Berger, R., Rethore, M., Archambault, L., Jérome, H., Thieffry, S., Aicardi, J., Broyer, M., Lafourcade, J., Cruveillier, J. & Turpin, R. (1964) Monosomie partielle pour un petit acrocentrique. *C.R. Acad. Sci.* 259, 4187.

Lejeune, J., Berger, R., Vidal, O.R. & Rethore, M.O. (1965) Un cas de translocation G~G en tandem. *Ann. Génét.* 8, 60.

Lejeune, J., Gautier, M. & Turpin, R. (1959a) Les chromosomes humains en culture de tissus. *C.R. Acad. Sci.* 248, 602.

Lejeune, J., Gautier, M. & Turpin, R. (1959b) Etudes des chromosomes somatiques de neuf enfants mongoliens. *C.R. Acad. Sci.* 248, 1721.

Lele, K.P. (1964) Personal communication.

Lelong, M, Borniche, P., Kreisler, L. & Baudy, R. (1949) Mongolien issu de mère mongolienne. *Arch. franç. Pédiat.* 6, 231.

Lennox, B., White, H. St C. & Campbell, J. (1962) The polymorph alkaline phosphatase in mongolism. *Lancet* 2, 991.

Lenz, W., Nowakowski, H., Prader, A. & Schirren, C. (1959) Die Ätiologie des Klinefelter-Syndromes. *Schweiz. med. Wschr.* 89, 727.

Lesch, M. & Nyhan, W.L. (1964) A familial disorder of uric acid metabolism and central nervous system function. *Amer. J. Med.* 36, 561.

Levan, A. & Hsu, T.C. (1959) The human idiogram. *Hereditas (Lund)* 45, 665.

Levan, A. & Hsu, T.C. (1960) The chromosomes of a mongoloid female, mother of a normal boy. *Hereditas (Lund)* 46, 770.

Levinson, A., Friedman, A. & Stamps, F. (1955) Variability of mongolism. *Pediatrics* 16, 43.

Lewis, E.B. & Gencarella, W. (1952) Claret and non-disjunction in *Drosophila melanogaster. Genetics* 37, 600.

Licznerski, G. & Lindsten, J. (1972) Trisomy 21 in man due to maternal nondisjunction during the first meiotic division. *Hereditas (Lund)* 70, 153.

Lilienfeld, A.M. (1969) *Epidemiology of mongolism.* Baltimore: John Hopkins Press.

Lind, J., Vuorenkoski, V., Rosberg, G., Partanen, T.J. & Wasz-Höckert O. (1970) Spectrographic analysis of vocal response to pain stimuli in infants with Down's syndrome. *Develop. Med. Child Neurol.* 12, 237.

Lindsten, J., Alvin, A., Gustavson, K.-H. & Fraccaro, M. (1962) Chromosomal mosaic in a girl with some features of mongolism. *Cytogenetics* 1, 20.

Littlefield, J.W., Milunsky, A. & Jacoby, L.B. (1971) Prenatal genetic diagnosis: present and future developments. *Proc. 4th Int. Congr. Hum. Genet., Paris.*

Liu, M.C. & Corlett, K. (1959) A study of congenital heart defects in mongolism. *Arch. Dis. Childh.* 34, 410.

Loeffler, F. & Smith, G.F. (1964) Unpublished observations.

Loesch-Mdzewska, D. (1968) Some aspects of the neurology of Down's syndrome. *J. ment. Defic. Res.* 12, 237.

Loftus, J. & Mellman, W.J. (1965) Chromosome studies performed at the cytogenetics laboratory, Children's Hospital of Philadelphia, 1964. *Human Chromosome Newsletter* 15, 14. (personal communication).

Loftus, J. & Mellman, W.J. (1966) Chromosome studies performed at the cytogenetics laboratory, Children's Hospital of Philadelphia, 1965. *Human Chromosome Newsletter* 18, 12. (personal communication).

Lopez, V. (1974) Serum IgE concentration in trisomy 21. *J. ment. Defic. Res.* 18, 111.

Lopez, V., Millar, A. & Thuline, H.C. (1973) Antibody deficiency in trisomy 21 (Abst.). *Clin. Res.* 21, 212.

Lopez, V., Ochs, H.D., Thuline, H.C., Davis, S.D. & Wedgwood R.J. (1975) Defective antibody response to bacteriophage $\emptyset$X 174 in Down's syndrome. *J. Pediat.* 86, 207.

Lötter, C.D. v E. (1955) Mongolism in the Bantu—report of a case. *S. Afr. med. J.* 29, 706.

Louw, J.H. (1952) Congenital duodenal stenosis and mongolism. *S. Afr. med. J.* 26, 521.

Lowe, R.F. (1949) The eyes in mongolism. *Brit. J. Ophthal.* 33, 131.

Lowrey, G.H., Beierwalters, W.H., Lampe, I. & Gomberg, H.J. (1949) Radioiodine uptake curve in humans. II. Studies in children. *Pediatrics* 4, 627.

Lu, K.H. (1968) An information and discriminant analysis of fingerprint patterns pertaining to identification of mongolism and mental retardation. *Amer. J. hum. Genet.* 20, 24.

Luder, J. & Musoke, L.K. (1955) Mongolism in Africans. *Arch. Dis. Childh.* 30, 310.

Lundin, L.G. & Gustavson, K.-H. (1962) Urinary BAIB excretion in Down's syndrome (mongolism). *Acta genet., Basel* 12, 156.

Luthardt, F.W. & Palmer, C.G. (1971) X chromosome long arm deletion in a patient with Down's syndrome. *J. med. Genet.* 8, 387.

Lyle, J.G. (1959) The effect of an institution environment upon the verbal development of imbecile children. I. Verbal intelligence. *J. ment. Defic. Res.* 3, 122.

Lyle, J.G. (1960) The effect of an institution environment upon the verbal development of imbecile children. II. Speech and language. *J. ment. Defic. Res.* 4, 1.

Lynch, M.R. (1960) *Our exceptional son, Chris.* Boston: Daughters of St. Paul.

McClure, H.M., Belden, K.H., Pieper, W.A. & Jacobson, C.B. (1969) Autosomal trisomy in a chimpanzee: resemblance to Down's syndrome. *Science* 165, 1010.

McCormick, D.P., Meyer, W.J. & Nesbit, M.E. (1971) Coexistence of Hodgkin's disease and Down's syndrome. *Amer. J. Dis. Child.* 122, 71.

McCoy, E.E. & Chung, S.I. (1964) The excretion of tryptophan metabolites following deoxypyridoxine administration in mongoloid and non-mongoloid patients. *J. Pediat.* 64, 227.

McCoy, E.E., Ebadi, M. & England, J. (1966) Steroid mediated changes of leucocyte alkaline phosphatase activity in Down's syndrome. *Pediatrics* 38, 996.

McCrea, M.G., Heston, J.F., Wood, H.F. & Sullivan, J.E. (1968) Milk precipitins: a serological survey of 932 individuals. *J. Amer. med. Ass.* 203, 557.

McDonald, A.D. (1964) Mongolism in twins. *J. med. Genet.* 1, 39.

McDonald, A.D. (1972a) Yearly and seasonal incidence of mongolism in Quebec. *Teratology,* 6, 1.

McDonald, A.D. (1972b) Thyroid disease and other maternal factors in mongolism. *Canad. med. Ass. J.* 106, 1085.

MacFarland, C. (1964) Personal communication.

Macgillivray, R.C. (1967) Epilepsy in Down's anomaly. *J. ment. Defic. Res.* 11, 43.

MacIntyre, M.N., Staples, W.I., Steinberg, A.G. & Hempel, J.M. (1962) Familial mongolism (trisomy—21 syndrome) resulting from a "15/21" chromosome translocation in more than three generations of a large kindred. *Amer. J. hum. Genet.* 14, 335.

MacKaye, L. (1936) Mongolism in non-identical twins. *Amer. J. Dis. Child.* 52, 141.

McMillan, R.S. & Kashgarian, M. (1916) Relation of human abnormalities of structure and function to abnormalities of the dentition. II. Mongolism. *J. Amer. dent. Ass.* 63, 368.

Maas, J.W. (1964) Some biochemical data on children with mongolism. *Int. Copenhagen Cong. Sci. Study Ment. Retard* 1, 211.

Makino, S. (1964) Chromosome studies in patients with congenital and hereditary diseases, developmental deficiencies and sexual abnormalities. *Cytologia (Tokyo)* 29, 125.

Makino, S., Tonomura, A. & Matsunaga, E. (1960) Chromosome studies in ten cases of mongolism. *Proc. Japan. Acad.* 36, 670.

Malamud, N. (1954) Recent trends in classification of neuropathological findings in mental deficiency. *Amer. J. ment. Defic.* 58, 438.

Malamud, N. (1972) Neuropathology of organic brain syndromes associated with aging. In *Aging and the Brain.* C.M. Gaits, ed. New York: Plenum Press.

Malpas, P. (1937) The incidence of human malformations. *J. Obstet. Gynaec. Brit. Emp.* 44, 434.

Malz, W. (1937) Ein Beitrag zur Frage des mongoloiden Idiotie: gibt es einen tatenten Mongolismus? *Mschr. Kinderheilk.* 70, 376.

Malzberg, B. (1950) Some statistical aspects of mongolism. *Amer. J. ment. Defic.* 54, 266.

Marden, P.M., Smith, D.W. & McDonald, M.J. (1964) Congenital anomalies in the newborn infant, including minor variations. *J. Pediat.* 64, 357.

Marks, J.F., Wiggins, K.M. & Spector, B.J. (1967) Trisomy 21—trisomy 18 mosaicism in a boy with clinical Down's syndrome. *J. Pediat.* 71, 126.

Marmol, J.G., Scriggins, A.L. & Vollman, R.F. (1969) Mothers of mongoloid infants in the Collaborative Project. *Amer. J. Obstet. Gynec.* 104, 533.

Marsden, H.B., Mackay, R.I., Murray, A. & Ward, H.E. (1966) Down's syndrome with a familial D/D reciprocal translocation and a G/G chromosome. *J. med. Genet.* 3, 56.

Martel, W. & Tishler, J.M. (1966) Observations on the spine in mongoloidism. *Amer. J. Roentgenol.* 97, 630.

Martel, W., Uyham, R. & Stimson, C.W. (1969) Subluxation of the atlas causing spinal cord compression in a case of Down's syndrome with a "manifestation of an occipital vertebra". *Radiology* 93, 839.

Martin, R. & Saller, K. (1958) *Lehrbuch der Anthropologie,* 5th ed. Stuttgart: Gustav Fischer.

Masland, R.L., Sarason, S.B. & Gladwin, T. (1958) *Mental subnormality.* New York: Basic Books Inc.

Massimo, L., Borrone, C., Vianello, M.G. & Dagna-Bricarelli, F. (1967) Familial immune defects. *Lancet* 1, 108.

Masterson, J.G., Law, E.M., Power, M.M., Stokes, B.M. & Murphy, D. (1970) Reproduction in two females with Down's syndrome. *Ann. Génét.* 13, 38.

Matsaniotis, N., Karpouzas, J. & Economou-Mavrou, C. (1967) Hypothyroidism and seminoma in association with Down's syndrome. *J. Pediat.* 70, 810.

Matsui, I., Nakagome, Y. & Higurashi, M. (1966) Dermatoglyphic study of Down's syndrome in Japan. *Paediat. Univ. Tokyo* 13, 43.

Matsunaga, E. (1964) Down's syndrome in Japan. *Ann. Rep. Nat. Inst. Genet.* 14, 128.

Matsunaga, E. (1967a) Parental age, live-birth order and pregnancy-free interval in

Down's syndrome in Japan. *Mongolism—Ciba Foundation Study Group No. 25,* p. 6. London: J. & A. Churchill Ltd.

Matsunaga, E. (1967b) General discussion. *Mongolism—Ciba Foundation Study Group No. 25,* p. 88. London: J. & A. Churchill Ltd.

Matsunaga, E. & Tonomura, A. (1972) Parental age and birth weight in translocation Down's syndrome. *Ann. hum. Genet.* 36, 209.

Matsuo, N., Oshima, M., Naganuma, M., Shimizu, K., Okada, R. & Sperling, D.R. (1972) Major and minor anomalies in Japanese children with Down's syndrome. *Jap. Heart J.* 13, 307.

Mattelaer, P.M. & Riley, H.D. (1964) Leukemia in the perinatal period. *Ann. paediat. (Basel)* 203, 124.

Mauer, I. & Noe, O. (1964) Triple stem-line chromosomal mosaicism in Down's syndrome (mongolism). *Lancet* 1, 666.

Mautner, H. (1950) Abnormal findings on the spine in mongoloids. *Amer. J. ment. Defic.* 55, 105.

Mayerhofer, E. (1939) Causal connection of curettage for abortion to mongolian idiocy. *Ann. Paediat.* 154, 57.

Medenis, R., Forbes, A. & Rosenthal, I.M. (1962). Mosaicism associated with mongolism. *Soc. Pediat. Res.,* 32nd Annual Meeting, p. 75 (abstr.).

Medovikoff, P.S. (1910) Mongolism of children. *Russk. Vrach. S. Peterb.* 9, 1589.

Méhes, K (1973) Paternal trisomy 21 mosaicism and Down's anomaly. *Humangenetik* 17, 297.

Mehregan, A.H. (1968) Elastosis perforans serpiginosa: a review of the literature and report of 11 cases. *Arch. Derm. (Chic.)* 97, 381.

Melartin, L. & Panelius, M. (1967) Occurrence of Australia antigen in Finnish mongolism patients. *Ann. Med. exp. Fenn.* 45, 157.

Mellman, W.J. (1962) Personal communication.

Mellman, W.J., Oski, F.A., Tedesco, T.A., Maciera-Coelho, A. & Harris, H. (1964) Leucocyte enzymes in Down's syndrome. *Lancet* 2, 674.

Mellman, W.J., Raab, S.O. & Oski, F.A. (1967) Abnormal granulocyte kinetics: an explanation of the atypical granulocyte enzyme activities observed in trisomy 21. *Mongolism—Ciba Foundation Study Group No. 25,* p. 77. London: J. & A. Churchill Ltd.

Mellman, W.J., Younkin, L.H. & Baker, D. (1970) Abnormal lymphocyte function in trisomy 21. *Ann. N.Y. Acad. Sci.* 171, 537.

Mellon, J.P., Pay, B.Y. & Green, D.M. (1963) Mongolism and thyroid auto-antibodies. *J. ment. Defic. Res.* 7, 31.

Melnyk, J., Thompson, H., Rucci, A.J., Vanasek, F. & Hayes, S. (1969) Failure of transmission of the extra chromosome in subjects with 47,XYY karyotype. *Lancet* 2, 797.

Melyn, M.A. & White, D.T. (1973) Mental and developmental milestones of noninstitutionalized Down's syndrome children. *Pediatrics* 52, 542.

Menghi, P. (1954) Osservazioni sull'etá scheletrica nel mongolismo. *Minerva pediat.* 6, 81.

Mengoli, V., Halfer, G., Montenovesi, P. & Lanzoni, E. (1957) Il mongolismo negli aspetti medici e sociali. *Atti XXV Cong. Soc. Ital. Ped., Palermo,* p. 705.

Menolascino, F.J. (1965) Psychiatric aspects of mongolism *Amer. J. ment. Defic.* 69, 653.

Merrit, D.H. & Harris, J.S. (1956) Mongolism and acute leukaemia: a report of four cases. *Amer. J. Dis. Child.* 92, 41.

Mertz, E.T., Fuller, R. W. & Concon, J.M. (1963) Serum uric acid in young mongoloids. *Science* 141, 353.

Meyer, A. & Jones, J. (1939) Histological changes in the brain in mongolism *J. ment. Sci.* 85, 206.

Michel, J.F. & Carney, R.J. (1964) Pitch characteristics of mongoloid boys. *J. Speech Dis.* 29, 121.

Migeon, B.R., Kaufmann, B.N. & Young, W.J. (1962) A chromosome abnormality with centric fragment in a paramongoloid child. *Amer. J. Dis. Child.* 104, 533.

Mikkelsen, M. (1964) Personal communication.

Mikkelsen, M. (1967a) Down's syndrome at young maternal age: cytogenetical and genealogical study of eighty-one families. *Ann. hum. Genet. Lond.* 31, 51.

Mikkelsen, M. (1967b) DNA replication analysis of six 13-15/21 translocation families. *Ann. hum. Genet. Lond.* 30, 325.

Mikkelsen, M. (1970) A Danish survey of patients with Down's syndrome born to young mothers. *Ann. N.Y. Acad. Sci.* 171, 370.

Mikkelsen, M. (1971) Down's syndrome. Current stage of cytogenetic research. *Humangenetik* 12, 1.

Mikkelsen, M. (1974) Rare translocation 47,XY,t(12;21) in Down's syndrome. *Hum. Hered.* 24, 160.

Milcu, St M. & Maicanesco, M. (1963) Syndrome de Klinefelter associe au mongolisme et à l'ectopie testiculaire bilatérale. *Path. et Biol.* 11, 1247.

Milham, S. & Gittelsohn, A.M. (1965) Parental age and malformations. *Hum. Biol.* 37, 13.

Miller, J. McC., Sherrill, J.G. & Hathaway, W.E. (1967) Thrombocythemia in the myeloproliferative disorder of Down's syndrome. *Pediatrics* 40, 847.

Miller, J.R., Dill, F.J., Corey, M.J. & Rigg, J.M. (1970) A rare translocation (47,XY,t(2p-;21q+),21+) associated with Down's syndrome. *J. med. Genet.* 7, 389.

Miller, M.E., Mellman, W.J., Cohen, M.M., Kohn, G. & Dietz, W.H. (1969) Depressed immunoglobulin G in newborn infants with Down's syndrome. *J. Pediat.* 75, 996.

Miller, M.E., Mellman, W.J., Kohn, G. & Dietz, W.H. (1970) Qualitative and quantitative deficiencies of immunoglobulin G(IgG) in newborns with Down's syndrome. *Ann. N.Y. Acad. Sci.* 171, 512.

Miller, M.E., Mellman, W.J., Oski, F.A. & Kohn, G. (1967) Immunoglobulins in Down's syndrome. *Lancet* 2, 257.

Miller, O.J., Breg, W.R., Schmickel, R.D. & Tretter, W. (1961) A family with an XXXXY male, a leukaemia male and two 21-trisomic mongoloid females. *Lancet* 2, 78.

Miller, O.J., Mittwoch, U. & Penrose, L.S (1960) Spermatogenesis in man with special reference to aneuploidy. *Heredity* 14, 456.

Miller, R.W. (1963) Down's syndrome (mongolism), other congenital malformations and cancers among the sibs of leukemic children. *New Engl. J. Med.* 268, 393.

Miller, R.W. (1964) Radiation, chromosomes and viruses in the etiology of leukemia. Evidence from epidemiologic research. *New Engl. J. Med.* 271, 30.

Miller, R.W. (1970) Neoplasia and Down's syndrome. *Ann. N.Y. Acad. Sci.* 171, 637.

Milunsky, A. (1968) Cystic fibrosis and Down's syndrome. *Pediatrics* 42, 501.

Milunsky, A. (1973) *The prenatal diagnosis of hereditary disorders.* Springfield, Ill.: C.C. Thomas.

Milunsky, A. & Fisher, J.H. (1968) Annular pancreas in Down's syndrome. *Lancet* 2, 575.

Milunsky, A., Littlefield, J.W., Kanfer, J.N., Kolodny, E.H., Shih, V.E. & Atkins, L. (1970) Prenatal genetic diagnosis. *New Engl. J. Med.* 283, 1370, 1441 & 1498.

Milunsky, A, & Neurath, P.W. (1968) Diabetes mellitus in Down's syndrome. *Arch. environm. Hlth.* 17, 372.

Mir, G.H. & Cumming, G.R. (1971) Response to atropine in Down's syndrome. *Arch. Dis. Childh.* 46, 61.

Mitchell, A. (1876) *see* Fraser, J. & Mitchell, A.

Mittwoch, U. (1952) The chromosome complement in a mongolian imbecile. *Ann. Eugen., Lond.* 17, 37.

Mittwoch, U. (1957) Some observations on the leucocytes in mongolism. *J. ment. Defic. Res.* 1, 26

Mittwoch, U. (1958a) The leucocyte count in children with mongolism. *J. ment. Sci.* 104, 457.

Mittwoch, U. (1958b) The polymorphonuclear lobe count in mongolism and its relation to the total leucocyte count. *J. ment. Defic. Res.* 2, 75.

Mittwoch, U. (1959) The relationship between the leucocyte count, the "shift to the left" and the incidence of drumsticks in mongolism. *Acta genet. med. (Roma)* Supp. 2, p. 131.

Mittwoch, U. (1964a) Personal communication.

Mittwoch, U. (1964b) Frequency of drumsticks in normal women and in patients with chromosomal abnormalities. *Nature, Lond.* 201, 317.

Mittwoch, U. (1967) DNA synthesis in cells grown in tissue culture from patients with mongolism. *Mongolism—Ciba Foundation Study Group No. 25*, p. 51. London: J. & A. Churchill Ltd.

Mittwoch, U. (1972) Mongolism and sex: a common problem of cell proliferation? *J. med. Genet.* 9, 92.

Miyoshi, I., Yoshimoto, S., Fujiwara, S., Hiraki, K & Kimura, S. (1974) Down's syndrome: establishment of lymphoblastoid cell lines with trisomy 21. *Cancer (Philad.)* 33, 739.

Molloy, J.S. (1972) *Trainable children: curriculum and procedures.* 2nd ed. New York: John Day Co.

Montague, J.C. & Hollien, H. (1973) Perceived voice quality disorders in Down's syndrome children. *J. Communic. Dis.* 6, 76.

Monteleone, P.L., Nadler, H.L., Pi, C.-S. & Hsia, D.Y.-Y. (1967) Isoenzymes in Down's syndrome. *Lancet* 2, 367.

Moore, B.C., Thuline, H.C. & Capes, L. (1968) Mongoloid and non-mongoloid retardates: a behavioral comparison. *Amer. J. ment. Defic.* 73, 433.

Moorhead, P.S., Mellman, W.J. & Wenar, C. (1961) A familial chromosome translocation associated with speech and mental retardation. *Amer. J. hum. Genet.* 13, 32.

de Moragas, J. (1958) Treatment of mongolism with dehydroepiandrosterone. *Rev. Esp. Ped.* 14, 493.

Morgan, T.H., Bridges, C.B. & Sturtevant, A.H. (1925) The genetics of *Drosophila. Bibliographica Genetica* 2, 1.

Mori, W. & Koike, M. (1971) Liver changes in Down's syndrome. *Acta hepato-splenol. (Stuttg.)* 18, 363.

Morić-Petrović, S. & Garzicić, B. (1970) Mother with Down's syndrome and her child. *J. ment. Defic. Res.* 14, 68.

Morić-Petrović, S., Marković, V., Kalicanin, P., Garzicić, B, Ziković, S., Soldatović, B., Marković, S., Despotović, M. & Laća, Z. (1971) Cytogenetic survey of Down's syndrome in Serbia (Yugoslavia): incidence of numerical and structural abnormalities. *J. ment. Defic. Res.* 15, 102.

Morris, R. (1971) Down's syndrome in New Zealand. *N.Z. med. J.* 73, 195.

Mortensson, W. & Hall, B. (1972) Abnormal pelvis in newborn infants with Down's syndrome. *Acta radiol(Stockh.)* 12, 847.

Mosier, H.D. (1965) Presence of the long-acting thyroid stimulator in serum in mongolism without hyperthyroidism. *J. clin. Endocr.* 25, 1005.

Mosier, H.D. (1967) The neck-thigh radioiodine ratio in mongolism. *J. ment. Defic. Res.* 11, 97.

Mosier, H.D. & Dingman, H.F. (1963) Exophthalmometry in mongolism. *J. ment. Defic. Res.* 7, 147.

Muir, J. (1903) An analysis of twenty-six cases of mongolism. *Arch. Pediat.* 20, 161.

Mullins, D.H., Estrada, W.R. & Gready, T.G. (1960) Pregnancy in an adult mongoloid female. *Obstet. Gynec.* 15, 781.

Murphy, M.M. (1956) Comparison of developmental patterns of three diagnostic groups of middle grade and low grade mental defectives. *Amer. J. ment. Defic.* 61, 164.

Murray, J.B., Sylvester, P.E. & Gibson, J. (1966) Rib absence in Down's syndrome. *Lancet* 1, 1375.

Mutton, D.E. (1973) Origin of the trisomic 21 chromosome. *Lancet* 1, 375.

Myers, C.R. (1938) An application of the control group method to the problem of the etiology of mongolism. *Proc. Amer. Ass. ment. Defic.* 43, 142.

Nadler, H.L. (1972) Prenatal detection of genetic disorders. In *Advances in human genetics.* H. Harris & K. Hirschhorn, eds. 3, 1. New York: Plenum Press.

Nadler, H.L., Inouye, T. & Hsia, D.Y.-Y. (1966) Enzymes in trisomy-18 syndrome. *Lancet* 1, 1270.

Nadler, H.L., Inouye, T., Justice, P. & Hsia, D.Y.-Y. (1967a) Enzymes in cultivated human fibroblasts derived from patients with Down's syndrome (mongolism). *Nature, Lond.* 213, 1261.

Nadler, H.L., Monteleone, P.L. & Hsia, D.Y.-Y. (1967b) Enzyme studies during lymphocyte stimulation with phytohemagglutinin in Down's syndrome. *Life Sci.* 6, 2003.

Nadler, H.L., Monteleone, P.L., Inouye, T. & Hsia, D.Y.-Y. (1967c) Lymphocyte and granulocyte enzyme activity in patients with Down's syndrome *Blood* 30, 669.

Nagao, T., Lampkin, B.C. & Hug, G. (1970) A neonate with Down's syndrome and transient abnormal myelopoiesis: serial blood and bone marrow studies. *Blood* 36, 443.

Naiman, J.L., Oski, F.A. & Mellman, W.J. (1965) Phosphokinase activity of erythrocytes in mongolism. *Lancet* 1, 821.

Nakamura, H. (1961) Nature of institutionalized adult mongoloid intelligence. *Amer. J. ment. Defic.* 66, 456.

Nakamura, H. (1965) An inquiry into systematic differences in the abilities of institutionalized adult mongoloids. *Amer. J. ment. Defic.* 69, 661.

Nankin, H.R., Talbott, J.B., Oshima, H., Fan, D.F., Pan, S.F. & Troen, P. (1974) Down and Klinefelter syndromes (48,XXY,G+) in a young man: cytogenetic, endocrine and testicular steroidogenesis studies. *Arch. int. Med.* 134, 352.

Nash, J.A. (1949) Quoted by C.E. Benda in *Mongolism and cretinism.* 2nd ed. New York: Grune & Stratton.

Nelson, T. (1961) Serum protein and lipoprotein fractions in mongolism. *Amer. J. Dis. Child.* 102, 115.

Nelson, T.L. (1964) Spontaneously occurring milk antibodies in mongoloids. *Amer. J. Dis. Child.* 108, 494.

Nelson, T.Y. (1963) Duodenal obstruction in infants and children. *Med. J. Austr.* 2, 709.

Neu, R.L., Bargman, G.J. & Gardner, L.I. (1969) Disappearance of a 47,XX,C+ leucocyte cell line in an infant who had previously exhibited 46,XX/47,XX,C+ mosaicism. *Pediatrics* 43, 623.

Neu, R.L., Scheuer, A.Q. & Gardner, L.I. (1971) A case of 48,XYY,21+ in an infant with Down's syndrome. *J. med. Genet.* 8, 533.

Neumann, H. (1899) Uber den mongoloiden Typus der Idiotie. *Berl. klin. Wschr.* 30, 210.

Neurath, P., De Remer, K., Bell, B., Jarvik, L. & Kato, T. (1970) Chromosome loss compared with chromosome size, age and sex of subjects. *Nature, Lond.* 225, 281.

Neville, J. (1959) Paranoid schizophrenia in a mongoloid defective: some theoretical considerations derived from an unusual case. *J. ment. Sci.* 105, 444.

Newcombe, H.B. & Tavendale, O.G. (1964) Maternal age and birth order correlations. *Mutat. Res.* 1, 446.

Newton, M.S., Cunningham, C., Jacobs, P.A., Price, W.H. & Fraser, I.A. (1972) Chromosome survey of a hospital for the mentally subnormal. Part 2: autosomal abnormalities. *Clin. Genet.* 3, 226.

Ng, W.G., Bergren, W.R. & Donnell, G.N. (1964) Galactose-1-phosphate uridyltransferase assay by use of radioactive galactose-1-phosphate. *Clin. chim. Acta* **10**, 337.

Nichols, W.W., Coriell, L.L., Fabrizio, D.P.A., Bishop, H.C. & Boggs, T.R. (1962) Mongolism with mosaic chromosome pattern. *J. Pediat.* **60**, 69.

Nicholson, D.N. & Keay, A.J. (1957) Mongolism in both of twins of opposite sex. *Arch. Dis. Childh.* **32**, 325.

Nicolis, F.B. & Sacchetti, G. (1963) A nomogram for the X-ray evaluation of some morphological anomalies of the pelvis in the diagnosis of mongolism. *Pediatrics* **32**, 1074.

Niebuhr, E. (1974) Down's syndrome. The possibility of a pathogenetic segment on chromosome No. 21. *Humangenetik* **21**, 99.

Nielsen, J. (1967) Inheritance in monozygotic twins. *Lancet* **2**, 717.

Norman, R.M. (1958) Malformations of the nervous system, birth injury and diseases of early life. *Neuropathology.* London: Edward Arnold & Co.

Novák, A. (1972) The voice of children with Down's syndrome. *Folia phoniat. (Basel)* **24**, 182.

Nowell, P.C. & Hungerford, D.A. (1960) A minute chromosome in human chronic granulocytic leukemia. *Science* **132**, 1497.

Nugent, C.A., MacDiarmid, W.D. & Tyler, F.H. (1962) Renal excretion of uric acid in leukemia and gout. *Arch. intern. Med.* **109**, 540.

O'Brien, D. & Groshek, A. (1962) The abnormality of tryptophan metabolism in children with mongolism. *Arch. Dis. Childh.* **37**, 17.

O'Brien, D., Haake, W. & Braid, B. (1960) Atropine sensitivity and serotonin in mongolism. *Amer. J. Dis. Child.* **100**, 873.

O'Brien, D., Zarins, B. & Jensen, C.B. (1962) The abnormality of tryptophan metabolism in children with mongolism: studies following 3-hydroxy-DL-kynurenine administration. *Proc. Cong. Amer. Soc. Ped. Res.,* p. 122.

O'Brien, R.L., Poon, P., Kline, E. & Parker, J.W. (1971) Susceptibility of chromosomes from patients with Down's syndrome to 7,12-dimethylbenz (a)anthracene-induced aberrations *in vitro. Int. J. Cancer* **8**, 202.

O'Connor, N. & Hermelin, B. (1961) Visual and stereognostic shape recognition in normal children and mongol and non-mongol imbeciles. *J. ment. Defic. Res.* **5**, 63.

O'Connor, N. & Hermelin, B. (1963) *Speech and thought in severe subnormality.* Oxford: Pergamon Press.

O'Donnell, J.J., Hall, B.D., Conte, F.A., Romanowski, J.C. & Epstein, C.J. (1975) Down's syndrome: localization of locus to distal portion of long arm of chromosome 21. *Ped. Res. Abst.* **9**, 315.

Ohara, P.T. (1972) Electron microscopical study of the brain in Down's syndrome. *Brain* **95**, 681.

O'Leary, W.D. (1931) Carbohydrate metabolism in mongoloid idiots as evidence of endocrine dysfunction. *Amer. J. Dis. Child.* **41**, 544.

Oliver, C.A. (1891) A clinical study of the ocular symptoms found in the so-called mongolian type of idiocy. *Trans ophthal. Soc. U.K.* **6**, 140.

Olson, M.I. & Shaw, C.-M. (1969) Presenile dementia and Alzheimer's disease in mongolism. *Brain,* **92**, 147.

Ong., B.H., Rosner, F., Mahanand, D., Houck, J.C. & Paine, R.S. (1967) Clinical, psychological and radiological comparisons of trisomic and translocation Down's syndrome. *Develop. Med. Child Neurol.* **9**, 307.

Oorthuys, A.M.A. & Doesburg, W.H. (1974) Dermatoglyphics in Down's syndrome. IV: Evaluation of the use of dermatoglyphic discriminants after the topological classification of constituent characters. *Clin. Genet.* **5**, 395.

Orel, H. (1927) Zur Klinik der mongoloiden Idiotie. *Z. Kinderheilk.* **44**, 449.

O'Riordan, M.L., Robinson, J.A., Buckton, K.E. & Evans, H.J. (1971) Distinguishing between the chromosomes involved in Down's syndrome (trisomy 21) and chronic myeloid leukaemia (Ph[1]) by fluorescence. *Nature, Lond.* **230**, 167.

Ormond, A.W. (1912) Notes on the ophthalmic condition of forty-two mongolian imbeciles. *Trans. ophthal. Soc. U.K.* 32, 69.

Orner, G. (1971) Congenitally absent permanent teeth among mongols and their sibs. *J. ment. Defic. Res.* 15, 292.

Orner, G. (1973) Eruption of permanent teeth in mongoloid children and their sibs. *J. dent. Res.* 52, 1202.

Orye, E. & Delire, C. (1967) Familial D/D and D/G₁ translocation. *Helv. paediat. Acta* 22, 36.

Osato, T., Kasahara, S. & Nakao, T. (1969) EB antibody levels in patients with Down's syndrome. *Igaku no Ayumi* 71, 119.

Øster, J. (1953) *Mongolism.* Copenhagen: Danish Science Press Ltd.

Øster, J. (1956) The causes of mongolism. *Dan. med. Bull.* 3, 158.

Øster, J., Mikkelsen, M. & Nielsen, A. (1964) The mortality and causes of death in patients with Down's syndrome (mongolism). *Int. Copenhagen Cong. Sci. Study Ment. Retard.* 1, 231.

O'Sullivan, J.B., Reddy, W.J. & Farrell, M.J. (1961) Adrenal function in mongolism. *Amer. J. Dis. Child.* 101, 37.

O'Sullivan, M.A. & Pryles, C.V. (1963) A comparison of leukocyte alkaline phosphatase determinations in 200 patients with mongolism and in 200 "familial" controls. *New Eng. J. Med.* 268, 1168.

Otermin Aguirre, J.A. (1973) Mogolismo y cirugia plastica (sindrome de Down) *Pren. méd. argent.* 60, 970.

Owens, D., Dawson, J.C. & Losin, S. (1971) Alzheimer's disease in Down's syndrome. *Amer. J. ment. Defic.* 75, 606.

Pabst, H.F., Pueschel, S. & Hillman, D.A. (1967) Etiologic interrelationship in Down's syndrome, hypothyroidism, and precocious sexual development. *Pediatrics* 40, 590.

Painter, T.S. (1921) The Y chromosome in mammals. *Science* 53, 503.

Painter, T.S. (1923) Studies in mammalian spermatogenesis. *J. exp. Zool.* 37, 291.

Palmer, C.G., Conneally, P.M. & Christian, J.C. (1969) Translocations of D chromosomes in two families: t(13q14q) and t(13q14q)+(13p14p). *J. med. Genet.* 6, 166.

Panizon, F. (1965) Neonatal jaundice in Down's syndrome. *Lancet* 2, 495.

Pantelakis, S.N., Karaklis, A.G., Alexiou, D., Vardas, E. & Valaes, T. (1970) Red cell enzymes in trisomy 21. *Amer. J. hum. Genet.* 22, 184.

Pantin, A.M. (1951) Blood groups of mental defectives and their maternal parents. *Nature, Lond.* 167, 76.

Paris Conference, 1971 (1972) Standardization in human cytogenetics. *Birth Defects Original Article Series,* Vol. 8, No. 7. New York: National Foundation.

Parker, G.F. (1950) The incidence of mongoloid imbecility in the newborn infant. *J. Pediat.* 36, 493.

Patau, K. (1963) The origin of chromosomal abnormalities. *Path. Biol.* 11, 1163.

Paulson, G.W. (1971) Failure of ambulation in Down's syndrome. A clinical survey. *Clin. Pediat.* 10, 265.

Pearce, F.H., Rankine, R. & Ormond, A.W. (1910) Notes on twenty-eight cases of mongolian imbeciles: with special reference to their ocular condition. *Brit. med. J.* 2, 186.

Pearse, J.J., Reiss, M. & Suwalski, R.T. (1963) Thyroid function in patients with mongolism. *J. clin. endocr.* 23, 311.

Pearson, H.A. (1967) Studies of granulopoiesis and granulocyte kinetics in Down's syndrome. *Pediatrics* 40, 92.

Pegg, P.J. (1964) Leucocyte life-span; leucocyte alkaline phosphatase and the 21st chromosome. *Lancet* 1, 557.

Péhu, M. & Gaté, J. (1937) Sur le mongolisme infantile. II. Mongolisme familial. Syphilis conjugale survenue après la naissance de quatre enfants mongoliens. *Rev. franç. Pédiat.* 13, 212.

Pelger, K. (1928) Demonstratie van een paar zeldzaam vorkomende typen van bloedlichampies en besprecking der patiënten. *Ned. T. Geneesk.* **72**, 1178.

Penrose, L.S. (1931) The creases on the minimal digit in mongolism. *Lancet* **2**, 585.

Penrose, L.S. (1932a) The blood grouping of mongolian imbeciles. *Lancet* **1**, 394.

Penrose, L.S. (1932b) On the interaction of heredity and environment in the study of human genetics, with special reference to mongolian imbecility. *J. Genet.* **25**, 407.

Penrose, L.S. (1933a) The relative effects of paternal and maternal age in mongolism. *J. Genet.* **27**, 219.

Penrose, L.S. (1933b) *Mental defect*. London: Sidgwick & Jackson Ltd.

Penrose, L.S. (1934a) The relative aetiological importance of birth order and maternal age in mongolism. *Proc. Roy. Soc. B.* **115**, 131.

Penrose, L.S. (1934b) A method of separating the relative aetiological effect of birth order and maternal age, with special reference to mongolian imbecility. *Ann. Eugen., Lond.* **6**, 108.

Penrose, L.S. (1938a) Some genetical problems in mental deficiency. *J. ment. Sci.* **84**, 693.

Penrose, L.S. (1938b) A clinical and genetic study of 1,280 cases of mental defect. *Spec. Rep. Ser. med. Res. Coun.* No. 229, London: H.M.S.O.

Penrose, L.S. (1939) Maternal age, order of birth and developmental abnormalities. *J. ment. Sci.* **85**, 1141.

Penrose, L.S. (1949a) *Biology of mental defect*. London: Sidgwick & Jackson Ltd.

Penrose, L.S. (1949b) Familial studies on palmar patterns in relation to mongolism. *Hereditas*, Supp. Vol., p. 412.

Penrose, L.S. (1949c) The incidence of mongolism in the general population. *J. ment. Sci.* **95**, 685.

Penrose, L.S. (1951) Maternal age in familial mongolism. *J. ment. Sci.* **97**, 738.

Penrose, L.S. (1953) Mongolian idiocy (mongolism) and maternal age. *Ann. N.Y. Acad. Sci.* **57**, 494.

Penrose, L.S. (1954a) The distal triradius *t* on the hands of parents and sibs of mongol imbeciles. *Ann. hum. Genet., Lond.* **19**, 10.

Penrose, L.S. (1954b) Observations on the aetiology of mongolism. *Lancet* **2**, 505.

Penrose, L.S. (1954c) Distance, size and shape. *Ann. Eugen., Lond.* **18**, 337.

Penrose, L.S. (1956) Some notes on heredity counselling. *Acta genet., Basel* **6**, 35.

Penrose, L.S. (1957) Similarity of blood antigens in mother and mongol child. *J. ment. Defic. Res.* **1**, 107.

Penrose, L.S. (1961a) Mongolism. *Brit. med. Bull.* **17**, 184.

Penrose, L.S. (1961b) Mongolism. *Clinical Aspects of Genetics*. London: Pitman Medical Publishing Co.

Penrose, L.S. (1962a) Paternal age in mongolism. *Lancet* **1**, 1101.

Penrose, L.S. (1962b) Chromosomes and natural selection. *Acta genet. med. (Roma)* **11**, 303.

Penrose, L.S. (1963a) Measurements of likeness in relatives of trisomics. *Ann. hum. Genet., Lond.* **27**, 183.

Penrose, L.S. (1963b) *Biology of mental defect* (3rd ed.). London: Sidgwick & Jackson Ltd.

Penrose, L.S. (1964a) Personal communication.

Penrose, L.S. (1964b) Genetical aspects of mental deficiency. *Int. Copenhagen Cong. Sci. Study Ment. Retard.* **1**, 165.

Penrose, L.S. (1964c) Review of "Abnormalities of the sex chromosome complement in man" by W.M. Court Brown *et al. Ann. hum. Genet., Lond.* **28**, 199.

Penrose, L.S. (1965a) Dermatoglyphics in mosaic mongolism and allied conditions. *Genetics Today* **3**, 973. Oxford: Pergamon Press.

Penrose, L.S. (1965b) Mongolism as a problem in human biology. *Symposium on the early conceptus, normal and abnormal*, p. 94. Dundee: D.C. Thomson Press Ltd.

Penrose, L.S. (1965c) The causes of Down's syndrome. *Advances in Teratology.* London: Logos Press.

Penrose, L.S. (1965d) Unpublished observations.

Penrose, L.S. (1967) Studies of mosaicism in Down's anomaly. In *Mental Retardation.* G.A. Jervis, ed. Springfield: Charles C. Thomas.

Penrose, L.S. (1968) Memorandum on dermatoglyphic nomenclature. *Birth Defects Original Article Series,* Vol. 4, No. 3. New York: National Foundation.

Penrose, L.S. & Berg, J.M. (1968) Mongolism and duration of marriage. *Nature, Lond.* 218, 300.

Penrose, L.S. & Delhanty, J.D.A. (1961a) Familial Langdon Down anomaly with chromosomal fusion. *Ann. hum. Genet., Lond.* 25, 243.

Penrose, L.S. & Delhanty, J.D.A. (1961b) Triploid cell cultures from a macerated foetus. *Lancet* 1, 1261.

Penrose, L.S. & Delhanty, J.D.A. (1962) Unpublished observation.

Penrose, L.S. & Ellis, J.R. (1961) Unpublished observation.

Penrose, L.S., Ellis, J.R. & Delhanty, J.D.A. (1960) Chromosomal translocations in mongolism and in normal relatives. *Lancet* 2, 409.

Penrose, L.S. & Loesch, D. (1967) A study of dermal ridge width in the second (palmar) interdigital area with special reference to aneuploid states. *J. ment. Defic. Res.* 11, 36.

Penrose, L.S. & Loesch, D. (1970a) Topological classification of palmar dermatoglyphics. *J. ment. Defic. Res.* 14, 111.

Penrose, L.S. & Loesch, D. (1970b) Comparative study of sole patterns in chromosomal abnormalities. *J. ment. Defic. Res.* 14, 129.

Penrose, L.S. & Loesch, D. (1971a) Dermatoglyphic patterns and clinical diagnosis by discriminant function. *Ann. hum. Genet., Lond.* 35, 51.

Penrose, L.S. & Loesch, D. (1971b) Diagnosis with dermatoglyphic discriminants. *J. ment. Defic. Res.* 15, 185.

Penrose, L.S. & Smith, G.F. (1966) *Down's anomaly.* London: J. & A. Churchill Ltd.

Penrose, M. & Penrose, L.S. (1933) The blood group distribution in the eastern counties of England. *Brit. J. exp. Path.* 14, 160.

Pepler, W.J., Smith, M. & van Niekerk, W.A. (1968) An unusual karyotype in a patient with signs suggestive of Down's syndrome. *J. med. Genet.* 5, 68.

Perry, T.L., Shaw, K.N.F. & Walker, D. (1959) Urinary excretion of β-amino*iso*-butyric acid in mongolism. *Nature, Lond.* 184, 1970.

Pfeiffer, R.A. (1963) The transmission of the G/G translocation. *Lancet* 1, 1163.

Pfeiffer, R.A. (1964) Doppelte Aneuploidie (Trisomie 21 und XXY) bei einem Säugling. *Arch. Kinderheilk.* 171, 69.

Pfeiffer, R.A. (1966) Résultats d'une étude cytogénétique et clinique de 312 mongoliens. Signification des translocations et mosaiques. *Ann. Génét.* 9, 94.

Philippe, C. & Oberthur, J. (1901) Etude histologique de deux cas d'idiotie type mongolien. *C.R. Bicêtre* 22, 148.

Phillips, J., Herring, R.M., Goodman, H.O. & King, J.S. (1967) Leucocyte alkaline phosphatase and erythrocyte glucose-6-phosphate dehydrogenase in Down's syndrome. *J. med. Genet.* 4, 268.

Pitt, D. (1974) *Your Down's syndrome child.* Arlington, Texas: National Association for Retarded Citizens.

Piussan, C., Faille, N. & van Poperinche, M. (1973) Un cas de thrombopenie congenitale au cours d'une trisomie 21. *Rev. Pédiat.* 9, 67.

Plato, C.C., Cereghino, J.J. & Steinberg, F.S. (1973) Palmar dermatoglyphics of Down's syndrome: revisited. *Pediat. Res.* 7, 111.

Pleydell, M.J. (1957) Mongolism and other congenital abnormalities: an epidemiological study in Northamptonshire. *Lancet* 1, 1314.

Pochedly, C. & Ente, G. (1968) Disseminated intravascular coagulation in a newborn with Down's syndrome. *J. Pediat.* 73, 298.

Pogue, M.E. (1917) A brief report of twenty-nine cases of mongolian idiocy, with special reference to the etiology from the standpoint of the clinical history, with presentation of three cases. *Illinois med. J.* **32**, 296.

Polani, P.E., Briggs, J.H., Ford, C.E., Clarke, C.M. & Berg, J.M. (1960) A mongol girl with 46 chromosomes. *Lancet* **1**, 721.

Polani, P.E., Hamerton, J.L., Giannelli, F. & Carter, C.O. (1965) Cytogenetics of Down's syndrome (mongolism). III. Frequency of interchange trisomics and mutation rate of chromosome interchanges. *Cytogenetics* **4**, 193.

Pollard, F.L., Zsako, S., Kelsall, M.A. & Kaplan, A.R. (1970) Antinuclear antibody factors and nuclear staining in mothers of children affected with Down's syndrome. *Acta Genet. med. (Roma)* **19**, 529.

Pongiglione, R. & Bezante, T. (1965) Mongolismo e diabete mellito. *Minerva pediat.* **17**, 178.

Popich, G.A. & Smith, D.W. (1970) The genesis and significance of digital and palmar hand creases: Preliminary report. *J. Pediat.* **77**, 1017.

Porter, I.H., Petersen, W. & Brown, C.D. (1969) Double autosomal trisomy (trisomy D+G) with mosaicism. *J. med. Genet.* **6**, 347.

Portius, W. (1941) Ein Grenzfall von Mongolismus mit familiärem Auftreten der Kleinfingerbeugefaltenanomalie. *Erbarzt* **9**, 83.

Pototzky, C. & Grigg, A.E. (1942) A reversion of the prognosis in mongolism. *Amer. J. Orthopsychiat.* **12**, 503.

Potts, W.A. (1909) The origin of the feeble-minded. *Birmingham med. Rev.* **65**, 121.

Pozsonyi, J., Gibson, D., & Zarfas, D.E. (1964) Skeletal maturation in mongolism (Down's syndrome). *J. Pediat.* **64**, 75

Price Evans, D.A., Donohoe, W.T.A., Bannerman, R.M., Mohn, J.F. & Lambert, R.M. (1966) Blood-group gene localization through a study of mongolism. *Ann. hum. Genet., Lond.* **30**, 49.

Priest, J.H. (1960) Atropine response of the eyes in mongolism. *Amer. J. Dis. Child.* **100**, 869.

Priest, J.H. (1969) Parental dermatoglyphs in age-dependent mongolism. *J. med. Genet.* **6**, 304.

Priest, J.H., Bryant, J.S. & Motulsky, A.G. (1963a) Down's syndrome: trisomy and a *de novo* translocation in a family. *Lancet* **2**, 411.

Priest, J.H., Thuline, H.C., Norby, D.E. & La Veck, G.D. (1963b) Reproduction in human autosomal trisomics—chromosome studies of a mongol mother, her nonmongol twins, and her family. *Amer. J. Dis. Child.* **105**, 31.

Priest, J.H., Verhulst, C. & Sirkin, S. (1973) Parental dermatoglyphics in Down's syndrome. A ten-year study. *J. med. Genet.* **10**, 328.

Prieto, F., Egozcue, J., Forteza, G. & Marco, F. (1970) Identification of the Philadelphia (Ph-[1]) chromosome. *Blood* **35**, 23.

Prieur, M., Dutrillaux, B., Carpentier, S., Berger, R., Raoul, O., Rethoré, M.-O. & Lejeune, J. (1972) Mosaique 45,X/47,XY,+21. *Ann. Génét.* **15**, 195.

Priscu, R., Moraru, I., Albu, A. & Sichitiu, S. (1974) Les taux des amino-acides libres dans le liquide cérébro-spinal chez les nourrissons trisomiques 21. *Humangenetik* **21**, 63.

Pritham, G.H., Appleton, M.D. & Fluck, E.R. (1963) Biochemical studies in mongolism. I. The influence of environment on the concentrations and mobilities of plasma proteins. *Amer. J. ment. Defic.* **67**, 517.

Pueschel, S.M. & O'Donnell, P. (1974) Unilateral partial adactyly in Down's syndrome. *Pediatrics* **54**, 466.

Punnett, H.H. & Di George, A.M. (1967) Down's/mosaic-Klinefelter's syndrome. *Lancet* **2**, 617.

Purtscher, E. (1958) Knotenförmige Verdichtungen im Irisstroma bei Mongolismus. *v. Graefes Arch. Ophthal.* **160**, 200.

Purvis-Smith, S.G. (1972) The Sydney line: a significant sign in Down's syndrome. *Aust. Paediat. J.* **8**, 198.

Raab, S.O., Mellman, W.J., Oski, F.A. & Baker, D. (1966) Abnormal leukocyte kinetics: an explanation for the enzyme abnormalities observed in trisomy-21 (Down's syndrome). *J. Pediat.* 69, 925.

Rabinowitz, J.G. & Moseley, J.E. (1964) The lateral lumbar spine in Down's syndrome: a new roentgen feature. *Radiology* 83, 74.

Rabinowitz, Y. (1964) Separation of lymphocytes, polymorphonuclear leukocytes and monocytes on glass columns, including tissue culture observations. *Blood* 23, 811.

Rapaport, I. (1957) Contribution à l'étude étiologique du mongolisme: role des inhibiteurs enzymatiques. *Encéphale,* 46, 468.

Rapaport, I. (1963) Oligophrénia mongolienne et caries dentaires. *Rev. Stomatol., Paris* 64, 207.

Rarick, L., Rapaport, I. & Seefeldt, V. (1964) Bone development in Down's disease. *Amer. J. Dis. Child.* 107, 7.

Rarick, G.L., Rapaport, I.F. & Seefeldt, V. (1966) Long bone growth in Down's syndrome. *Amer. J. Dis. Child.* 112, 566.

Rarick, G.L. & Seefeldt, V. (1974) Observations from longitudinal data on growth in stature and sitting height of children with Down's syndrome. *J. ment. Defic. Res.* 18, 63.

Rasmussen, J.E. (1972) Disseminated elastosis perforans serpiginosa in four mongoloids. *Brit. J. Derm.* 86, 9.

Record, R.G. & Smith, A. (1955) Incidence and sex distribution of mongoloid defectives. *Brit. J. prev. soc. Med.* 9, 10.

Redman, R.S., Shapiro, B.L. & Gorlin, R.J. (1965) Measurements of normal and reportedly malformed palatal vaults. III. Down's syndrome (trisomy 21, mongolism). *J. Pediat.* 67, 162.

Reed, T.E., Borgaonkar, D.S., Conneally, P.M., Yu, P., Nance, W.E. & Christian, J.C. (1970) Dermatoglyphic nomogram for the diagnosis of Down's syndrome. *J. Pediat.* 77, 1024.

Rehn, A.T. & Thomas, E. (1957) Family history of a mongolian girl who bore a mongolian child. *Amer J. ment. Defic.* 62, 496.

Reinwein, H., Wolf, U. & Ising, H.J. (1966) Bericht über 3 Mosaikfälle mit G_1-Trisomie (Mongolismus). *Halv. paediat. Acta* 21, 300.

Reisman, L., Shipe, D. & Williams, R.D.B. (1966) Mosaicism in Down's syndrome: studies in a child with an unusual chromosome constitution. *Amer. J. ment. Defic.* 70, 855.

Reiss, J.A., Lovrien, E.W. & Hecht, F. (1971) A mother with Down's syndrome and her chromosomally normal infant. *Ann. Génét.* 14, 225.

Renkonen, K.O. & Donner, M. (1964) Mongoloids, their mothers and sibships. *Ann. Med. exp. Fenn.* 42, 139.

Renkonen, K.O., Donner, M. & Valkeakari, T. (1968) Down's syndrome and erythoblastosis. *Lancet* 2, 102.

Rethoré, M., Lafourcade, J., Prieur, M., Caille, B., Cruveillier, J., Tanzy, M. & Lejeune, J. (1970) Mére et fille Trisomiques 21 libres. *Ann. Génét.* 13, 42.

Reuben, M.S. & Klein, S. (1926) Mongolian idiocy in both twins. *Arch. Pediat.* 43, 552.

Ricci, N., Ventimiglia, B. & Dallapiccola, B. (1967) Studio citogenetico di 140 pazienti affetti da sindrome di Down. *Acta Genet. med. (Roma)* 16, 376.

Ricci, N., Ventimiglia, B. & Preto, G. (1968) Transmission d'un petit chromosome surnuméraire dans une famille avec deux cas de trisomie 21. *Ann. Génét.* 11, 114.

Richards, B.W. (1969) Mosaic mongolism. *J. ment. Defic. Res.* 13, 66.

Richards, B.W. (1970) Observations on mosaic parents of mongol propositi. *J. ment. Defic. Res.* 14, 342.

Richards, B.W. & Stewart, A. (1962) Mosaicism in a mongol. *Lancet* 1, 275.

Richards, B.W. & Stewart, A. (1965) D/D translocation. *Lancet* 1, 1076.

Richards, B.W., Stewart, A. & Sylvester, P.E. (1965a) Reciprocal translocation and mosaicism in a mongol. *J. ment. Defic. Res.,* 9, 118.

Richards, B.W., Stewart, A., Sylvester, P.E. & Jasiewicz, V. (1965b) Cytogenetic survey of 225 patients diagnosed clinically as mongols. *J. ment. Defic. Res.* 9, 245.

Richards, B.W. & Sylvester, P.E. (1969) Mortality trends in mental deficiency institutions. *J. ment Defic. Res.* 13, 276.

Ridler, M.A.C. (1971) Banding patterns of metaphase chromosomes in Down's syndrome. *Lancet* 2, 603.

Ridler, M.A.C., Pendrey, M.J., Faunch, J.A. & Berg, J.M. (1969) Association of D/D translocation with mongolism. *J. ment. Defic. Res.* 13, 89.

Ridler, M.A.C. & Shapiro, A. (1959) The longitudinal study of the leucocyte count in infants with mongolism. *J. ment. Defic. Res.* 3, 96.

Ridler, M.A.C., Shapiro, A., Delhanty, J.D.A. & Smith, G.F. (1965) A mosaic mongol with normal leucocyte chromosomes. *Brit. J. Psychiat.* 111, 183.

Rigas, D.A., Elsasser, P. & Hecht, F. (1970) Impaired *in vitro* response of circulating lymphocytes to phytohemagglutinin in Down's syndrome: dose- and time-response curves and relation to cellular immunity. *Int. Arch. Allergy* 39, 587.

Rigrodsky, S., Prunty, F. & Glovsky, L. (1961) A study of the incidence, types and associated etiologies of hearing loss in an institutionalized mentally retarded population. *Trng. Sch. Bull.* 58, 30.

Rittner, Ch. & Rittner, B. (1973) Studies in Down's syndrome. IV. Investigations on the "Xh" factor. *Clin. Genet.* 4, 407.

Rittner, Ch. & Schwinger, E. (1973) Studies in Down's syndrome. II. Association studies with blood, serum and enzyme groups, and with the Au/SH antigen. *Clin. Genet.* 4, 398.

Roberts, J.A.F. (1963) *An introduction to medical genetics.* Oxford University Press.

Roberts, N. & Roberts, B. (1968) *David.* Richmond, Virginia: John Knox Press.

Robertson, W.R.S. (1916) Chromosome studies I. *J. Morph.* 27, 178.

Robinson, A. (1973) Personal communication.

Robinson, A. & Puck, T.T. (1965) Sex chromatin in newborns: presumptive evidence for external factors in human non-disjunction. *Science* 148, 83.

Robinson, A. & Puck, T.T. (1967) Studies on chromosomal nondisjunction in man. II. *Amer. J. hum Genet.* 19, 112.

Roche, A.F. (1961) Clinodactyly and brachymesophalangia of the fifth finger. *Acta Paediat.* 50, 387.

Roche, A.F. (1964) Skeletal maturation rates in mongolism. *Amer. J. Roentgenol.* 91, 979.

Roche, A.F. (1965) The stature of mongols. *J. ment. Defic. Res.* 9, 131.

Roche, A.F. & Barkla, D.H. (1964) The eruption of deciduous teeth in mongols. *J. ment. Defic. Res.* 8, 54.

Roche, A.F., Roche, P.J. & Lewis, A.B. (1972) The cranial base in trisomy 21. *J. ment. Defic. Res.* 16, 7.

Roche, A.F., Seward, F.S. & Sunderland, S. (1961a) Growth changes in the mongoloid head. *Acta paediat.* 50, 133.

Roche, A.F., Seward, F.S. & Sunderland, S. (1961b) Non-metrical observations on cranial roentgenograms in mongolism. *Amer. J. Roentgenol.* 85, 659.

Roche, A.F. & Sunderland, S. (1960) Postmortem observations on mongoloid crania. *J. Neuropath. exp. Neurol.* 19, 554.

Rogers, D.E. (1963) *Angel unaware.* Westwood, New Jersey: Fleming H. Revell Co.

Rohmer, A., Ruch, J.V., Schneegans, E. & Clavert, J. (1970) Jumeaux dizygotes, l'un 47,XX,21+ et cliniquement mongolien, l'autre 46,XX/47,XX,21+ et cliniquement non mongolien. *Arch franç Pediat.* 27, 667.

Rollin, H.R. (1946) Personality in mongolism with special reference to the incidence of catatonic psychosis. *Amer. J. ment. Defic.* 51, 219.

Romanski, B. & Walczynski, Z. (1966) Study on frequency of allergic manifestations and skin reactivity in children with Down's syndrome. *Bull. pol. med. Hist. Sci.* 9, 74.

Root, A.W., Bongiovanni, A.M., Breibart, S. & Mellman, W.J. (1964) Double aneuploidy: trisomy 21 and X0/XX sex chromosome mosaicism. *J. Pediat.* **65**, 937.

Rosanoff, A.J. & Handy, L.M. (1934) Etiology of mongolism with special reference to its occurrence in twins. *Amer. J. Dis. Child.* **48**, 764.

Rosecrans, C.J. (1968) The relationship of normal/21-trisomy mosaicism and intellectual development *Amer. J. ment. Defic.* **72**, 562.

Rosen, R.B. & Nishiyama, H. (1965) Leucocyte life-span and leucocyte alkaline phosphatase. *Lancet* **1**, 554.

Rosenberg, L. (1924) Die späteren Schicksale der mongoloiden Kinder. *Wien. med. Wschr.* **74**, 2503.

Rosenquist, G.C., Sweeney, L.J., Amsel, J. & McAllister, H.A. (1974) Enlargement of the membranous ventricular septum: an internal stigma of Down's syndrome. *J. Pediat.* **85**, 490.

Rosner, F. & Kozinn, P.J. (1972) Leucocyte function in Down's syndrome. *Lancet* **2**, 283.

Rosner, F. & Lee, S.L. (1972) Down's syndrome and acute leukemia: myeloblastic or lymphoblastic? Report of forty-three cases and review of the literature. *Amer. J. Med.* **53**, 203.

Rosner, F. & Ong, B.H. (1967) Dermatoglyphic patterns in trisomic and translocation Down's syndrome (mongolism). *Amer. J. med. Sci.* **253**, 556.

Rosner, F., Ong, B.H., Paine, R.S. & Mahanand, D. (1965) Blood-serotonin activity in trisomic and translocation Down's syndrome. *Lancet* **1**, 1191.

Ross, J.D. & Atkins, L. (1962) Chromosomal anomaly in a mongol with leukaemia. *Lancet* **2**, 612.

Ross, J.D., Moloney, W.C. & Desforges, J.F. (1963) Ineffective regulation of granulopoiesis masquerading as congenital leukaemia in a mongoloid child. *J. Pediat.* **63**, 1

Routil, R. (1933) Uber die Wertigkeit der Blutgruppenbefunde in Vaterschaftsprozessen. *Z. Rassen-physiol.* **6**, 70.

Rowe, M.J., Agranoff, B.W. & Tourtellotte, W.W. (1966) Immunoelectrophoretic study of serum proteins in mongolism. *Neurology (Minneap.)* **16**, 714.

Rowe, R.D. & Uchida, I.A. (1961) Cardiac malformations in mongolism: a prospective study of 184 mongoloid children. *Amer. J. Med.* **31**, 726.

Rowley, J.D. (1973) Chromosomal patterns in myelocytic leukemia. *New Engl. J. Med.* **289**, 220.

Ruhräh, J (1935) Cretin or mongol or both together. *Amer. J. Dis. Child.* **49**, 477.

Rundle, A.T. (1973) Theoretical implications of the application of polymorphic protein systems to gene location on a trisomic chromosome, and its application to the haptoglobin phenotype frequencies in Down's syndrome. *Clin. Genet.* **4**, 520

Rundle, A.T., Clothier, B. & Sudell, B. (1971) Serum IgD levels and infections in Down's syndrome. *Clin. chim. Acta.* **35**, 389.

Rundle, A.T., Coppen, A. & Cowie, V. (1961) Steroid excretion in mothers of mongols. *Lancet* **2**, 846.

Rundle, A.T., Donoghue, E.C., Abbas, K.A. & Krstić, A. (1972) A catch-up phenomenon in skeletal development of children with Down's syndrome. *J. ment. Defic. Res.* **16**, 41.

Rundle, A.T., Dutton, G. & Gibson, J. (1959) Endocrinological aspects of mental deficiency. I. Testicular function in mongolism. *J. ment. Defic Res.* **3**, 108.

Rundle, A.T. & Sylvester, P.E. (1962) Endocrinological aspects of mental deficiency. II. Maturational status of adult males. *J. ment. Defic. Res.* **6**, 87.

Runge, G.H. (1959) Glucose tolerance in mongolism. *Amer. J. ment. Defic.* **63**, 822.

Russell, L.B. (1964) Experimental studies on mammalian chromosome aberrations. *Mammalian cytogenetics and related problems in radiobiology.* p. 61 Oxford: Pergamon Press.

Russell, P.M.G. (1933) Mongolism in twins. *Lancet* **1**, 802.

Ruvalcaba, R.H.A., Ferrier, P.E. & Thuline, H.C. (1969) Incidence of goiter in patients with Down's syndrome. *Amer. J. Dis. Child.* **118**, 451.

Sachdeva, S., Wodnicki, J. & Smith, G.F. (1971) Fluorescent chromosomes of a tandem translocation in a mongol patient. *J. ment. Defic. Res.* **15**, 181.

Salzer, G., Stur, O. & Zweymüller, E. (1961) Erfolgreich operiertes Pankreas anulare bei einem neugeborenen Mongoloid. *Arch. Kinderheilk.* **164**, 152.

Sandberg, A.A., Ishihara, T., Miwa, T. & Hauschka, T.S. (1961) The *in vivo* chromosome constitution of marrow from 34 human leukemias and 60 non-leukemic controls. *Cancer Res.* **21**, 678.

Sandrucci, M.G. & Piccotti, M.L. (1958) La funzionalita cortico-surrenalica nel mongolismo. *Minerva pediat.* **9**, 1368.

Sands, V.E. (1969) Short arm enlargement in acrocentric chromosomes. *Amer. J. hum. Genet.* **21**, 293.

Sasaki, M. (1965) Meiosis in a male with Down's syndrome *Chromosoma (Berl.)* **16**, 652.

Sasaki, M. & Hara, Y. (1973) Paternal origin of the extra chromosome in Down's syndrome. *Lancet* **2**, 1257.

Sasaki, M. & Obara, Y. (1969) Hypersensitivity of lymphocytes in Down's syndrome by mixed leukocyte culture experiments. *Nature Lond.* **222**, 596.

Sasaki, M. & Tonomura, A. (1969) Chromosomal radiosensitivity in Down's syndrome. *Jap. J. hum. Genet.* **14**, 81.

Sasaki, M., Tonomura, A. & Matsubara, S. (1970) Chromosome constitution and its bearing on the chromosomal radiosensitivity in man. *Mutation Res.* **10**, 617.

Sawyer, G.M. (1949) Case report: reproduction in a mongoloid. *Amer. J. ment. Defic.* **54**, 204.

Sawyer, G.M. & Shafter, A.J. (1957) Reproduction in a mongoloid: a follow-up. *Amer. J. ment. Defic.* **61**, 793.

Schachter, M. (1947) Arriération mongolienne et syndrome d'Ehlers-Danlos. *Arch. franç. Pédiat.* **4**, 37.

Schachter, M. (1956) Les convulsions chez les mongoliens. *Méd. infant.* **63**, 5.

Schärer, K. (1962) Personal communication.

van der Scheer, W.M. (1919a) Verschiedene gevallen van mongoloide idiotie in een gezin. *Ned. T. Geneesk.* **1**, 328.

van der Scheer, W.M. (1919b) Cataracta lentis bei mongoloider Idiotie. *Klin. Mbl. Augenheilk.* **62**, 155.

van der Scheer, W.M. (1927) Beiträge zur Kenntnis der mongoloiden Missbildung. *Abh. aus der Neur., Psychiat., Psychol. und Grenzgebieten* **41**, 1.

Schendel, S.A. & Gorlin, R.J. (1974) Frequency of cleft uvula and submucous cleft palate in patients with Down's syndrome. *J. dent. Res.* **53**, 840.

Schlaug, R. (1958) A mongolian mother and her child. *Acta genet.,* Basel **7**, 533.

Schön, M. (1828) In *Hand, patholog. Ant. des menschl. Auges* (quoted by J. Sichel (1851).

Schönenberg, H. & Pfeiffer, R. (1966) Gliedmassenfehlbildungen (Perodaktylie, Symbrachydaktylie) bei 2 Säuglingen mit Down-Syndrom. *Ann. paediat. (Basel)* **207**, 172.

Schröder, H. (1940) Zur Frage der ovariellen Insufficienz bei mongoloidenmuttern. *Z. ges Neurol. Psychiat.* **170**, 148.

Schröder, J., Lydecken, K. & de la Chapelle, A. (1971) Meiosis and spermatogenesis in G-trisomic males. *Humangenetik* **13**, 15.

Schuh, B.E., Korf, B.R. & Salwen, M.J. (1974) A 21/21 tandem translocation with satellites on both long and short arms. *J. med. Genet.* **11**, 297.

Schuler, D., Dobos, M., Fekete, G., Machai, T. & Nemerskeri, A. (1972) Down-syndrome und Malignität. *Orv. Hetil.* **113**, 2631.

Schull, W.J. & Neel, J.V. (1962) Maternal radiation and mongolism. *Lancet* **1**, 537.

Schultze-Jena, B.S. (1959) Röntgenologische Merkmale des Beckens bei Mongolismus im Säuglingsalter. *Kinderärztl. Prax.* 27, 141.

Schunk, G.J. & Lehman, W.L. (1954) Mongolism and congenital leukaemia. *J. Amer. med. Ass.* 155, 250.

Schwarzmeier, J.D., Rett, A., Moser, K. & Andrle, M. (1973) Erythrozytenenzyme und substrate bei Kindern mit Down-Syndrom. *Wien. klin. Wschr.* 85, 33.

Schwinger, E., Roers, H. & Rittner, Ch. (1971) Studien an Patienten mit Down-Syndrom. III. Fluorescenzmikroskopische Untersuchungen. *Z. Kinderheilk.* 111, 217.

Séguin, E. (1846) *Le traitement moral, l'hygiène et l'éducation des idiots.* Paris: J.B. Baillière.

Séguin, E. (1866) *Idiocy and its treatment by the physiological method.* New York: William Wood & Co.

Seiler, A. (1938) Zur Verbreitung und Vererbung der Faltenzunge (lingua plicata). *Arch. J. Klaus. Stift.* 11, 18.

Sénéze, J., Lafourcade, J., Lejeune, J. & Thoyer-Rozat, J. (1964) Double aneuploide: trisomie-21 et syndrome de Klinefelter chez un couple de jumeaux monozygotes. *Bull. Féd. Soc. Gynéc. Obstét.* 16, 529.

Seppäläinen, A.M. & Kivalo, E. (1967) EEG findings and epilepsy in Down's syndrome. *J. ment. Defic. Res.* 11, 116.

Sergovich, F.R. (1962) Personal communication.

Sergovich, F.R. (1963) Personal communication.

Sergovich, F.R., Luce, A. & Carr, D.H. (1967) Chromosome aneuploidy in the father of a mongol. *Amer. J. Dis. Child.* 114, 407.

Sergovich, F.R., Soltan, H.C. & Carr, D.H. (1962) A 13–15/21 translocation chromosome in carrier father and mongol son. *Canad. med. Ass. J.* 87, 852.

Sergovich, F.R., Soltan, H.C. & Carr, D.H. (1964a) Twelve unrelated translocation mongols: cytogenetic, genetic and parental age data. *Cytogenetics* 3, 34.

Sergovich, F.R., Valentine, G.H., Carr, D.H. & Soltan, H.C. (1964a) Mongolism (Down's syndrome) with atypical clinical and cytogenetic features. *J. Pediat.* 65, 197.

Serrano Rios, M., San Roman Cos Gayon, C., Sordo, M.T. & Rodriquez Minon, J.L. (1973a) Insulin secretion in Down's syndrome. *Diabetologia* 9, 50.

Serrano Rios, M., Mato, J., Oya, M., Larrodera, L., Hawkins, F. & Escobar, F. (1973b) Failure to find IgG insulin antibodies in Down's syndrome. *Hormone Metab. Res. (Stuttg.)* 5, 57.

Sever, J.L., Gilkeson, M.R., Chen, T.C., Ley, A.C. & Edmonds, D. (1970) Epidemiology of mongolism in the Collaborative Project. *Ann. N.Y. Acad. Sci.* 171, 328.

Seward, F.S., Roche, A.F. & Sunderland, S. (1961) The lateral cranial silhouette in mongolism. *Amer. J. Roentgenol.* 85, 653.

Shaher, R.M., Farina, M.A., Porter, I.H. & Bishop, M. (1972) Clinical aspects of congenital heart disease in mongolism. *Amer. J. Cardiol.* 29, 497.

Shapiro, A. (1949) The differential leucocyte count in mongols. *J. ment. Sci.* 95, 689.

Shapiro, B.L. (1970) Prenatal dental anomalies in mongolism: comments on the basis and implications of variability. *Ann. N.Y. Acad. Sci.* 171, 562.

Shapiro, B.L., Gorlin, R.J., Redman, R.S. & Bruhl, H.H. (1967) The palate and Down's syndrome. *New Engl. J. Med.* 276, 1460.

Shapiro, L.R. & Farnsworth, P.G. (1972) Down's syndrome in twins. *Clin. Genet.* 3, 364.

Share, J., Koch, R., Webb, A. & Graliker, B. (1964) The longitudinal development of infants and young children with Down's syndrome (mongolism). *Amer. J. ment. Defic.* 68, 685.

Shaw, M.W. (1962a) Segregation ratios and linkage studies in a family with six translocation mongols. *Lancet* 1, 1407.

Shaw, M.W. (1962b) Familial mongolism. *Cytogenetics* 1, 141.

Shaw, M.W. & Gershowitz, S. (1962) A search for autosomal linkage in a trisomic population: blood group frequencies in mongols. *Amer. J. hum. Genet.* 14, 317.

Shaw, M.W. & Gershowitz, S. (1963) Blood group frequencies in mongols. *Amer. J. hum. Genet.* 15, 495.

Shelley, W.B. & Butterworth, T. (1955) The absence of the apocrine glands and hair in the axilla in mongolism and idiocy. *J. invest. Derm.* 25, 165.

Shih, L.-Y. & Hsia, D.Y.-Y. (1966) Enzymes in Down's syndrome. *Lancet* 1, 155.

Shih, L.-Y., Wong, P., Inouye, T., Makler, M. & Hsia, D.Y.-Y. (1965) Enzymes in Down's syndrome. *Lancet* 2, 746.

Shipe, D., Reisman, L.E., Chung, C.-Y., Darnell, A. & Kelly, S. (1968) The relationship between cytogenetic constitution, physical stigmata, and intelligence in Down's syndrome. *Amer. J. ment. Defic.* 72, 789.

Shipe, D. & Shotwell, A.M. (1965) Effect of out-of-home care on mongoloid children: a continuation study. *Amer. J. ment. Defic* 69, 649.

Shotwell, A.M. & Shipe, D. (1964) Effect of out-of-home care on the intellectual and social development of mongoloid children. *Amer. J. ment. Defic.* 68, 693.

Shuttleworth, G.E. (1883) Physical features of idiocy in relation to classification and prognosis. *Liverpool med. chir. J.* 3, 282.

Shuttleworth, G.E. (1886) Clinical lecture on idiocy and imbecility. *Brit. med. J.* 1, 183.

Shuttleworth, G.E. (1895) *Mentally deficient children.* London: H.K. Lewis.

Shuttleworth, G.E. (1906) Comments on R. Langdon Down's paper. *J. ment. Sci.* 52, 189.

Shuttleworth, G.E. (1909) Mongolian imbecility. *Brit. med. J.* 2, 661.

Shuttleworth, G.E. & Beach, F. (1899) Idiocy and imbecility. Allbutt's *A system of medicine*, Vol. 8. London: Macmillan & Co.

Sichel, J. (1851) Mémoire sur l'épicanthus et sur une espèce particulière et non encore décrite de tumeur lacrymale. *Ann. Oculist.* 26, 29.

Sichitiu, S., Sinet, P.M., Lejeune, J. & Frézal, J. (1974) Surdosage de la forme dimérique de l'indolphenoloxydase dans la trisomie 21, secondaire au surdosage génique. *Humangenetik* 23, 65.

Siegel, M. (1948) Susceptibility of mongoloids to infection. I. Incidence of pneumonia, influenza A and Shigella dysenteriae (Sonne). *Amer. J. Hyg.* 48, 53.

Siegert, F. (1906) Zur Diagnosis des Mongolismus und des infantilen Myxödems. *Verhandl. 22 Kong. Inn. Med., Wiesbaden* 33, 675.

Siegert, F. (1910) Der Mongolismus. *Ergebn inn. Med. Kinderheilk.* 6, 565.

Sigler, A.T., Lilienfeld, A.M., Cohen, B.H. & Westlake, J.E. (1965a) Parental age in Down's syndrome (mongolism). *J. Pediat.* 67, 631.

Sigler, A.T., Lilienfeld, A.M., Cohen, B.H. & Westlake, J.E. (1965b) Radiation exposure in parents of children with mongolism (Down's syndrome). *Bull. Johns Hopk. Hosp.* 117, 374.

Silimbani, C. (1962) Contributions to the study of dental anomalies in mongolian idiocy. *Panminerva Med.* 4, 532.

Silverstein, A.B. (1964) An empirical test of the mongoloid stereotype. *Amer. J. ment. Defic.* 68, 493.

Simon, A., Ludwig, C., Gofman, J. & Crook, G. (1954) Metabolic studies in mongolism: serum protein-bound iodine, cholesterol and lipoprotein. *Amer. J. Psychiat.* 111, 139.

Simon, E., Gedalia, I., Shapiro, S. & Margolin, V. (1968) Citrate content of blood and saliva in relation to periodontal disease in man. *Arch. oral Biol.* 13, 1243.

Sinet, P.-M., Allard, D., Lejeune, J. & Jérôme, H. (1974) Augmentation d'activité de la superoxyde dismutase érythrocytaire dans la trisomie pour le chromosome 21. *C.R. Acad. Sci.* 278, 3267.

Sinet, P.-M., Allard, D., Lejeune, J. & Jérôme, H. (1975) Gene dosage effect in trisomy 21. *Lancet* 1, 276.

Singer, J., Sachdeva, S., Smith, G.F. & Hsia, D.Y.-Y. (1972) Triple X female and a Down's syndrome offspring. *J. med. Genet.* **9**, 238.

Sinson, J. & Wetherick, N.E. (1973) Short-term retention of colour and shape information in mongol and other severely subnormal children. *J. ment. Defic. Res.* **17**, 177.

Skeller, E. & Øster, J. (1951) Eye symptoms in mongolism. *Acta ophthal.* **29**, 149.

Slavin, R.E., Kamada, N. & Hamilton, H.B. (1967) A cytogenetic study of Down's syndrome in Hiroshima and Nagasaki. *Jap. J. hum. Genet.* **12**, 17.

Slavitt, D.R. (1973) *The outer mongolian.* New York: Doubleday Co.

Smith, A. (1973) Origin of the extra chromosome in Down's syndrome. *Lancet* **2**, 1449.

Smith, A. & McKeown, T. (1955) Pre-natal growth of mongoloid defectives. *Arch. Dis. Childh.* **30**, 257.

Smith, A. & Record, R.G. (1955) Maternal age and birth rank in the aetiology of mongolism. *Brit. J. prev. soc. Med.* **9**, 51.

Smith, D.W., Patau, K. & Therman, E. (1961) Autosomal trisomy syndromes. *Lancet* **2**, 211.

Smith, D.W., Therman, E., Patau, K. & Inhorn, S.L. (1962) Mosaicism in mother of two mongoloids. *Amer. J. Dis. Child.* **104**, 534.

Smith, D.W. & Wilson, A.A. (1973) *The child with Down's syndrome (mongolism).* Philadelphia: W.B. Saunders Co.

Smith, G.F. (1964a) Unpublished observations.

Smith, G.F. (1964b) Dermatoglyphic patterns on the fourth interdigital area of the sole in Down's syndrome. *J. ment. Defic. Res.* **8**, 125.

Smith, G.F. (1964c) Qualitative genetics of the patterns of the hallucal area of the sole. *Ann. hum. Genet., Lond.* **28**, 181.

Smith, G.F. (1973) Unpublished observations.

Smith, G.F. (1974) Evaluation of cosmetic surgery in Down's syndrome. Unpublished observations.

Smith, G.F. (1975) Present approaches to therapy in Down's syndrome. In *Down's syndrome: research, prevention and management.* (Ed. R. Koch & F. de la Cruz). New York: Brunner/Mazel Inc.

Smith, G.F., Bat-Miriam, M. & Ridler, M.A.C. (1966) Dermal patterns on the fingers and toes in mongolism. *J. ment. Defic. Res.* **10**, 105.

Smith, G.F. & Berg, J.M. (1974) The biological significance of mongolism. *Brit. J. Psychiat.* **125**, 537.

Smith, G.F. & Sachdeva, S. (1973) Origin of extra chromosome in trisomy 21. *Lancet* **1**, 487.

Smith, G.F., Sachdeva, S., Becker, N. & Justice, P. (1975) Enzyme levels in long-term cultured lymphocytes in Down's syndrome. *Proc. 3rd Cong. int. Assoc. sci. Study ment Defic., The Hague.* **2**, 47. Warsaw: Polish Medical Publishers.

Smith, G.F. & Turral, G.M. (1965) Dermal configurations: a study of the hallucal area of the sole in mongoloids, non-mongoloids, mental defectives and a control series. *Genetics Today* **3**, 128. Oxford: Pergamon Press

Smith, G.S., Tips, R.L. & Howard, H. (1965) Autosomal mosaicism occurring in conjunction with Down's syndrome. *Amer. J. ment. Defic.* **70**, 218.

Smith, G.S., Warren, S.A. & Turner, D.R. (1963) Hair characteristics in mongolism (Down's syndrome). *Amer. J. ment. Defic.* **68**, 362.

Smith, T.T. (1896) A peculiarity in the shape of the hand in idiots of the mongol type. *Pediatrics* **2**, 315.

Snedeker, D.M. (1948) A study of the palmar dermatoglyphics of mongoloid imbeciles. *Hum. Biol.* **20**, 146.

Sobel, A.E., Strazzulla, M., Sherman, B.S., Elkan, B., Morgenstern, S.W., Marius, N. & Meisel, A. (1958) Vitamin A absorption and other blood composition studies in mongolism. *Amer. J. ment. Defic.* **62**, 642.

Solitaire, G.B. (1969) The spinal cord of the mongol. *J. ment. Defic. Res.* **13**, 1.

Solitaire, G.B. & Lamarche, J.B. (1966) Alzheimer's disease and senile dementia as seen in mongoloids: neuropathological observations. *Amer. J. ment. Defic.* **70**, 840.

Solitaire, G.B. & Lamarche, J.B. (1967) Brain weight in the adult mongol. *J. ment. Defic. Res.* **11**, 79.

Solnitzky, O. (1962) Disorder associated with chromosomal aberration. *Georgetown med. Bull.* **15**, 276.

Solomons, G., Zellweger, H., Jahnke, P.G. & Opitz, E. (1965) Four common eye signs in mongolism. *Amer. J. Dis. Child.* **110**, 46.

Soltan, H.C. & Clearwater, K. (1965) Dermatoglyphics in translocation Down's syndrome *Amer. J. hum. Genet.* **17**, 476.

Soltan, H.C., Wiens, R.G. & Sergovich, F.R. (1964) Genetic studies and chromosomal analyses in families with mongolism (Down's syndrome) in more than one member. *Acta genet., Basel* **14**, 251.

Sommer, A. & Eaton, A.P. (1970) Achondroplasia and Down's syndrome. *J. med. Genet.* **7**, 63.

Soudek, D., Laxova, R. & Adamek, R. (1968) Pericentric inversion in a family with a 21/22 translocation. *Cytogenetics* **7**, 108.

Soukup, S.W., Passarge, E., Becroft, D.M.O., Shaw, R.L. & Young, L.G. (1969) Familial translocation (3?-;G?q+) and nondisjunction of chromosome in group G in two unrelated families. *Cytogenetics* **8**, 315.

Sparkes, R.S. & Motulsky, A.G. (1963) Hashimoto's disease in Turner's syndrome with isochromosome X. *Lancet* **1**, 947.

Sparkes, R.S., Muller, H.M. & Veomett, I.C. (1970) Inherited pericentric inversion of a human Y chromosome in trisomic Down's syndrome. *J. med. Genet.* **7**, 59.

Spellman, M.P. (1966) Mongolism: survey in Cork City and County. *J. Irish med. Ass.* **59**, 12.

Spencer, D.A. (1973) A white lock in Down's syndrome. *Lancet* **1**, 729.

Spinelli-Ressi, F. & Bergonzi, F. (1963) Red cell triiodothyronine uptake as a measure of thyroid function in mongolism. *Acta paediat.* **52**, 575.

Spitzer, R. & Quilliam, R.L. (1958) Observations on congenital anomalies in teeth and skull in two groups of mental defectives (a comparative study). *Brit. J. Radiol.* **31**, 596.

Spitzer, R., Rabinowitch, J.Y. & Wybar, K.C. (1961) A study of the abnormalities of the skull, teeth and lenses in mongolism. *Canad. med. Ass. J.* **84**, 567.

Spitzer, R. & Robinson, M.I. (1955) Radiological changes in teeth and skull in mental defectives. *Brit. J. Radiol.* **28**, 117.

Stahlecker, L.V. (Ed.) (1967) *Occupational information for the mentally retarded: selected readings.* Springfield, Illinois: Charles C. Thomas.

Stark, C.R. & Fraumeni, J.F. (1966) Viral hepatitis and Down's syndrome. *Lancet* **1**, 1036.

Stark, C.R. & Mantel, N. (1967) Lack of seasonal or temporal-spatial clustering of Down's syndrome births in Michigan. *Amer. J. Epidem.* **86**, 199.

Stearns, P.E., Droulard, K.E. & Sahhar, F.H. (1960) Studies bearing on fertility of male and female mongoloids. *Amer. J. ment. Defic.* **65**, 37.

Stedman, D.J. & Eichorn, D.H. (1964) A comparison of the growth and development of institutionalized and home-reared mongoloids during infancy and early childhood. *Amer. J. ment. Defic.* **69**, 391.

Steggerda, M. (1942) Inheritance of short metatarsals. *J. Hered.* **33**, 233.

Stene, J. (1970a) Statistical inference on segregation ratios for D/G- translocations, when the families are ascertained in different ways. *Ann. hum. Genet. Lond.* **34**, 93.

Stene, J. (1970b) Detection of higher recurrence risk for age-dependent chromosome abnormalities with an application to trisomy G_1 (Down's syndrome). *Hum. Hered.* **20**, 112.

Stene, J. (1970c) A statistical segregation analysis of (21q22q)- translocations. *Hum. Hered.* **20**, 465.

Stephens, M.C. & Menkes, J.H. (1969) Cerebral lipids in Down's syndrome. *Develop. Med. Child Neurol.* 11, 346.

Stern, E.N., Campbell, C.H. & Faulkner, H.W. (1973) Conservative management of congenital eversion of the eyelids. *Amer. J. Ophthal.* 75, 319.

Stern, J. (1964) Personal communication.

Stern, J. & Lewis, W.H.P. (1957a) Serum proteins in mongolism. *J. ment. Sci.* 103, 222.

Stern, J. & Lewis, W.H.P. (1957b) The serum cholesterol level in children with mongolism and other mentally retarded children. *J. ment. Defic. Res.* 1, 96.

Stern, J. & Lewis, W.H.P. (1958) Calcium, phosphate and phosphatase in mongolism. *J. ment. Sci.* 104, 880.

Stern, J. & Lewis, W.H.P. (1959) The serum lipoproteins of mentally retarded children. *J. ment. Sci.* 105, 1012.

Stern, J. & Lewis, W.H.P. (1960) Blood magnesium in children with mongolism and other mentally retarded children. *Amer. J. ment. Defic.* 64, 972.

Stern, J. & Lewis, W.H.P. (1962) Serum esterase in mongolism. *J. ment. Defic. Res.* 6, 13.

Sternlicht, M. & Wanderer, Z.W. (1962) Nature of institutionalized adult mongoloid intelligence. *Amer. J. ment. Defic.* 67, 301.

Stevens, H.C. (1915) Mongolian idiocy and syphilis. *J. Amer. med. Ass.* 64, 1936.

Stevens, H.C. (1916) The spinal fluid in mongolian idiocy. *J. Amer. med. Ass.* 66, 1373.

Stevenson, A.C., Johnston, H.A., Stewart, M.I.P. & Golding, D.R. (1966) Congenital malformations. A report of a study of series of consecutive births in 24 centres. *Bull. Wld. Hlth. Org. (Suppl.)* 34.

Stevenson, A.C., Mason, R. & Edwards, K.D. (1970) Maternal diagnostic X-irradiation before conception and the frequency of mongolism in children subsequently born. *Lancet* 2, 1335.

Stewart, A.M. (1961) Aetiology of childhood malignancies: congenitally determined leukaemias. *Brit. med. J.* 1, 452.

Stewart, A.M., Webb, J. & Hewitt, D. (1958) A survey of childhood malignancies. *Brit. med. J.* 1, 1495.

Stickland, C.A. (1954) Two mongols of unusually high mental status. *Brit. J. med. Psychol.* 27, 80.

Stiehm, E.R. & Fudenberg, H.H. (1966) Serum levels of immune globulins in health and disease: a survey. *Pediatrics* 37, 715.

Stiles, K.A. (1958) Reproduction in a mongoloid imbecile. *Proc. X Int Cong. Genetics, Montreal* 2, 276.

Stiles, K.A. & Goodman, H.O. (1961) Reproduction in a mongoloid. *Acta Genet. med. (Roma)* 50, 457.

Stoeltzner, W. (1919) Zur Ätiologie des Mongolismus. *Münch. med. Wschr.* 66, 1943.

Stoller, A. & Collmann, R.D. (1965a) Incidence of infective hepatitis followed by Down's syndrome nine months later. *Lancet,* 2, 1221.

Stoller, A. & Collmann, R.D. (1965b) Virus aetiology of Down's syndrome (mongolism). *Nature (Lond.)* 208, 903.

Stoller, A. & Collmann, R.D. (1966) Area relationship between incidences of infectious hepatitis and of the births of children with Down's syndrome nine months later. *J. ment. Defic. Res.* 10, 84.

Stoller, A., Judge, C., Krupinski, J. & Wallace, L. (1973) Cancer, leukaemia, congenital abnormalities and Down's syndrome in Victoria, Australia. *J. ment. Defic. Res.* 17, 263.

Stransky, E. (1968) Perinatale leukämie. *Arch. Kinderheilk.* 178, 8.

Strauss, L. (1953) Congenital cardiac anomalies associated with mongolism. *Trans. Amer. Coll. Cardiol.* 3, 214.

Strazzulla, M. (1953) Speech problems of the mongoloid child. *Quart Rev. Pediat.* 8, 268.

Sturtevant, A.H. (1929) The "claret" mutant type of *Drosophila simulans*. A study of chromosome elimination and of cell lineage. *Z. wiss. Zool.* 135, 325.

Šubrt, I. (1970) A further example of familial Gp+ associated with trisomy G. *Humangenetik* 9, 86.

Šubrt, I., Blehová, B. & Kučera, J. (1968) Aberrant chromosome 13-15 in a patient with Down's syndrome, diabetes mellitus and hyperthyroidism and in his father. *Acta genet. (Basel)* 18, 38.

Šubrt, I. & Prchlíková, H. (1970) An extra chromosomal centric fragment in an infant with stigmata of Down's syndrome. *J. med. Genet.* 7, 407.

Sutherland, G.A. (1899) Mongolian imbecility in infants. *Practitioner* 63, 632.

Sutherland, G.A. (1900) Differential diagnosis of mongolism and cretinism. *Lancet* 1, 23.

Sutherland, G.R., Fitzgerald, M.G. & Danks, D.M (1972) Difficulty in showing mosaicism in the mother of three mongols. *Arch. Dis. Childh.* 47, 790.

Sutherland, G.R. & Wiener, S. (1972) Cytogenetics of 271 mongols. *Austr. paediat. J.* 8, 90.

Sutnick, A.I., London, W.T. & Blumberg, B.S. (1969) Effects of host and environment on immunoglobulins in Down's syndrome. *Arch. int. Med.* 124, 722.

Swallow, J.N. (1964) Dental disease in children with Down's syndrome. *J. ment. Defic. Res.* 9, 102.

Sweet, L.K. (1934) Mongoloid imbecility in the Mongolian races. Report of two cases in Chinese children. *J. Pediat.* 5, 352.

Sznajder, N., Carraro, J.J., Otero, E. & Carranza, A. (1968) Clinical periodontal findings in trisomy 21 (mongolism). *J. periodont. Res.* 3, 1.

Tada, K., Uesaki, T., Isshiki, G. & Oura, T. (1972) Activities of hypoxanthine-guanine phosphoribosyltransferase and adenine phosphoribosyltransferase in erythrocytes from patients with Down's syndrome. *Tohoku J. exp. Med.* 108, 197.

Tagher, P. & Reisman, C.E. (1966) Reproduction in Down's syndrome (mongolism): chromosomal study of mother and normal child. *Obstet. Gynec.* 27, 182.

Taillens, M. (1908) L'idiotie mongolienne. *Rev. méd. Suisse rom.* 28, 242.

Taktikos, A. (1964) Association of retinoblastoma with mental defect and other pathological manifestations. *Brit. J. Ophthal.* 48, 495.

Talbot, F.B. (1924) Studies in growth III. Growth of untreated mongolian idiots. *Amer. J. Dis. Child.* 27, 152.

Tan, C.V., Rosner, F. & Feldman, F. (1973) Nitroblue tetrazolium dye reduction in various hematologic disorders. *N.Y. St. J. Med.* 73, 952.

Tan, Y.H., Schneider, E.L., Tischfield, J., Epstein, C.J. & Ruddle, F.H. (1974) Human chromosome 21 dosage: effect on the expression of the interferon-induced antiviral state. *Science* 186, 61.

Tan, Y.H., Tischfield, J. & Ruddle, F.H. (1973) The linkage of genes for the human interferon-induced antiviral protein and indophenol oxidase-B traits to chromosome G-21. *J. exp. Med.* 137, 317.

Tanaka, K. & Okada, M. (1969) Case of mongolism presenting leukemia-like symptoms. *Jap. J. clin Med.* 27, 1539.

Tandon, R. & Edwards, J.E. (1973) Cardiac malformations associated with Down's syndrome. *Circulation* 47, 1349.

Taylor, A.I. (1968) Cell selection *in vivo* in normal/G trisomic mosaics. *Nature, Lond.* 219, 1028.

Taylor, A.I. (1970) Further observations of cell selection *in vivo* in normal/G trisomic mosaics. *Nature, Lond.* 227, 163.

Taylor, A.I. & Moores, E.C. (1967) A sex chromatin survey of newborn children in two London hospitals. *J. med. Genet.* 4, 258.

Taysi, K., Kohn, G. & Mellman, W.J. (1970) Mosaic mongolism. II. Cytogenetic studies. *J. Pediat.* 76, 880.

Tennies, L.G. (1943) Some comments on the mongoloid. *Amer. J. ment. Defic.* **48**, 46.

Tettenborn, U., Gropp, A., Murken, J.-D., Tinnefeld, W., Fuhrmann, W. & Schwinger, E. (1970) Meiosis and testicular histology in XYY males. *Lancet* **2**, 267.

Thelander, H.E. & Pryor, H.B. (1966) Abnormal patterns of growth and development in mongolism. An anthropometric study. *Clin. Pediat.* **5**, 493.

Therkelsen, A.J. (1964) Enlarged short arm of a small acrocentric chromosome in grandfather, mother and child, the latter with Down's syndrome. *Cytogenetics* **3**, 441.

Thom, H. & McKay, E. (1972) Gm antigenic titres in adults with Down's syndrome (mongolism), non-mongoloid mental defectives and healthy blood donors. *Clin. exp. Immunol.* **12**, 515.

Thompson, H., Melnyk, J. & Hecht, F. (1967) Reproduction and meiosis in XYY. *Lancet* **2**, 831.

Thompson, M.W. (1961) Reproduction in two female mongols. *Canad. J. Genet. Cytol.* **3**, 351.

Thompson, M.W. (1962) 21-trisomy in a fertile female mongol. *Canad. J. Genet. Cytol.* **4**, 352.

Thompson, M.W. & Bandler, E. (1973) Finger pattern combinations in normal individuals and in Down's syndrome. *Hum. Biol.* **45**, 563.

Thompson, W.H. (1939) A study of the frequency of mongolianism in negro children in the United States. *Proc. Amer. Ass. ment. Def.* **44**, 91.

Thomson, J. (1898) On the diagnosis and prognosis of certain forms of imbecility in infancy. *Scot. med. surg. J.* **3**, 203.

Thomson, J. (1907) Notes on the peculiarities of the tongue in mongolism and on tongue-sucking in their causation. *Brit. med. J.* **1**, 1051.

Thores, O.A. & Philion, J. (1973) Down's syndrome in British Columbia Indians. *Canad. med. Ass. J.* **109**, 1108.

Thuline, H.C. & Islam, A.R. (1966) Absence of a rib in Down's syndrome. *Lancet* **1**, 1156.

Thuline, H.C. & Priest, J.H. (1961) Pregnancy in a 14-year-old mongoloid. *Lancet* **1**, 1115.

Thursfield, H. (1921) Notes on mongolism. *Brit. J. Child. Dis.* **18**, 18.

Timme, W. (1921) The mongolian idiot. *Arch. Neurol. Psychiat.* **5**, 568.

Timson, J., Harris, R., Gadd, R.L., Ferguson-Smith, M.E. & Ferguson-Smith, M.A. (1971) Down's syndrome due to maternal mosaicism, and the value of antenatal diagnosis. *Lancet* **1**, 549.

Tips, R.L., Smith, G.S. & Meyer, D.L. (1963) Paternal transmission of a 15/21 translocation. *Amer. J. Dis. Child.* **106**, 630.

Tishler, J. & Martel, W. (1965) Dislocation of the atlas in mongolism. *Radiology* **84**, 904.

Tizard, J. (1960) Residential care of mentally handicapped children. *Brit. med. J.* **1**, 1041.

Tjio, J.H. & Levan, A. (1956) The chromosome number of man. *Hereditas (Lund)* **42**, 1.

Todaro, G.J. & Martin, G.M. (1967) Increased susceptibility of Down's syndrome fibroblasts to transformation by SV_{40}. *Proc. Soc. exp. Biol. Med.* **124**, 1232.

Tolksdorf, M., Lehmann, W., Hansen, H.G. & Wiedermann, H.-R. (1965) Edwards-Syndrom mit aussergewöhnlichem chromosomalen Befund. *Z. Kindeheilk.* **93**, 55.

Tonomura, A. & Karita, T. (1964) Triple chromosome mosaicism in a Japanese child with Down's syndrome *Acta. genet., Basel* **14**, 67.

Tonomura, A., Oishi, H., Matsunaga, E. & Kurita, T. (1966) Down's syndrome: a cytogenetic and statistical survey of 127 Japanese patients. *Jap. J. hum. Genet.* **11**, 1.

Tough, I.M., Court Brown, W.M., Baikie, A.G., Buckton, K., Harnden, D.G., Jacobs,

P.A., King, M. & McBride, J.A. (1961) Cytogenetic studies in chronic myeloid leukaemia and acute leukaemia associated with mongolism. *Lancet* 1, 411.

Townes, P.L. (1968) Latent aneuploidy in father and grandfather of doubly aneuploid child: mongolism in a child with 48 chromosomes. *J. Pediat.* 73, 97.

Tredgold, A.F. (1908) *Mental deficiency (amentia)*. London: Baillière, Tindall & Cox.

Tricomi, V., Valenti, C. & Hall, J.E. (1964) Ovulatory patterns in Down's syndrome. *Amer. J. Obstet. Gynec.* 89, 651.

Trubowitz, S., Kirman, D. & Masek, B. (1962) The leucocyte alkaline phosphatase in mongolism. *Lancet* 2, 486.

Tsuang, M.-T. (1964) Personal communication.

Tsuang, M.-T. & Lin, T.-L. (1964) A clinical and family study of Chinese mongol children. *J. ment. Defic. Res.* 8, 84.

Tsuboi, T., Inouye, E. & Kamide, H. (1968) Chromosomal mosaicism in two Japanese children with Down's syndrome. *J. ment. Defic. Res.* 12, 162.

Tsunemitsu, A. (1963) Blood citrates in severe early destructive periodontal disease. *J. dent. Res.* 42, 783.

Tumpeer, I.H. (1922) Mongolian idiocy in a Chinese boy. *J. Amer. med. Ass.* 79, 14.

Turkel, H. (1963) Medical treatment of mongolism. *Proc. 2nd Int. Cong. Ment. Retard., Vienna* 1, 409.

Turnbull, A.C., Gregory, P.J. & Laurence, K.M. (1973) Antenatal diagnosis of foetal abnormality with special reference to amniocentesis. *Proc. roy. Soc. Med.* 66, 1115.

Turner, B., den Dulk, G.M. & Watkins, G. (1964) The 17–18 trisomy and 21 trisomy syndromes in siblings. *J. Pediat.* 64, 601.

Turner, J.H. (1963) *The mongoloid phenotype: its incidence, etiology and association with leukemia and other neoplastic diseases.* Thesis, University of Michigan (University Microfilms No. 63-7539).

Turner, J.H., Kaplan, S. & Tomley, J. (1966) Mosaicism and mongoloid stigmata in the mother of a Down's syndrome child. *Human Chromosome Newsletter* No. 20, p. 31. (personal communication).

Turpin, R. & Bernyer, G. (1947) De l'influence de l'hérédité sur la formule d'Arneth. *Rev. Hémat.* 2, 189.

Turpin, R., Bernyer, G. & Teissier, C. (1947) Mongolisme et stigmates familiaux de la série mongolienne. *Presse méd.* 53, 597.

Turpin, R. & Caratzali, A. (1933) Conclusions d'une étude génétique de la langue plicaturée. *C.R. Acad. Sci., Paris* 196, 2040.

Turpin, R. & Caratzali, A. (1934) Remarques sur les ascendants et les collatéraux des sujets atteints de mongolisme. *Presse méd.* 42, 1186.

Turpin, R. & Caspar-Fonmarty (1945) La dactyloscopie des mongoliens. *Sem. Hôp., Paris* 13, 341.

Turpin, R. & Lejeune, J. (1953) Etude dermatoglyphique des paumes des mongoliens et de leurs parents et germains. *Sem. Hôp., Paris* 76, 3955.

Turpin, R. & Lejeune, J. (1965) *Les chromosomes humains.* Paris: Gauthier-Villars.

Turpin, R., Thoyer-Rozat, J., Lafourcade, J., Lejeune, J., Caille, B. & Kesseler, A. (1964) Coincidence de mongolisme et de syndrome de Klinefelter chez l'un et l'autre jumeaux d'une paire monozygote. *Pédiatrie (Lyon)* 19, 43.

Uchida, I.A. (1970) Epidemiology of mongolism: the Manitoba study. *Ann. N.Y. Acad. Sci.* 171, 361.

Uchida, I.A. (1973) Paternal origin of the extra chromosome in Down's syndrome. *Lancet* 2, 1258.

Uchida, I. & Curtis, E.J. (1961) A possible association between maternal radiation and mongolism. *Lancet* 2, 848.

Uchida, I.A., Ray, M. & Duncan, B.P. (1966) 21 trisomy with an XYY sex chromosome complement. *J. Pediat.* 69, 295.

Usher, C.H. (1935) The Bowman Lecture on a few hereditary eye affections. *Trans. ophthal. Soc. U.K.* **55**, 164.

Vacher, L.B., Garcia, W.M. & Palacio, A.G. (1956) Enfermedad de Hirschsprung et un mongólico de 38 dias de nacido. *Rev. cuba. Pediat.* **28**, 473.

Valencia, J.I., de Lozzio, C.B. & de Coriat, L.F. (1963) Heterosomic mosaicism in a mongoloid child. *Lancet* **2**, 488.

Valentine, W.N. & Beck, W.S. (1951) Biochemical studies on leucocytes. I. Phosphatase activity in health, leucocytosis and myelotic leukemia. *J. Lab. clin. Med.* **38**, 39.

Vamos-Hurwitz, E., Arya, S., Boggs, T.R. & Nichols, W.W. (1967) Familial enlargement of the short arm of a small acrocentric chromosome. *Hereditas (Lund)* **57**, 185.

Vas, J. (1925) Beiträge zur Pathogenese und Therapie der Idiotia mongoliana. *Jb. Kinderheilk.* **111**, 51.

Veall, R.M. (1974) The prevalence of epilepsy among mongols related to age. *J. ment. Defic. Res.* **18**, 99.

Verresen, H. & van den Berghe, H. (1965) 21-trisomy and XYY. *Lancet* **1**, 609.

Verresen, H., van den Berghe, H. & Creemers, J. (1964) Mosaic trisomy in phenotypically normal mother of mongol. *Lancet* **1**, 526.

Vertrella, M., Barthelmai, W. & Matsuda, H. (1969) Kongenitale amegakaryocytäre Thrombocytopenie mit finaler Pancytopenie bei Trisomie 21 mit cyticer Pankreas fibrose. *Z. Kinkderheilk.* **107**, 210.

Vincent, P.C., Sinha, S., Neate, R., den Dulk, G. & Turner, B. (1963) Chromosome abnormalities in a mongol with acute myeloid leukemia. *Lancet* **1**, 1328.

Vogel, W. (1972) Identification of G-group chromosomes involved in a G/G tandem-translocation by Giemsa-band technique. *Humangenetik* **14**, 255.

Vogel, W. & Löning, B. (1973) Identification of a familial 19/21 translocation by Q and G band patterns. *Humangenetik* **18**, 219.

Vogel, W., Reinwein, H. & Engel, W. (1970) Tandem chromosomen (G/G) mit Satelliten am kurzen und langen Arm bei einem Patienten mit Translokations-trisomie G₁. *Humangenetik* **9**, 361.

Vrydagh-Laoureaux, S. (1967) Le pli palmaire transverse dans une population belge normale et chez 86 mongoliens. *Bull. Soc. roy. belge. Anthrop. Prehist.* **78**, 237.

Waardenburg, P.J. (1932) *Das menschliche Auge und seine Erbanlagen.* Haag: Martinus Nijhoff.

Wagner, H.R. (1962) Mongolism in orientals. *Amer. J. Dis. Child.* **103**, 706.

Wahrman, J. & Fried, K. (1970) The Jerusalem prospective newborn survey of mongolism. *Ann. N.Y. Acad. Sci.* **171**, 341.

Wald, N., Borges, W.H., Li, C.C., Turner, J.H. & Harnois, M.C. (1961) Leukaemia associated with mongolism. *Lancet* **1**, 1228.

Walker, A. & Garrison, M. (1966) The reticulocyte count in mongols. *Amer. J. ment. Defic.* **70**, 509.

Walker, F.A. & De Mars, R. (1966) Enzyme alterations in fibroblasts derived from patients with Down's syndrome. *3rd Int. Cong. Hum. Genet., Chicago.* (Abstr.), p. 103. Baltimore: Johns Hopkins Press.

Walker, F.A. & Ising, R. (1969) Mosaic Down's syndrome in a father and daughter. *Lancet* **1**, 374.

Waller, H. & Waller, M. (1973) Chromosomenmosaik 46,XY,D-,t(DqGq)+/92,XYXY, 2D-,2t(DqGq)+ bei einen Säugling mit Down-Syndrom. *Humangenetik* **17**, 99.

Wallin, J.E.W. (1949) Mongolism among schoolchildren. *Amer. J. Orthopsychiat.* **14**, 104.

Wallis, H.R.E. (1951) The significance of Brushfield's spots in the diagnosis of mongolism in infancy. *Arch. Dis. Childh.* **26**, 495.

Wallis, H.R.E. (1954) Mongolian blue spots. *Brit. med. J.* **1**, 457.

Wallis, H.R.E. (1955) The diagnosis of mongolism in infancy: small auditory meatus. *Brit. med. J.* **1**, 30.

Wallis, H.R.E. (1962) "Mongolian blue spots". *Lancet* 1, 163.

Walter, R.D., Yeager, C.L. & Rubin, H.K. (1955) Mongolism and convulsive seizures. *Arch. Neurol. Psychiat. (Chic.)* 74, 559.

Warkany, J., Passarge, E. & Smith, L.B. (1966) Congenital malformations in autosomal trisomy syndromes. *Amer. J. Dis. Child.* 112, 502.

Warkany, J., Schubert, W.K. & Thompson, J.N. (1963) Chromosome analyses in mongolism (Langdon Down syndrome) associated with leukemia. *New Engl. J. Med.* 268, 1.

Warkany, J. & Soukup, S.W. (1963) A chromosomal abnormality in a girl with some features of Down's syndrome (mongolism). *J. Pediat.* 62, 890.

Warkany, J., Weinstein, E.D., Soukup, W., Rubinstein, J.H. & Curless, M.C. (1964) Chromosome analyses in a children's hospital. *Pediatrics* 33, 454.

Waxman, S.H. & Arakaki, D.T. (1966) Familial mongolism by a G/G mosaic carrier. *J. Pediat.* 69, 274.

Weaver, D.D. & Lyons, R.B. (1968) Leucocyte-alkaline-phosphatase isoenzymes. *Lancet* 1, 1196.

Weber, W.W., Mittwoch, U. & Delhanty, J.D.A. (1965) Leucocyte alkaline phosphatase in Klinefelter's syndrome. *J. med. Genet.* 2, 112.

Wegelius, R., Väänanen, I. & Koskela, S.-L. (1967) Down's syndrome and transient leukaemia-like disease in a newborn. *Acta Paediat. (Uppsala)* 56, 301.

Weinberg, B. & Zlatin, M. (1970) Speaking fundamental frequency characteristics of five- and six-year-old children with mongolism. *J. Speech Res.* 13, 418.

Weinberger, M.M. & Oleinick, A. (1970) Congenital marrow dysfunction in Down's syndrome. *J. Pediat.* 77, 273.

Weinstein, E.D. & Rucknagel, D.L. (1964) Quantitative studies on sickle and fetal hemoglobins in negroes with Down's syndrome (mongolism). *Amer. Soc. Hum. Genet. Mtg., Colorado.*

Weinstein, E.D., Rucknagel, D.L. & Shaw, M.W. (1965) Quantitative studies on A_2, sickle cell and fetal hemoglobins in negroes with mongolism, with observations on translocation mongolism in negroes. *Amer. J. hum. Genet.* 17, 443.

Weinstein, E.D. & Warkany, J. (1963) Maternal mosaicism and Down's syndrome (mongolism). *J. Pediat.* 63, 599.

Weise, P., Koch, R., Shaw, K.N.F. & Rosenfeld, M.J. (1974) The use of 5-HTP in the treatment of Down's syndrome. *Pediatrics* 54, 165.

Weiss, L. & Wolf, C.B. (1968) Familial C/G translocation causing mitotic nondisjunction. *Amer. J. Dis. Child.* 116, 609.

Weiss, N.S. & Grolnick, M. (1967) Allergy survey of children with Down's syndrome. *N.Y. State J. Med.* 67, 1871.

Welch, B.L. (1939) Note on discriminant functions. *Biometrika* 31, 218.

Weninger, M. (1947) Zur Vererbung der Hautleistenmuster am Hypothenar de menschlichen Hand. *Mitt. öst. Ges. Anthropol.* 73–77, 55.

West, J.P. (1901) A note on the little finger of the mongolian idiot and of normal children. *Arch. Pediat.* 18, 918.

Wetterberg, L., Gustavson, K.-H., Bäckström, M., Ross, S.B. & Frödén, O. (1972) Low dopamine-β-hydroxylase activity in Down's syndrome. *Clin. Genet.* 3, 152.

Whang-Peng, J., Freireich, E.J., Oppenheim, J.J., Frei, E. & Tjio, J.H. (1969) Cytogenetic studies in 45 patients with acute lymphocytic leukemia. *J. nat. Cancer Inst.* 42, 881.

White, D. & Kaplitz, S.E. (1964) Treatment of Down's syndrome with a vitamin-mineral-hormonal preparation. *Int. Copenhagen Cong. Sci. Study Ment. Retard.* 1, 224.

White, M.J.D. (1954) *Animal cytology and evolution.* Cambridge University Press.

van Wijck, J.A.M., Blankenborg, G.J. & Stolte, L.A.M. (1964) XO/XX mosaicism and mongolism in the same person. *Lancet* 1, 171.

Wilder, I.W. (1930) The morphology of the palmar digital triradii and main lines. *J. Morphol.* 49, 153.

Williams, E.J., McCormick, A.Q. & Tischler, B. (1973) Retinal vessels in Down's syndrome. *Arch. Ophthal.* **89,** 269.

Williams, J.D., Summitt, R.L., Martens, P.R. & Kimbrell, R.A. (1975) Familial Down syndrome due to t(10;21) translocation: evidence that the Down phenotype is related to trisomy of a specific segment of chromosome 21. *Amer. J. hum. Genet.* **27,** 478.

Wilmarth, S.W. (1890) Report on the examination of one hundred brains of feeble-minded children. *Alienist and Neurologist* **11,** 520.

Wilson, M.G., Fujimoto, A. & Alfi, O.S. (1974) Double autosomal trisomy and mosaicism for chromosomes No. 8 and No. 21. *J. med. Genet.* **11,** 96.

Winer, R.A. & Cohen, M.M. (1961) Dental caries in institutionalized mongoloid patients. *J. dent. Res.* **40,** 661.

Winer, R.A. & Cohen, M.M. (1962) Dental caries in mongolism. *Dent. Progr.* **2,** 217.

Winer, R.A. & Feller, R.P. (1972) Composition of parotid and submandibular saliva and serum in Down's syndrome. *J. dent. Res.* **51,** 449.

Woillez, M. & Dansaut, C. (1960) Les manifestations oculaires dans le mongolisme. *Arch. Ophtal. (Paris)* **20,** 810.

Wolcott, J.G. & Chun, R.W.M. (1973) Myoclonic seizures in Down's syndrome. *Develop. Med. Child Neurol.* **15,** 805.

Wolf, H.G. & Zweymüller, E. (1962) Mongolismus und aganglionäres Megacolon. *Wien. klin. Wschr.* **74,** 219.

Wolf, U., Baitsch, H., Künzer, W. & Reinwein, H. (1964) Familiäres Auftreten eines Anomalen D-Chromosoms.*Cytogenetics* **3,** 112.

Wolf, U., Brehme, H., Baitsch, H., Künzer, W. & Reinwein, H. (1963) Aplasia of the dermal ridge patterns in mongolism (G-trisomy). *Lancet* **2,** 887.

Wolff, C. & Rollin, H.R. (1942) The hands of mongolian imbeciles in relation to their personality groups. *J. ment. Sci.* **88,** 415.

de Wolff, E. (1964) Etude clinique de 134 mongoliens. *Ann. Paediat.* **202,** Suppl.

de Wolff, E., Scharer, K. & Lejeune, J. (1962) Contribution à l'étude des jumeaux mongoliens. Un cas de monozygotisme hétérokaryote. *Helv. paediat. Acta* **17,** 301.

Wood, J. (1909) Mongolian imbecility. *Australian Med. Cong., Melbourne* **3.**

Wood, W.J. (1962) "Mongolian blue spots". *Lancet* **1,** 538.

Woodford, F.P. & Bearn, A.G. (1970) A critical examination of some reported biochemical abnormalities in mongolism. *Ann. N.Y. Acad. Sci.* **171,** 551.

Woods, L.K., Moore, G.E., Bainbridge, C.J., Huang, C.C., Huzella, C. & Quinn, L.A. (1973) Lymphoid cell lines established from peripheral blood of persons with Down's syndrome. *N.Y. St. J. Med.* **73,** 869.

Workman, G.W. (1939) *A study of the palmar dermatoglyphics of mongolian idiots.* Thesis, University of Toronto.

Wright, S.W., Day, R.W., Mosier, H.D., Koons, A. & Mueller, H. (1963) Klinefelter's syndrome, Down's syndrome (mongolism), and twinning in the same sibship. *J. Pediat.* **62,** 217.

Wright, S.W., Day, R.W., Muller, H. & Weinhouse, R. (1967) The frequency of trisomy and translocation in Down's syndrome. *J. Pediat.* **70,** 420.

Wright, S.W. & Fink, K. (1957) The excretion of beta-aminoisobutyric acid in normal, mongoloid and non-mongoloid defective children. *Amer. J. ment. Defic.* **61,** 530.

Wunderlich, C. & Braun-Falco, O. (1965) Mongolismus und Alopecia areata. *Med. Welt.* **1,** 477.

Wunsch, W.L. (1957) Some characteristics of mongoloïds evaluated in a clinic for children with retarded mental development. *Amer. J. ment. Defic.* **62,** 122.

Würth, A. (1937) Die Entstehung der Beugefurchen der menschlichen hohlhand. *Z. Morphol. Anthropol.* **36,** 187.

Ying, K.L. (1973) Sporadic (GqGq) translocations in Down's syndrome. *Canad. J. Genet. Cytol.* **15,** 309.

Yunis, J.J. (1965) *Human chromosome methodology.* New York and London: Academic Press.

Yunis, J.J., Hook, E.B. & Alter, M. (1964) XXX 21-trisomy. *Lancet* 1, 437.

Yunis, J.J., Hook, E.B. & Mayer, M. (1965) Identification of the mongolism chromosome by DNA replication analysis. *Amer. J. hum. Genet.* 17, 191.

Zaetz, J.L. (1971) *Organization of sheltered workshop programs for the mentally retarded adult.* Springfield, Illinois: Charles C. Thomas.

Zappella, M. & Cowie, V. (1962) A note on time of diagnosis in mongolism. *J. ment. Defic. Res.* 6, 82.

Zeaman, D. & House, B.J. (1962) Mongoloid M.A. is proportional to log C.A. *Child development* 33, 481.

Zeligman, I. & Scalia, S.P. (1954) Dermatologic manifestations of mongolism. *Arch. Derm. Syph.* 69, 342.

Zellweger, H. (1968a) Is Down's syndrome a modern disease? *Lancet* 2, 458.

Zellweger, H. (1968b) Familial aggregates of the 21-trisomy syndrome. *Ann. N.Y. Acad. Sci.* 155, 784.

Zellweger, H. & Abbo, G. (1963) Chromosomal mosaicism and mongolism. *Lancet* 1, 827.

Zellweger, H. & Abbo, G. (1965) Familial mosaicism attributable to a new gene. *Lancet* 1, 455.

Zellweger, H. & Abbo, G. (1967) Double trisomy and double trisomic mosaicism. *Amer. J. Dis. Child.* 113, 329.

Zellweger, H., Abbo, G., Nielsen, K. & Wallwork, K. (1966a) Cytogenetics in a pediatric department. *Human Chromosome Newsletter* 19, 40. (personal communication).

Zellweger, H., Abbo, G., Nielsen, M.K. & Wallwork, K. (1966b) Mosaic mongolism with normal chromosomal complement in the white cells. *Humangenetik* 4, 323.

Zellweger, H. & Mikamo, K. (1961) Autosomal cytogenetics. *Helv. paediat. Acta* 16, 670.

Zellweger, H., Mikamo, K. & Abbo, G. (1963) An unusual translocation in mongolism. *J. Pediat.* 62, 225.

Zellweger, H. & Simpson, J. (1973) Is routine prenatal karyotyping indicated in pregnancies of very young women? *J. Pediat.* 82, 675.

Zergollern, L. (1974) Three generations and seven family members with a t(21q22q) chromosome. *J. med. Genet.* 11, 378.

Zergollern, L. & Hoefnagel, D. (1964) X-chromosome mosaicism with trisomy-21. *Lancet* 1, 1108.

Zergollern, L., Hoefnagel, D., Benirschke, K. & Corcoran, P.A. (1964) A patient with trisomy 21 and a reciprocal translocation in 13–15 group. *Cytogenetics* 3, 148.

Zeuthen, E. & Nielsen, J. (1973) Prevalence of chromosome abnormalities among males examined for military service. *Clin. Genet.* 4, 422.

Zsako, S. & Kaplan, A.R. (1969) Titres of antistreptolysin 0 in mothers of children affected with Down's syndrome. *Nature, Lond.* 223, 1281.

Zuelzer, W.W. & Brown, A.K. (1961) Neonatal jaundice: a review. *Amer. J. Dis. Child.* 101, 87.

Index

Abdomen, 37–8, 40, 152
Abilities, 8, 60, 62, 65–6, 71, 149, 275–8
ABO blood groups, 3, 7, 105–8, 148
  distribution, 7, 105–7
  immunization, 105
  loci, 106-7
Abortions, 191, 193, 195, 220–1, 223,
    231, 233, 238, 248, 271–3
    (see also Miscarriages)
Accidents, 246
Acetabular angle, 52–4, 159
Achondroplasia, 43
Acrocephaly, 44
Acrocyanosis, 39, 156
Acromicria, 12
Actinic factors, 14
Actinomycin, 137
Adactyly, 58
Adenoids, 15
Adolase, 135
Adrenal gland
  damage, 5
  function, 130–1
  hormones, 123, 130–1
  hypoplasia, 5, 36, 41
Aetiology (see Causes)
Age
  grandparental, 165, 168, 202, 223–4
  maternal, 2–9, 11, 37, 106–7, 118,
    150, 163, 165, 168, 176–8,
    180–1, 185–6, 188, 190,
    199, 200, 202–3, 207–9,
    211–3, 220–5, 228, 231–2,
    235–7, 246–65, 267–71, 273
  paternal, 6, 177–8, 180, 188, 190,
    200, 202–3, 207–8, 212–3,
    220–1, 248–9, 251, 256,
    260, 263–4, 271
Ageing, 43, 143, 262
Agglutinins, 143
Alanine, 127
Albumin, 120–1, 147
Alcoholism, 4
Allergies, 39, 148
Alopecia, 39
Altitudinal index, 47

Alveolar process, 17, 47
Alzheimer's disease, 62–3, 75
Amenorrhea, 40, 220
Amiability, 73–4
Amino acids, 125–7
Amniocentesis, 219, 230–3, 265, 272–4
Anmiotic sac, 5
Amylase, 140
Aneuploidy (see Chromosomes)
  relatives with, 217–22
Angiocardiography, 34, 37
Ankles, 38–9
Anoxia, 5, 18, 66
Anthranilic acid, 126
Antibiotics, 210, 241
Antibodies, 120, 130–1, 141–7, 228, 258
  auto-, 130, 144–5
  milk, 146–7
  responses, 142–4
  thyroid, 130–1, 145, 228, 258
  titres, 142–3
Antigenic stimulation, 142
Antigens, 142–4, 146–7 (see also Blood
    groups)
  Australia, 144, 146
  milk, 146–7
Antihelix, prominent, 32 (see also Ears)
Antimongolism (see Chromosomes,
    monosomy)
Antitoxin titre, 143
Antiviral protein, 138, 230
Anus, 38, 212
Aorta, coarctation of, 36
Apocrine glands, 40
Areola, 41
Arms, 39, 60, 159
Art, works of, 1
Articulation (see Voice)
Asphyxia, 244
Asteatosis (see Xerosis)
Asthma, 148
Asynapsis, 175
Atmospheric pollution, 258
Atopic disease, 142
Atrioventricularis communis, 34–6
Atropine, 140

Attention span, 64
Auditory meatus, external, 32
Autoimmune disease, 123, 144–6, 258
Autopsy studies, 33, 40, 61, 109, 114, 128–9, 212
Autoradiography, 171–2, 174, 178, 209, 214
Avitaminosis, 14

β-aminoisobutyric acid, 127
β-glucoronidase, 135, 137
Bacteriophage ØX174, 143
Banding, 171–5, 178, 188–9, 192, 195, 205–6, 214, 225–7, 249, 271–2
    fluorescence, 171–2, 174–5, 178, 188–9, 192, 195, 214, 225–6, 249, 271–2
    Giemsa, 171–4, 214, 271
Barr body (see Chromatin)
Basophilis, 102
Bathing, 66
B.C.G., 143
Beard, 40
Behaviour (see Personality)
    ratings, 73–5
Bibliography, 30
Bicarbonate, 120
Biliary papilla, 38
Bilirubin, 104–5
Bimodality, 254
Binet-Simon test, 67
Biochemical studies, 7, 41, 119–40
Bioflavonids, 109
Biogenic amines, 132
Birth
    length, 155
    order, 4, 6, 107, 248–50, 263
    weight, 37, 43, 101, 149, 154–5, 159
Bitangentiality, 254
Bivalents, 183, 227, 262
Bladder training, 65–6
Blastogenesis, 223
Blindness, 30
Blood
    antibodies, 144
    cells, 100–5, 109, 113 (see also Leukaemia)
    chemistry, 7, 18, 101, 109, 119–26, 129–30, 135, 138–42
    circulation, 18, 64, 142
    culture, 10, 116–8, 144–5, 178, 187–8, 200–4, 207, 209, 214, 220–1, 228, 232, 258
    enzymes, 130–1, 133–7

Blood (continued)
    precipitins, 146–7
    vessels, 27, 30, 34, 36–7, 61, 63, 104, 109
Blood groups
    ABO, 3, 7, 105–8, 148
    incompatibility, 5, 105, 107, 114
    loci, 106–8
    other than ABO, 107–8, 148
Bones, 42–59 (see also Skeletal)
    age, 42–3
    facial, 14, 18–20, 22, 48–50
    hypoplastic, 53
    limbs, 36, 42–3, 51–2, 54–9
    marrow, 8, 9, 101, 104, 109, 118, 169, 202, 207, 220
    ossification centres, 42–3
    pelvic, 7, 51–4, 156
    ribs, 36, 51
    skull, 14, 45–50
    spine, 50–1
    sternum, 43
Bowel
    absorption, 125
    malrotation, 38
    training, 65–6
Brachycephaly, 1, 2, 44, 48–9
Brachymesophalangia, 56
Brachyoxycephaly, 45
Brain, 2, 7, 29, 61–4, 75, 116, 140
    chemistry, 63, 140
    oxygen consumption and utilization, 7, 63, 140
    sensory areas, 64
    -stem, 61
    temperature control, 64
    tumours, 116
    weight, 61–2
Breast, 40–1
Brushfield's spots, 22–4, 152, 156, 164
Buccal smear, 209 (see also Chromatin)
Bühler-Hetzer test, 67

Calcium, 7, 119–20
Cancer, 115–6, 244, 246
Candida albicans, 147
Canthal ligaments, 30
Capillary fragility, 109
Carbohydrates, 122–4, 140, 144
Carcinogens, 229–30
Cardiac defects (see Heart)
Carriers (see Chromosomes and Translocation)
Catalase, 135
Cataracts (see also Eyes and Lens)
    congenital, 25–6

Cataracts (*continued*)
   types, 26, 28
Catecholamines, 131–2
Catheterization, cardiac, 37
Cattell test, 71
Causation, early ideas on, 3–5
Causes, maternal age dependent, 176,
      232, 235, 246, 248, 253–4,
      258–64, 268
   oocyte deterioration, 253–4,
      258–64
Causes, maternal age independent, 226,
      232, 237–8, 248, 251,
      254–8, 264, 270, 272
   environmental, 237–8, 251, 254,
      257–8, 264
   genes, 251, 256–7, 264, 270, 272
   parental translocation, 251, 255–6,
      264
   secondary non-disjunction (*see* Non-
      disjunction)
Causes of death, 33–7, 242–6
Central nervous system, 30, 60–5, 126,
      226 (*see also* Brain)
Centric fusion (*see* Translocation)
Cephalic index, 44, 47, 156, 161
Cephalin flocculation test, 125
Cerebellum, 61–2
Cerebral palsy (*see* Limbs, paralysis of)
Cerebro-spinal fluid, 127
Cerebro-vascular accidents, 63, 244, 246
Cheeks, 29, 164
Chest, 153
Chiasma formation, 175, 225, 262
Chin, 19, 215
Chlorides, 120
Cholesterol, 124–5
Chromatid separation, 175, 182, 229
Chromatin, 8, 209, 211, 217, 220
Chromomere patterns, 174
Chromosomes, 8–11, 37, 53, 63, 72, 74,
      84, 98, 115–8, 132–3,
      137–8, 145, 149–50, 164–5,
      169–233, 251, 256, 258, 261,
      264, 271–2
   breaks, 116, 118, 176, 229, 258,
      261
   deletions, 195–6, 205–6, 208,
      215–7, 225, 229, 272
   duplications, 256
   enlarged arms, 196–7, 204, 208–9,
      215, 272
   fragility, 118
   fragments, 116, 189, 210, 221, 264
   inversions, 192–4, 196, 208, 215,
      251, 256, 264, 272

Chromosomes (*continued*)
   iso-, 9, 188, 191–2, 208, 210, 215,
      217, 227, 256, 271
   losses in culture, 228–9
   marker, 196, 204, 208, 215, 225–6
   monosomy, 117, 183, 215–7
   multiple aberrations, 116–8
   numbers, 8, 116–7, 176, 187
   pairing, 256, 264, 272
   partial trisomy, 149, 171, 205–6,
      211, 229
   Philadelphia, 132–3, 174
   radiosensitivity, 229
   ring, 215, 217, 229
   satellites, 170–1, 192, 194, 196,
      200, 215, 221, 225, 256, 272
   secondary constrictions, 272
   tandem, 188, 192, 194–5, 211
Circulation, 18, 64, 142
Cirrhosis, 109, 114
Citric acid, 18
Cleft palate, 15, 36
Clinodactyly (*see* Fingers)
Clitoris, 40
Clones, hybrid, 230
Coagulation, intravascular, 104
Coitus, 262
Colon, 38
Common bile duct, 36
Comparative studies, 10–1
Conjunctiva, 1, 30
Connective tissue, 30, 60, 109
Consanguinity, 255, 257
Contraceptives, 5, 276
Convulsions (*see* Epilepsy *and* Seizures)
Cornea, (*see also* Eyes)
   hydrops of, 30
Corpus callosum, 36
Cortex, 29, 61–2 (*see also* Brain)
Corticoids, 131
Corticotropin, 131
Coxa valga, 51, 53
Cranial capacity, 44, 47
Cranium (*see* Head)
Creatinine, 138–40
Cretinisim, 1, 4, 5, 33, 128, 266
Cribriform plate, 50
Cruciate ligament, 50
Cryptorchidism, 40, 152
Curettage, 5
Cystic fibrosis, 37

Dark adaptation, 30
Darwin, Charles, 3
Datura stramonium, 10
Deafness (*see* Hearing loss)

Dehydroepiandrosterone, 266
Dehydrogenases, 133–7
Dementia, 62
Denver classification, 170, 174
Deoxypyridoxine, 126
Dermatoglyphs, 4, 7, 67, 76–99, 149, 156, 159–68, 177, 199, 204, 213–6, 255, 264
  effects of mosaicism, 84, 96–8
  effects of translocation, 98, 177
  finger-tips, 76–81, 85, 89, 96–9, 149, 161–3, 165–7
  hereditary influences, 76–8, 81–2, 84, 88, 93, 95
  indices, 95–6, 98
  nomogram, 96
  palms, 81–9, 96–8, 159, 162–3, 165–7, 199, 215–6
  ridge-counts, 77–8, 80, 82, 88–9, 93–4, 98
  ridge size, 76, 89
  soles, 88, 91–8, 160–3, 165–7, 216
  toes, 89–91, 96
Dermatomyositis, 20
Desynapsis, 175
Developmental
  patterns, 65–6
  quotient, 67–70, 130
Diabetes mellitus, 123–4, 144
Diagnosis (see also Discriminative methods)
  combination of traits in, 7, 149–50, 152–4, 161, 163–4, 166
  discriminative indices in, 7, 53–4, 95–6
  informing parents of, 150
  in infancy, 150–7, 234
  of partial Down's syndrome, 163–8
  prenatal (see Amniocentesis)
  single traits in, 157–62, 165
Diakinesis, 8, 183–4, 189, 226, 262
Diaphysis, 56
Diastasis recti, 38, 152
Dicarboxylic acid, 127
Dictytene, 260
Diet, 109
Diploë, 45, 48
Diplotene, 260
Discriminative methods
  clinical, 7, 57, 149–68
  cytological (see Chromosomes)
  dermatoglyphic, 7, 84, 89, 95–6, 156, 159–63, 165–7
  radiological, 7, 53–4, 163
Dislocation
  of atlas, 50–1

Dislocation (continued)
  of hips, 36, 53
DNA
  binding, 172
  damage, 230
  polymerase activity, 145
  synthesis, 145, 228, 230
Dolicocephaly, 45
Dopamine-β-hydroxylase, 131
Drawing, 8
Dressing, 66
Drosophila melanogaster, 10–1, 217, 256
Drug susceptibility, 140
Drumsticks (see Neutrophils)
Ductus arteriosus, patent, 34, 36–7
Duodenal
  bands, 38
  obstruction, 38, 156
  stenosis or atresia, 38
Dysentery, 245

Ears, 31–3, 152–3, 156, 212, 217
  auditory meatus, 32
  helix and anti-helix, 31–2, 152, 156
  lobes, 31–2, 152, 156
  location, 32, 212, 217
  pinna, 32
  projecting, 32, 152
  tragus and anti-tragus, 31
Ectodermal defects, 20
Eczema, 39, 148
Education, 30, 65–7, 238, 265, 275–8
Ehlers-Danlos syndrome, 39
Eisenmenger's complex, 36
Elastosis perforans serpiginosa, 39
Elbows, 39
Electroencephalography, 7, 63, 75, 266
Electronmicroscopy, 62, 71
Electrophoretic mobility, 142
Embryonic development, 155, 182, 191
Emotional disturbance, 62, 73–5
  maternal, 4, 258, 273
Encephalon, 45
Endocrine dysfunction, 5, 28, 41, 125, 143, 244, 262, 266
Endotoxins, 109
Enolase, 135
Environment (see also Living conditions)
  home, 18, 65–6, 68, 74, 120, 141, 150, 245, 275–6
  institutional, 18, 33, 66–8, 71, 74–5, 112, 120, 141, 144, 146, 239, 243–5, 275–6
Environmental causes (see Causes)

Enzymes
  activity, 100, 109, 122–4, 127, 130, 136,145, 229–30
  inhibitors, 18, 125–6
  iso-, 132, 136
  levels, 113, 131–7
  loci, 122, 133, 135, 137
Eosinophils, 102, 131
Epicanthic variations, 20–2 (see also Eyes)
Epilepsy, 4, 63, 126, 220, 266
Epinephrine, 131
Epiphyses, 45, 56–7
Epstein-Barr virus, 143, 228
Equatorial plate, 8
Erythroblastosis, 105
Erythrocytes
  counts, 100
  enzymes, 100, 130–7, 230
  fragility, 100
  life-span, 104–5
  magnesium, 120
  precursors, 101
  size, 100, 132
  triiodothyronine uptake, 129–30
  volume, 100
Erythroproliferative disorders, 101
Escherichia coli, 143
Euthyroid cases, 128–30
Evolution, 3
Exophthalmos, 29
Eyelids, 1, 21–2, 30, 156
Eyes, 1–2, 7, 11, 20–30, 116, 140, 152, 154, 156, 164, 215, 217, 266
  canthal ligaments, 30
  cataract, 25–8, 30
  conjunctiva, 1, 30
  cornea, 30
  epicanthic folds, 11, 20–2, 29–30, 152, 156, 164
  iris, 22–4, 152, 156, 164
  lens, 25–30
  nystagmus, 29–30, 152
  optic nerve, 30
  palpebral fissures, 20, 29, 152, 154, 156, 215
  pupil, 23, 140
  retina, 30
  slant of, 20, 29, 217
  strabismus, 29, 152, 266
  tumours, 116

Face, 14, 18–22, 47, 114, 149, 151–2, 154, 156, 164, 215–7, 266–7
Fallot's tetralogy, 34, 36

Familial
  incidence, 3, 6–9, 57, 84, 98, 112, 150, 165, 167, 180–1, 187, 190–1, 194–5, 198–9, 201–3, 206, 219, 223–7, 251–7, 263–4, 267–9, 273
  transmission of t(Dq21q), 9, 84, 112, 179, 180–7
  transmission of t(Gq21q), 179–80, 186, 188–92
  transmission of other translocations, 194–5
Feeding, 66, 157, 244 (see also Diet)
Feet, 58–60, 153, 156
  dermatoglyphs (see Dermatoglyphs)
  plantar furrow, 153
Fertility (see Reproduction)
Fertilization
  delayed, 262
  post-cleavage, 148
Fetus, abnormal, 12, 218, 220–2, 233, 238, 258, 271 (see also Abortions and Zygotes)
Fibroblast
  culture, 8–10, 117–8, 187–9, 200–4, 213–4, 221, 223, 228, 230, 270
  enzymes, 135, 230
Fingers, 1–2, 36, 54–9, 153–4, 156, 215
  clinodactyly, 2, 54–7, 153, 156
  flexion creases, 55, 57–8, 153, 156
Fits (see Epilepsy)
Fluorescence, quinacrine (see Banding)
Fluorine, 18, 258
Fontanelles, 45, 152, 156
Forearm, 58, 212
Forehead, 45, 156

Gait (see Locomotion)
Galactosaemia, 133
Galactose tolerance, 122
Gametes, 176, 180–3, 190–1, 202, 223, 225–6, 256
Gaussian distributions, 157–8
Genes, 11, 78, 81, 106–7, 119, 133, 135, 137–8, 148, 171, 195, 230, 251, 255–7, 264, 270, 272 (see also Hereditary influences)
  antiviral protein, 138, 230
  dominant, 107
  frequencies, 106–7
  indophenol oxidase, 138, 230
  recessive, 11
  sticky, 11, 257

Genetic counselling (see Amniocentesis and Genetic prognosis)
Genetic prognosis, 269-72 (see also Recurrence risks)
Geneva conference, 233
Genitalia, 40, 132, 152, 156
Gesell test, 69-70
Gestation period, 4, 155, 159
Gingivitis, 18
Glabella, 45, 156
Globulins, 120-1, 125, 128-9, 141-2, 147
Glottis, 19
Glucose, 122
  tolerance curves, 122-4
Glutamic acid, 266
Glycine, 127
Glycogen, 123
Gnathic index, 47
Goitre (see Thyroid gland)
Graffian follicle, 260
Grandparental age (see Age)
Granulocytes, 102, 109, 113-4, 136-7
Granulomatous disease, 147
Graves' disease, 130
Growth
  prenatal, 155
  rate, 11, 130
Gums, 16-8

Haematocrit, 101, 104
Haematological studies, 100-18
Haemodynamics, 37
Haemoglobins, 100-1, 104, 107-8, 134, 230
Haemolytic disease, 105, 113
Hair, 33, 38-40, 132, 138, 263
  axillary, 40
  colour, 39, 263
  direction, 39
  line, 33
  pubic, 40, 132
  texture, 39
Hands, 42-3, 54-9, 153-4, 156, 162-3, 165-7
  dermatoglyphs (see Dermatoglyphs)
Haptoglobins, 121-2
Hare lip, 15, 36, 180-1
Hassal corpuscles (see Thymus gland)
Hay fever, 148
Head, 1-2, 28, 33, 39, 43-9, 60, 149, 152, 156-60, 163, 215
  control, 65
  dimensions, 28, 44-7, 149, 156-60, 163

Head (continued)
  shape, 1-2, 33, 44-5, 48-9, 152, 156, 215
Hearing, 64
  loss, 33
Heart, congenital defects of, 2, 4, 11, 33-7, 65, 114, 156, 212, 217, 242-6
  frequency of, 33-5
  mortality from, 33-7, 242-6
  types of, 34-6
Heart-rate, 140
Height (see Stature)
  sitting, 60
  quotient, 60
Helix (see also Ears)
  overlapping (folded), 32, 152, 156
Hemiplegia, 63
Hepatitis, 125, 146
  neonatal, 109
Hereditary influences, 5-8, 11, 16, 22, 76-8, 81-2, 84, 88, 93, 95, 105, 109, 127, 164, 185, 217, 251-2, 268, 272 (see also Genes)
Hernia
  diaphragmatic, 36-7
  umbilical, 37, 152
Hips, 36, 51-4, 153, 156
  dislocation, 36, 53
Hirschsprung's disease, 38
Histamine, 148
Histidine, 127
HL-A phenotypes, 148
Hodgkin's disease, 116
Homatropine, 140
Hormones
  adrenal, 123, 130-1
  corticotropic, 123
  testicular, 40, 132, 258
  therapy, 14, 40, 227, 265-6
  thyroid, 129
Hostility, 73-5
Humour, 72-3
Hunger, 64, 157
Hydrocephaly, 36, 45, 269
Hydrocoele, 36
5-Hydroxytryptamine, 126, 226
5-Hydroxytryptophan, 126, 226
Hyperbilirubinaemia, 104-5
Hyperflexibility, 57, 153-4, 156
Hypermetropia, 30
Hypertelorism, 28-9, 212
Hyperthyroidism (see Thyroid gland)
Hypertonia, 60, 214
Hypoparathyroidism, 119

Hypothyroidism (see Thyroid gland)
Hypotonia, 11, 19, 30, 37, 60, 63, 65, 73, 126, 153–4, 156
Hysteria, 75

I^{131}, 128–30
Idiocy
    ethnic classification of, 3–4
    Kalmuck, 2, 11
    mongolian, 1, 11
    mongoloid, 11
    Tartar, 11
Ileum, 38
Iliac
    angle, 52–4
    index, 53
    spine, 54
Illegitimacy, 263
Imbecility, 11
Immune responses, 143–5
Immunization, 143–4
Immunoglobulins, 141–4
Immunological studies, 141–8
Incidence of Down's syndrome
    and parental age, 6, 150, 163, 231–7, 246–7, 251–4, 267–70, 273
    at birth, 5–6, 150, 155, 168, 209, 234–8
    at conception, 238
    cycles of, 236–7
    distribution curves, 236
    familial (see Familial, incidence)
    in abortuses (see also Abortions)
    in different populations, 5–6, 10, 234–5, 237
    seasonal, 237
Incoordination, 3
Independence, 276
Indoleacetic acid, 125–6
Indophenol oxidase, 138, 230
Infections, 5, 18, 37, 101–2, 113–4, 120, 141–2, 145–7, 231, 237–8, 244–6, 257–8, 261–2, 264
Infectious hepatitis, 238, 258
Influenza vaccine, 143
Inheritance (see Hereditary influences)
Inoculation, 142–3
Insanity (see Mental illness)
Insulin, 123–4
    antibodies, 144
    tolerance test, 122
Intelligence, 10, 43, 62, 66–72, 159, 164, 200, 204, 213, 216, 220, 265, 276–7 (see also Mental retardation)

Intelligence (continued)
    and mosaicism, 10, 71–2, 164, 200, 204
    deterioration of, 71
    longitudinal studies, 69–71
    quotient, 66–72, 164, 204, 213, 216, 265
    range, 66–72
Intelligence, and related, tests
    Binet-Simon, 67, 159, 164
    Bühler-Hetzer, 67
    Cattell, 71
    Gesell, 69–70
    Leiter, 71
    Merrill-Palmer, 71
    Psyche-Cattell, 68, 70
    Stanford-Binet, 68–71, 213
    Vineland, 71
    Wechsler, 71
Interdental papillae, 18
Interferon, human, 230
Interpupillary distance, 28–9, 159
Intervertebral discs, 50–1
Intestines (see Bowel)
Iodine levels
    butanol-extractable, 128
    protein-bound, 128–30
Ionized air, 5
Iris (see also Eyes)
    colour, 24–5
    hypoplasia, 24
    speckled, 22–4, 152, 156, 164
Islets of Langerhans, 144
Isochromatid exchanges, 229
Isofluorophate, 137
Isomerases, 135

Jaundice, 104–5, 114, 146
Jejunum, 38
Joints, 50, 57, 153
Jordaens, Jacob, 1

Karyotypes (see Chromosomes)
Keratoconus, 30
17-Ketosteroids, 131–2
Kidneys, 36, 119, 212, 244
Kinases, 133–6
Kinetochore, 107
Kinurenines, 125–6
Klinefelter's syndrome, 8, 103, 136, 208–9, 212, 218–20, 231, 239, 261–2, 269
    combined with Down's syndrome, 9, 169, 206–10
Knuckles, 39
Kyphosis, 153

Labia, 40, 156
Landau reaction, 60
Larynx, 19
Leiter test, 71
Lens (see also Eyes)
  fibres, 28
  opacities, 25–30
Leptotene, 260
Leucocytes, 7, 101–3, 109, 113, 118, 132–8, 147, 159
  bactericidal abilities, 147
  count, 101–2
  enzymes, 132–7
  life-span, 137
  lobulation, 7, 102–3, 113, 159
  nicotinic acid amine dinucleotide, 118
  nitrobluetetrazolium reducing capacity, 147
  periodic acid/Schiff activity, 147
  peroxidase activity, 147
  regulation, 137
Leucokinetic studies, 109, 137
Leukaemia, 7, 109–18, 132, 137–8, 146, 156, 219, 244, 246
  chromosome findings in, 116–8
  incidence of, 110, 112, 115
  in mosaics, 112
  in translocation cases, 112
  mortality from, 110–2, 115–6, 244, 246
  spontaneous remissions, 113–4, 117
  surveys of, 110, 116
  transient, 111, 113–5
  types of, 110–3
Leukaemoid reaction, 110, 112, 114–5
Libido, 40
Lichenification, 39
Lichen simplex chronicus, 39
Life expectancy, 3, 33–7, 62, 155, 209, 212, 233, 239–45, 275, 277
  secular changes, 239–41, 244
Life tables, 239–45
Limbs, 39, 59–60, 159, 212
  paralyses of, 53, 63, 128
Linkage, 106–7, 137, 194, 230 (see also Genes)
Lipids, 63, 124–5
Lipoproteins, 125
Lips, 1, 14–5, 19, 152, 156, 164
  scaling and crusting, 14
  vertical fissuring, 14–5, 152
Liver abnormalities, 109, 114, 123, 125, 146, 238
  chirrhosis, 109, 114
  hepatitis, 109, 125, 146, 238

Living conditions, 237, 241, 243–4, 249–50, 265, 275–8 (see also Environment)
Locomotion, 60, 64–6
Log ratio tests, 122
Lungs
  abnormal lobation, 36–7
  emboli, 244
  explants, 187
  fibroblasts, 8
  hypoplasia, 37
  infections, 37, 114, 244–6
Lycine, 127
Lymph nodes, 114, 116
Lymphoblastoid cell lines, 228
Lymphocytes, 101–2, 113, 118, 127–8, 136, 144–5, 148, 228–30
  microtoxicity test, 148
  Phytohaemagglutinin stimulation, 127–8, 136, 144–5
  surface antigenicity, 148
  transformation, 144–5
  tritiated thymidine uptake, 144–5

Macrocytosis, 100, 132
Magnesium, 120
Maize, 11, 257
Mandible, 9, 48, 50
Mantegna, Andrea, 1, 5
Marmoration, 39
Marriage duration, 262
Maternal age (see Age)
Maturation, 265
Maturity age, 69–70
Maxilla, 14, 19, 48, 50
Megakaryocytes, 104
Meiosis 11, 106–7, 171, 175–6, 182–3, 189, 191, 196–8, 225–7, 256, 260–4
Menarche, 40
Meninges, 61
Meningocoele, 36
Menopause, 236
Menstruation, 40
Mental age (see Intelligence)
Mental illness, 4, 62, 75
Mental retardation, 7, 30, 40, 63, 65, 150, 198, 204, 206, 214, 217, 220, 223–4, 234, 239, 250
  in mosaics, 10, 71–2, 164, 200, 204
  in relatives, 4
Merrill-Palmer test, 71
Metabolism, 28, 105, 119–40
Metacarpals, 54–7
Methionine, 127
Methylating ability, 138

Microcephaly, 44–7
Microsymptoms, 3, 15, 164–5, 200, 204, 206, 255 (see also Mosaicism)
Mimicry, 8, 72–3
Miscarriages, 180–1, 185, 219, 271 (see also Abortions)
Mischievousness, 73
Mitosis, 11, 144–5, 191, 201, 205, 227, 257–8, 264
Mobility, 60 (see also Locomotion)
Mongolian spots, 39
Monoamine oxidase, 126–7
Monocytes, 103
Moro reflex, 60, 153–4, 156
Mortality from
    cancer, 244, 246
    cardiac defects, 33–7, 242–6
    cerebro-vascular accidents, 244, 246
    endocrine disorders, 244
    gastro-intestinal disease, 244–5
    infections, 37, 141, 244–6
    leukaemia, 110–2, 115–6, 244, 246
    renal disease, 244
    respiratory tract disease, 37, 141, 244–6
    trauma, 246
Mosaicism
    and behaviour, 74
    and clinical findings (see Microsymptoms)
    and dermatoglyphs, 84, 96–8, 164, 167, 204
    and intelligence, 10, 71–2, 164, 200, 204
    and leukaemia, 112, 118
    incidence of, 98, 167–8, 201, 232, 255
    in Down's syndrome, 10, 12, 63, 71, 118, 149, 151, 163–5, 167–8, 175, 200–6, 208, 212–4, 222–3, 229, 233, 257, 272
    in sex chromosome disorders, 9–10, 201–2, 207–9, 212, 215, 218–20
    maternal, 10, 72, 84, 97–8, 165–8, 199–200, 202, 218, 221, 225, 232–3, 251, 254–5, 265, 267, 270–1, 273
    paternal, 98, 168, 187–8, 203, 221, 232, 251, 254–5, 263–5, 270–1, 273
Motor skills, 276
Mouse, 11, 101, 155, 185, 230, 262
Mouth, 14–5, 19, 152, 156

Multiple sclerosis, 146
Multivalents, 227
Muramidase, 109
Muscles, 37, 50, 60, 64–5, 126, 153, 156, 266
Musical sense, 8, 64
Mutagens, chemical, 11
Mutation, 180, 255–6
Mydriasis (see Pupil)
Myelofibrosis, 110
Myeloproliferative disorders, 104
Myopia, 29–30
Myxoedema, 130

N_1-methyl-6-pyridone-5-carboxamide, 138
Nares, 20
Nasopharynx, 15
Nausea, 64
Neck, 19, 33, 36, 38–9, 49, 152–4, 156
    webbing, 33, 36, 156
Neuropathological changes, 61–3
Neutrophils, 102–4, 147
    adhesiveness, 147
    count, 102–3
    nuclear appendages (drumsticks), 103–4
    nuclear lobes, 102–3
    phagocytic ability, 147
Niacins, 126
Nicotinamide, 138
Nicotinic acid, 118, 138
Nipples, 41, 153
Nomenclature, 11–2, 171, 174
Non-disjunction, 8, 10–1, 107, 175–6, 182–3, 192, 196–9, 201–2, 205, 223, 225–6, 251, 254–62, 264–5, 270, 272
    secondary (inevitable), 10, 202, 223, 225, 251, 254–5, 264
Nose, 1, 19–20, 22, 48–9, 64, 152, 156, 164, 215
    bones, 19–20, 22, 48–9
    bridge, 19, 152, 156
    discharge, 20
    mucosa, 20, 64
    obstruction, 19
Nucleolar organizers, 261
Nucleo-protein breakdown, 138
Nutrition, 18, 43, 124
Nystagmus (see also Eyes)
    pseudo-, 29

Object identification tests, 62
Obstinacy, 73
Occipital flattening, 33, 44–5, 49, 152, 156

Oestriol, 258
Oestrogen, 227
Offspring
    of mosaic and fully affected Down's
        syndrome females, 3, 6, 10,
        72, 97, 165, 167–9, 200,
        202–3, 223–5, 232, 251,
        254–5, 264
    of mosaic Down's syndrome males,
        187–8, 203, 254–5, 263–4
Oocytes, 202, 253–4, 258–64
Oogenesis, 225, 255–7, 264
Oogonia, 255, 260
Optic nerve, 30
Oral cavity (see Mouth)
    hygiene, 18
Orbits, 20, 47–50
Osseous development (see Bones)
Ossification, 42–3, 45
Ostium (see also Heart)
    primum, 34–5
    secundum, 36
Otitis media, 33, 114
Ovaries, 40
    dysfunction, 5
Ovulation, 41
Ovum, 5, 185, 203, 219, 253–5, 261–2
Oxygen consumption and utilization,
    cerebral (see Brain)

Pachytene, 174, 226–7, 260
Pain
    sensation, 64
    stimuli, 19
Palate, 14–5, 19, 36, 48, 152, 156
Palmar crease, 57–8
    single transverse, 4, 7, 55, 57, 153–4,
        156–7, 161–2, 166
Palpebral fissures (see also Eyes)
    in different populations, 20
Pancreas
    agenesis, 36
    annular, 38
Panencephalitis, subacute sclerosing, 63
Pan troglodytes, 11
Paramongoloid, 12
Paraplegia, 53
Paredrine hydrobromide, 140
Parent associations, 275
Pareses, 53, 63
Paris classification, 174–5, 206
Parity, 250
Partial Down's syndrome, 6, 12, 95, 149,
    163–8 (see also Mosaicism)
Paternal age (see Age)
Pelger-Huët anomaly, 103

Pelvis, 7, 51–4, 153–4, 156, 163
    angles, 7, 163
    index, 54
Penis, 40, 65, 152, 156
    ejaculation, 65
    erection, 65
Penrose, L.S., 12–3
Periodontal disease, 17–8
Peristatic amentia, 12
Pernicious anaemia, 146
Perodactyly, 58
Personality, 7, 8, 58, 72–5, 156–7, 275
Phalanges (see Fingers and Toes)
Phenylalanine, 127
Phenylketonuria, 66
Pheochromocytoma, 116
Philadelphia chromosome, 132–3, 174
Phosphatase
    acid, 120, 133–7
    alkaline, 7, 120, 132–3, 135–7
Phosphates, 119–20, 124, 135
Phosphoglycerate mutase, 135
Phospholypids, 125
Pituitary gland
    dysfunction, 5, 41, 119
    fossa, 50
    hormones, 123
    therapy, 266
Placenta, 155, 231
Placing reaction, 60
Plantar furrow, 153
Plants, 175, 177
Plasma viscosity, 101
Platelets, 104, 109, 113, 126–7, 135
    enzymes, 135
    5-hydroxytryptamine binding, 126
    mono-amine oxidase, 126–7
    serotonin, 126
Play activities, 276
Polar body, 260
Polycythaemia, 101, 114
Polydactyly, 36, 58
Posture, 11, 60
Potassium, 120
Prausnitz-Kustner reaction, 148
Precipitins, 146–7
Prednisolone, 137
Pregnancy intervals, 250
Prematurity, 155, 212
Prevalance, 237–9
Prevention, 265–9, 278 (see also Amnio-
    centesis and Genetic prog-
    nosis)
Primordium, 17
Probabilities, statistical, 158–63,
    165–7, 259–60

Progesterone, 137
Prognathism (see Chin)
Prognosis, 149
Proteins, serum, 101, 120–2, 125, 130,
    140–1
Protein synthesis, 127–8, 137, 148
Pseudocholinesterase, 7
Psyche-Cattell test, 68, 70
Psychosis, 75
Puberty, 41, 43
Pupil (see also Eyes)
    dilation, 140
    irregularity, 64
    margin, 24
    vasculature, 27
Puromycin, 137

Quadrivalents, 189

Radiation effects, 229, 257–8, 264
Random mating, 107
Rat, 132
Reading, 276
Rectum, 38
Recurrence risks, 231–2, 267–72 (see
    also Genetic counselling)
Reductases, 135
Reflexes
    accommodation, 29
    convergence, 29
    mandibular, 64
    Moro, 60, 153–4, 156
    palmar grasp, 60
    patellar, 60
    plantar grasp, 60
Refraction, 30
Regression, 4
Regression curves, 228
Renal function, 119, 244
Reproduction, 3, 6, 10–1, 40, 72, 97,
    202–3, 223–5 (see also Off-
    spring)
Reproductive period, 255
Research, trends of recent, 5–8
Respiration, 19, 37
Reticulocyte count, 100–1
Retinal vessels, 30
Retinoblastoma, 116
Reversion, 4, 22
Rhagades, 14
Rhesus incompatibility, 107, 114
Rheumatoid factor titres, 147
Rhythm, 8, 64
Riboflavin, 138
Ribosomes, 127–8
Ribs, 36, 51

RNA synthesis, 137, 228
Robertsonian translocation (see Trans-
    location)

Saliva, 14, 108, 140
Schizophrenia, 75
Schmorl's nodes, 51
Schooling (see Education)
Scleroderma, 20
Scrotum, 40, 126, 135, 152, 156
Seizures (see also Epilepsy)
    grand and petit mal, 63
    myoclonic, 63
Self-help skills, 276
Sella turcica, 50
Semen, 40
Seminoma, 116
Sensory
    nerves, 64
    organs, 64
    responses, 63–5
Septal defects (see also Heart)
    atrial, 34
    ventricular, 34–7, 212
Serotonin, 126, 135, 140, 266
Serum (see Blood)
Sex
    behaviour, 276
    differences, 32, 43, 51, 55–6, 59, 67,
        76, 78–80, 83, 90, 93–6,
        100–3, 122, 129, 139,
        154–5, 204, 239, 242–5
    precocious, 40
    ratio, 5
    relationships, 276
    secondary characteristics, 40–1, 220
    sensations, 65
Sheltered workshops, 277
Shoulders, 33, 38
Siccacell therapy, 266
Sickle cell trait, 107–8
Sight (see Vision)
Simian crease (see Palmar crease)
Sinuses, 48–50
Sitting, 65–6
Skeletal
    development, 59 (see also Bones)
    maturation, 42–3
    quotient, 42
Skin, 1, 14, 20, 33, 38–9, 58, 76, 138,
    148, 152–4, 156
Skull, 3, 14–5, 20, 45–50, 61, 156
    diploë, 45, 48
    measurements, 46–50
    sutures, 45, 48–9, 156
    weight, 47

Sleep, 157
Smell sensations, 64
Social
    competence, 71–4, 275–8
    opportunities, 275–8
    quotient, 71, 265
Sociological observations, 3
Sodium, 120
Spectacles, 30
Spectrographic analysis, 19
Speech, 1, 65–6, 75, 198
Speech therapy, 277
Sperm, 40, 185, 203, 219, 223, 255, 260, 270
    count, 40
Spermatocytes, 8, 174, 226
Spermatogenesis, 8, 189, 226–7
Spermatogonia, 226–7
Spinal
    column, 39, 50–1
    cord, 51, 62
    curvature, 50, 153
    fusion, 50
    vertebrae, 50–1
Spindle mechanism, 261
Spleen, 114
Squint (see Strabismus)
Standing, 66
Stanford-Binet test, 68–71
Stature, 42, 45, 59–60, 89, 148, 159, 239
Steffen's test, 130
Stenosis
    common bile duct, 36
    duodenal, 36
    oesophageal, 38
    pulmonary, 34
    pyloric, 38
Sterility, 227
Sternum, 43, 212
Steroids, 131–2
Stillbirths, 185, 191, 221, 223–4, 256, 263
Strabismus (see Eyes)
Subclavian artery, aberrant, 34, 36
Sugar, blood (see Carbohydrates)
Suicide, 246
Superoxide dismutase, 138, 230
Surgery
    cardiac, 36, 110, 241, 266
    cosmetic, 267
    gastro-intestinal, 266
Survival (see Life expectancy)
Sweat
    glands, 76
    uric acid, 139

Sydney line, 57
Synbrachydactyly, 58
Synchondrosis, 50
Syndactyly, 36, 58–9, 217
Syphilis, 4

Talipes, 36, 59, 212
Taste sensations, 64
Teeth
    absent, 17
    carious, 18
    deciduous, 16–8
    enamel aplasia, 17
    eruption, 16–8
    irregular development, 16–9, 48
    microdontia, 17, 152
    permanent, 16–7
    roots, 17
    spacing, 19, 152
    X-rays, 17
Temperament (see Personality)
Temperature sensation, 64
Termination of pregnancy (see Abortions)
Testes
    biopsy, 183, 198, 203, 227
    hormones, 40, 132
    size, 8, 40, 239
    tumours, 116, 246
    undescended, 40, 152
Tetanus toxoid, 142–3
Texts of general interest, 12, 276
Therapy (see Treatment)
Thiamine, 138
Thighs, 39
Thirst, 64
Thrombocytopenia, 104
Thymus gland
    deficiency, 4, 41
    Hassal corpuscles, 41
    therapy, 266
Thyroid gland
    antibodies, 130–1, 145, 228, 258
    dysthyroidism, maternal, 5
    function, 4, 7, 41, 119, 125, 128–30
    goitre, 5, 41, 130
    hormone, 129
    hyperthyroidism, 5, 41, 128, 130
    hypothyroidism, 39–41, 266
    lyophilized, 130
    neck/thigh ratios, 129
    therapy, 5, 128, 130, 265–6
Thyroid stimulator, long-acting, 130
Thyroxine (see Thyroid gland)
Tibial length, 143
Toes, 58–9, 153, 156, 215, 217

Toes (*continued*)
dermatoglyphs (*see* Dermatoglyphs)
retroposition, 58
wide space between first two, 58, 153, 156
Tongue, 1, 6, 14–6, 19, 64, 152, 156, 161, 266
furrowed (fissured), 6, 15–6, 64, 152, 161
papillary hypertrophy, 16, 64
protrusion, 14–5, 152, 156, 266
sucking, 16
Tonsils, 15–6
Touch sensation, 64
Training (*see* Education)
Transaminases, 100, 125, 135
Transferases, 131–7
Transferrins, 120–1
Translocations, 9, 53, 63, 72, 74, 84, 98, 106, 112, 117–8, 126, 133–6, 154–5, 171, 175–203, 206–11, 214–5, 219–22, 227, 232, 249, 251–2, 255–6, 263–73
Dq21q type, 9, 63, 84, 98, 112, 117–8, 171, 176–87, 189, 198–200, 203, 207, 210, 214, 227, 252, 255–6, 263, 267–8, 270–3
Gq21q type, 9, 112, 117–8, 171, 179–180, 186–93, 203, 210, 214, 220–22, 227, 249, 256, 263, 267–8, 271, 273
other types, 194–9, 201, 206, 208, 211, 214–5, 219, 221, 256
transmission of (*see* Familial)
Transposition of great vessels, 36
Treatment
antibiotics, 110, 241
educational, 65, 265, 275–8
glutamic acid, 266
hormonal, 5, 14, 40, 128, 130, 227, 265–6
5-hydroxytrypthophan, 126, 266
iodine, 266
Siccacell, 266
surgical, 36, 110, 241, 266–7
vitamin, 14, 266
Trigonocephaly, 45
Triiodothyronine, 129–30
Triple X syndrome, 103, 209, 218, 220, 231, 261–2
combined with Down's syndrome, 10, 207–12
Triploidy, 218, 221–2

Trisomy, other than *21* (*see also* Chromosomes)
comparative, 10–1
8, combined with Down's syndrome, 208, 214
13–15, 37, 183, 209, 218, 220, 230–1,
combined with Down's syndrome, 10, 208–9, 211, 213–4
18, 37, 136, 209, 218, 220–1, 228, 230–1,
combined with Down's syndrome, 10, 208–9, 212–3
22, 174, 208
X (*see* Triple X syndrome)
Trivalents, 174, 183–4, 226–7
Trunk, 59
Tryptophan, 125–6, 266
Tuberculin, 145
Tuberculosis, 4, 245–6
Tumours, 116, 246 (*see also* Cancer)
Turner's syndrome, 209, 217–8, 220
combined with Down's syndrome, 10, 208–9, 211–2
Twins
concordant, 6, 141, 148, 207, 222–3
discordant, 6, 10, 99, 117, 148, 219–23
dizygotic, 6, 78, 141, 148, 219–22
monozygotic, 6, 10, 78, 88, 98–9, 148, 207, 222–4
Typhoid vaccine, 142
Tyrosine, 127

Ultrasound scanning, 231
Ultraviolet light, 230, 258
Umbilical cord, 220
Univalents, 226–7, 262
Uric acid, 138–40
Uridine disphosphate glucose-4-epimerase, 135
Urinary
acids, 125–7, 139, 266
carboxamide, 138
creatinine, 138–9
epinephrine, 131
hormones, 131–2, 258
I^{131}, 128, 130
kinurenines, 125–6
nicotinamide, 138
Uterine selection, 262
Uterus, 40
Uvula, bifid, 15

Vaginal smears, 41
Valine, 127

Valvular defects, 36 (see also Heart)
Vertabral column (see Spinal column)
Vineland test, 71
Viruses
 Epstein-Barr, 143, 228
 infectious hepatitis, 238, 258
 SV40, 118, 228
Vision, 30, 64
Visual retention tests, 62
Visuomotor tests, 64
Vital statistics, 234-50
Vitamins
 A, 30, 138
 B_6, 125-6
 C, 109, 138
 deficiency, 14, 138
 nicotinic acid, 138
 riboflavin, 138
 therapy, 14, 266
 thiamine, 138
Vitiligo, 39, 145
Vocabulary (see Speech)
Voice, 1, 19, 66
 characteristics, 19
 defects, 66

Walking (see Locomotion)
Wechsler test, 71
Weight, 59
 sensations, 64
Work skills, 8, 277

Wrists, 38-9, 42-3
 flexion creases, 82
Writing, 8, 276

Xanthurenic acid, 125-6, 266
Xeroderma (see Xerosis)
Xerosis, 39
X-rays
 feet and toes, 57
 hands and fingers, 42-3, 54-7
 long bones, 43
 lymphocytes, 229
 pelvic, 7, 51-4, 156, 163
 ribs, 51
 skull, 15, 45, 49-50
 spine, 50
 teeth, 17
 tongue, 16
 wrists, 42-3
XO female (see Turner's syndrome)
XXX female (see Triple X syndrome)
XXXX female, 218, 220
XXY male (see Klinefelter's syndrome)
XXXXY male, 113, 217-9
XYY male, 209, 212, 218, 220, 227, 231, 239
 combined with Down's syndrome, 10, 207-12

Zygotene, 175-6, 260
Zygotes, 182-3, 185, 190-1, 202, 205, 219, 223, 226, 255-7, 272